Epicardial Interventions in Electrophysiology

Guest Editors

KALYANAM SHIVKUMAR, MD, PhD, FHRS
NOEL G. BOYLE, MD, PhD, FHRS

CARDIAC ELECTROPHYSIOLOGY CLINICS

www.cardiacEP.theclinics.com

Consulting Editors

RANJAN K. THAKUR, MD, MPH, FHRS
ANDREA NATALE, MD, FACC, FHRS

March 2010 • Volume 2 • Number 1

SAUNDERS an imprint of ELSEVIER, Inc.

W.B. SAUNDERS COMPANY
A Division of Elsevier Inc.

1600 John F. Kennedy Boulevard • Suite 1800 • Philadelphia, Pennsylvania 19103-2899

http://www.theclinics.com

CARDIAC ELECTROPHYSIOLOGY CLINICS Volume 2, Number 1
March 2010 ISSN 1877-9182, ISBN-13: 978-1-4377-1798-3

Editor: Barbara Cohen-Kligerman
Developmental Editor: Donald Mumford

Cardiac Electrophysiology Clinics (ISSN 1877-9182) is published quarterly by Elsevier Inc., 360 Park Avenue South, New York, NY 10010-1710. Months of issue are March, June, September, and December. Subscription prices are $167.00 per year for US individuals, $250.00 per year for US institutions, $84.00 per year for US students and residents, $187.00 per year for Canadian individuals, $279.00 per year for Canadian institutions, $239.00 per year for international individuals, $299.00 per year for international institutions and $120.00 per year for Canadian and international students/residents. To receive student/resident rate, orders must be accompanied by name of affilliated institution, date of term, and the signature of program/residency coordinator on institution letterhead. Orders will be billed at individual rate until proof of status is received. Foreign air speed delivery is included in all Clinics subscription prices. All prices are subject to change without notice. **POSTMASTER:** Send address changes to Cardiac Electrophysiology Clinics, Elsevier Health Sciences Division, Subscription Customer Service, 3251 Riverport Lane, Maryland Heights, MO 63043. **Customer Service: 1-800-654-2452 (US and Canada). From outside of the US and Canada, call 314-477-8871. Fax: 314-447-8029. E-mail: JournalsCustomerService-usa@elsevier.com (for print support); JournalsOnlineSupport-usa@elsevier.com (for online support).**

Reprints. For copies of 100 or more of articles in this publication, please contact the Commercial Reprints Department, Elsevier Inc., 360 Park Avenue South, New York, NY 10010-1710. Tel.: 212-633-3812; Fax: 212-462-1935; E-mail: reprints@elsevier.com.

Printed and bound in the United Kingdom
Transferred to Digital Print 2011

The cover illustration depicts the following: *Left Panel*: Epicardial access in the LAO view with guide wire following outline of heart border. *Center Panel*: Ventricular tachycardia with epicardial focus. *Right Panel*: LAO view showing a Meditech balloon expanded in pericardial space to protect the left phrenic nerve during epicardial VT ablation.

Contributors

CONSULTING EDITORS

RANJAN K. THAKUR, MD, MPH, FHRS
Professor of Medicine, and Director, Arrhythmia Service, Thoracic and Cardiovascular Institute, Sparrow Health System, Michigan State University, Lansing, Michigan

ANDREA NATALE, MD, FACC, FHRS
Executive Medical Director of the Texas Cardiac Arrhythmia Institute at St David's Medical Center, Austin, Texas; Consulting Professor, Division of Cardiology, Stanford University, Palo Alto, California; Clinical Associate Professor of Medicine, Case Western Reserve University, Cleveland, Ohio; Senior Clinical Director, EP Services, California Pacific Medical Center, San Francisco; Department of Biomedical Engineering, University of Texas, Austin, Texas

GUEST EDITORS

KALYANAM SHIVKUMAR, MD, PhD, FHRS
Professor of Medicine and Radiological Sciences; Director, UCLA Cardiac Arrhythmia Center & EP Programs, Ronald Reagan UCLA Medical Center, David Geffen School of Medicine at UCLA, Los Angeles, California

NOEL G. BOYLE, MD, PhD, FHRS
Professor of Medicine; Director, Cardiac Electrophysiology Labs, UCLA Cardiac Arrhythmia Center, Ronald Reagan UCLA Medical Center, David Geffen School of Medicine at UCLA, Los Angeles, California

AUTHORS

SAMUEL J. ASIRVATHAM, MD, FHRS
Professor of Medicine, Division of Cardiovascular Diseases and Internal Medicine; Division of Pediatric Cardiology, Department of Pediatrics and Adolescent Medicine, Mayo Clinic College of Medicine, Rochester, Minnesota

BERNARD BELHASSEN, MD
Director, Cardiac Electrophysiology Laboratory, The Department of Cardiology, Tel Aviv Sourasky Medical Center and the Sackler Faculty of Medicine, Tel Aviv University, Tel Aviv, Israel

NOEL G. BOYLE, MD, PhD, FHRS
Professor of Medicine; Director, Cardiac Electrophysiology Labs, UCLA Cardiac Arrhythmia Center, Ronald Reagan UCLA Medical Center, David Geffen School of Medicine at UCLA, Los Angeles, California

CHARLES J. BRUCE, MD
Division of Cardiovascular Diseases and Internal Medicine, Mayo Clinic, Rochester, Minnesota

ERIC BUCH, MD
Director, Specialized Program for AF, UCLA Cardiac Arrhythmia Center, David Geffen School of Medicine at UCLA, Los Angeles, California

TRACI BUESCHER, RN
Division of Cardiovascular Diseases and Internal Medicine, Mayo Clinic College of Medicine, Rochester, Minnesota

J. DAVID BURKHARDT, MD
Staff, Texas Cardiac Arrhythmia Institute at St David's Medical Center, Austin, Texas; Stereotaxis, St Louis, Missouri

YONG-MEI CHA, MD
Division of Cardiovascular Diseases and Internal Medicine, Mayo Clinic College of Medicine, Rochester, Minnesota

KEVIN CHRISTENSEN, BA
Mayo Medical School, Mayo Clinic, Rochester, Minnesota

ANDREW DANIELSEN, MS
Mayo Clinic Health Solutions, Mayo Clinic, Rochester, Minnesota

LUIGI DI BIASE, MD
Texas Cardiac Arrhythmia Institute at St David's Medical Center, Austin, Texas; Department of Biomedical Engineering, University of Texas, Austin, Texas; Department of Cardiology, University of Foggia, Foggia, Italy

SABINE ERNST, MD, FESC
Consultant Cardiologist/Electrophysiologist, Honorary Senior Lecturer, Cardiology Department, Royal Brompton and Harefield Hospital; National Heart and Lung Institute, Imperial College London, London, United Kingdom

PAUL A. FRIEDMAN, MD, FHRS, FACC
Professor of Medicine, Division of Cardiovascular Diseases, Department of Medicine, Mayo Clinic College of Medicine, Rochester, Minnesota

NAGA VAMSI GARIKIPATI, MD, MPH
Research Fellow, Clinical Electrophysiology, The Al-Sabah Arrhythmia Institute, St Luke's and Roosevelt Hospitals Center, Columbia University College of Physicians & Surgeons, New York, New York

KASTURI K. GHIA, MD
Department of Cardiovascular Medicine, William Beaumont Hospital, Oakland University William Beaumont School of Medicine, Royal Oak, Michigan

ALEXANDER I. GREEN, MD
Department of Cardiology, Cardiovascular Institute, Loyola University Medical Center, Maywood, Illinois

DAVID E. HAINES, MD
Chairman, Department of Cardiovascular Medicine, William Beaumont Hospital, Oakland University William Beaumont School of Medicine, Royal Oak, Michigan

SIEW YEN HO, PhD, FRCPath
Professor of Cardiac Morphology, Cardiac Morphology Unit, Imperial College London; Cardiac Morphology Unit, Royal Brompton and Harefield Hospital, London, United Kingdom

RODNEY HORTON, MD
Texas Cardiac Arrhythmia Institute at St David's Medical Center, Austin, Texas; Akron General Hospital, Department of Cardiology, Akron, Ohio; Department of Biomedical Engineering, University of Texas, Austin, Texas

MATHEW D. HUTCHINSON, MD
Assistant Professor of Medicine, Cardiovascular Division, Department of Medicine, University of Pennsylvania, The Hospital of the University of Pennsylvania, Philadelphia, Pennsylvania

G. NEAL KAY, MD
Professor of Medicine, Division of Cardiovascular Disease, University of Alabama at Birmingham, Birmingham, Alabama

NIRUSHA LACHMAN, PhD
Department of Anatomy, Mayo Clinic, Rochester, Minnesota

FRANCIS E. MARCHLINSKI, MD
Professor of Medicine, Cardiovascular Division, Department of Medicine, University of Pennsylvania, The Hospital of the University of Pennsylvania, Philadelphia, Pennsylvania

JENNIFER A. MEARS, BS
Division of Cardiovascular Diseases and Internal Medicine, Mayo Clinic College of Medicine, Rochester, Minnesota

YOAV MICHOWITZ, MD
The Department of Cardiology, Tel Aviv Sourasky Medical Center and the Sackler Faculty of Medicine, Tel Aviv University, Tel Aviv, Israel; UCLA Cardiac Arrhythmia Center, Ronald Reagan UCLA Medical Center, David Geffen School of Medicine at UCLA, Los Angeles, California

SUNEET MITTAL, MD
Director, Electrophysiology Laboratory, The Al-Sabah Arrhythmia Institute, St Luke's-Roosevelt Hospitals Center, Columbia University College of Physicians & Surgeons, New York, New York

THOMAS M. MUNGER, MD
Division of Cardiovascular Diseases and Internal Medicine, Mayo Clinic College of Medicine, Rochester, Minnesota

SHIRO NAKAHARA, MD
UCLA Cardiac Arrhythmia Center, David Geffen School of Medicine at UCLA, Los Angeles, California

ANDREA NATALE, MD
Executive Medical Director of the Texas Cardiac Arrhythmia Institute at St David's Medical Center, Austin, Texas; Consulting Professor, Division of Cardiology, Stanford University, Palo Alto, California; Clinical Associate Professor of Medicine, Case Western Reserve University, Cleveland, Ohio; Senior Clinical Director, EP Services, California Pacific Medical Center, San Francisco; Department of Biomedical Engineering, University of Texas, Austin, Texas

VIJAYAPRAVEENA PARUCHURI, MD
Research fellow, Clinical Electrophysiology, The Al-Sabah Arrhythmia Institute, St Luke's and Roosevelt Hospitals Center, Columbia University College of Physicians & Surgeons, New York, New York

DAMIAN SANCHEZ-QUINTANA, MD, PhD
Professor of Anatomy, Departamento de Anatomía Humana, Facultad de Medicina, University of Extremadura, Badajoz, Spain

MAURICIO SCANAVACCA, MD, PhD
Electrophysiologist of the Cardiac Arrhythmia and Pacemaker Unit and Associated Professor in the Heart Institute (INCOR) do Hospital das Clínicas da Faculdade de Medicina da Universidade de São Paulo, São Paulo, Brazil

ROBERT A. SCHWEIKERT, MD
Chief of Cardiology, Akron General Medical Center, Akron, Ohio; Associate Professor of Internal Medicine, Northeast Ohio Universities College of Medicine, Rootstown, Ohio

KALYANAM SHIVKUMAR, MD, PhD, FHRS
Professor of Medicine and Radiological Sciences; Director, UCLA Cardiac Arrhythmia Center & EP Programs, Ronald Reagan UCLA Medical Center, David Geffen School of Medicine at UCLA, Los Angeles, California

EDUARDO SOSA, MD, PhD
Director of the Cardiac Arrhythmia and Pacemaker Unit and Associated Professor in the Heart Institute (INCOR) do Hospital das Clínicas da Faculdade de Medicina da Dr. Stanton Universidade de São Paulo, São Paulo, Brazil

CHRISTOPHER M. STANTON, MD
Division of Cardiovascular Diseases and Internal Medicine, Mayo Clinic, Rochester, Minnesota

WILLIAM G. STEVENSON, MD
The Cardiovascular Division, Department of Medicine, Brigham and Women's Hospital; Professor of Medicine, Harvard Medical School, Boston, Massachusetts

FAISAL SYED, MBChB
Department of Internal Medicine, Mayo Clinic, Rochester, Minnesota

USHA TEDROW, MD, MSc
The Cardiovascular Division, Department of Medicine, Brigham and Women's Hospital; Instructor of Medicine, Harvard Medical School, Boston, Massachusetts

DAVID J. WILBER, MD
Department of Cardiology, Cardiovascular Institute, Loyola University Medical Center, Maywood, Illinois

TAKUMI YAMADA, MD, PhD
Instructor of Medicine, Division of Cardiovascular Disease, University of Alabama at Birmingham, Birmingham, Alabama

Contents

up and running, so this is a good opportunity to review the indications, the risks that are inherent in the procedure, and the infrastructure necessary in the electrophysiology laboratory and institution to perform the procedure safely and effectively.

Energy Sources for Ablation in the Pericardial Space **45**

Kasturi K. Ghia and David E. Haines

Catheter ablation has been widely used for the management of cardiac arrhythmias. Transvenous endocardial catheter ablation successfully eliminates or modifies the critical substrate for most arrhythmias. Most arrhythmias can be eliminated with conventional endocardial mapping and radiofrequency energy delivery, but some critical arrhythmic substrates are not accessible via endocardial access and this has led to epicardial mapping and ablation in addition to traditional endocardial mapping techniques. This article reviews current approaches to epicardial ablation and discusses the specialized tools that increase ablation efficacy and safety.

Epicardial Ablation of Ventricular Tachycardia in Chagas Heart Disease **55**

Mauricio Scanavacca and Eduardo Sosa

Chagas heart disease is a chronic diffuse inflammatory cardiomyopathy with focal aspects. A wide spectrum of cardiac involvement can be found over time and these pathologic aspects determine different clinical presentations of the disease. The peculiar progress of the anatomic substrate may predispose the patient to a progressive cardiomyopathy, complex arrhythmias, and thromboembolic phenomena. Chagas ventricular tachycardia is a reentrant and scar-related tachycardia, and epicardial circuits are frequently found that substrate predominantly related to the inferior and lateral basal walls. Combining endocardial and epicardial mapping and ablation could improve the results of conventional endocardial ventricular tachycardia ablation.

Epicardial Ablation of Ischemic Ventricular Tachycardia **69**

Usha Tedrow and William G. Stevenson

Endocardial catheter ablation for ventricular arrhythmias in patients with ischemic cardiomyopathy decreases ventricular tachycardia (VT) episodes, and painful implantable defibrillator shocks and can be lifesaving in the context of VT storm. Unfortunately, up to approximately one-third of postinfarction VTs are not accessible for ablation from the endocardium. Percutaneous access to the epicardial space has allowed ablation of a portion of these circuits, although anatomic barriers, such as the phrenic nerve, coronary arteries, and intramural circuits, still limit success in some cases. Adhesions, most often due to prior cardiac surgery, frequently necessitate a surgical approach to the pericardial space.

Epicardial Ablation of Idiopathic Ventricular Tachycardia **81**

Alexander I. Green and David J. Wilber

Epicardial ventricular tachycardia (VT) is an increasingly recognized arrhythmia in clinical practice. Electrocardiographic algorithms to identify epicardial VT should be used with the understanding that they are an initial guide to localization and do not exclude an epicardial origin of VT, particularly when endocardial approaches are unsuccessful. Ablation using a transvenous approach or direct epicardial access may produce favorable results, although care must be taken to avoid coronary artery

or phrenic nerve injury. A subset of patients require a combined endocardial and epicardial approach to eliminate VT. Although these ablation strategies are generally well tolerated, they should be limited to patients with highly symptomatic arrhythmias or those in whom myocardial depression is thought to be related to prolonged tachycardia or repetitive ventricular ectopy.

Epicardial Ablation of VT in Patients with Nonischemic LV Cardiomyopathy **93**

Mathew D. Hutchinson and Francis E. Marchlinski

The past decade has seen a remarkable period of discovery and refinement of ventricular tachycardia (VT) ablation in patients with left ventricular cardiomyopathy (LVCM). Patients with LVCM presenting with VT have a common substrate distribution involving predominantly the basal or perivalvular LV, which is often more dramatic on the LV epicardium. They typically present with multiple and often unstable tachycardias due to scar-based reentry. Percutaneous intrapericardial access can be safely performed in the electrophysiology laboratory and has greatly enhanced the efficacy of VT ablation in this setting by allowing detailed mapping. Epicardial ablation incurs unique procedural considerations that must be understood to safely and effectively perform the procedure.

Epicardial Ablation of Supraventricular Tachycardia **105**

Robert A. Schweikert

Epicardial catheter-based mapping and ablation of a variety of supraventricular tachycardias is feasible, safe, and effective. Supraventricular tachycardia substrates are not uncommonly epicardial, and approaches with percutaneous epicardial instrumentation or via the epicardial venous structures, such as the coronary sinus, are becoming more widely accepted. These techniques are an important treatment option as an alternative to a more invasive surgical approach or to allowing patients to suffer from an ongoing arrhythmia. New technologies and innovative techniques are being developed that hold great potential to improve the efficacy and safety of the epicardial catheter-based approach to these challenging arrhythmias.

Epicardial Catheter Ablation of Atrial Fibrillation **113**

Eric Buch, Shiro Nakahara, Noel G. Boyle, and Kalyanam Shivkumar

Atrial fibrillation (AF) can cause significant symptoms despite control of ventricular rate, and for some patients a rhythm-control strategy is more appropriate. Because antiarrhythmic drugs have limited efficacy for treating AF and can cause significant side effects, nonpharmacologic therapy has found a growing role in the treatment of this arrhythmia. While endocardial catheter ablation has shown superior results over drug therapy, long-term clinical outcomes are still disappointing, especially for persistent AF. This article discusses percutaneous epicardial catheter ablation, the rationale for using this approach to treat AF, anatomy relevant to the approach, challenges in performing such procedures, and finally, the potential future directions in this promising new field.

Remote Navigation and Electroanatomic Mapping in the Pericardial Space **121**

J. David Burkhardt, Luigi Di Biase, Rodney Horton, Robert A. Schweikert, and Andrea Natale

Mapping and ablation in the pericardial space has been shown to be beneficial for the treatment of different supraventricular and ventricular arrhythmias. The

Cardiac Electrophysiology Clinics

FORTHCOMING ISSUES

June 2010

Advances in Arrhythmia Analyses: A Case-Based Approach
Melvin Scheinman, MD, and
Masood Akhtar, MD, *Guest Editors*

September 2010

Arrhythmogenic Right Ventricular Cardiomyopathy/Dysplasia
Domenico Corrado, MD, PhD, Cristina Basso, MD, PhD, and Gaetano Thiene, MD,
Guest Editors

December 2010

Advances in Antiarrhythmic Drug Therapy
Peter R. Kowey, MD, and
Gerald V. Naccarelli, MD,
Guest Editors

RECENT ISSUE

December 2009

Sudden Cardiac Death
Ranjan K. Thakur, MD, MPH, FHRS, and
Andrea Natale, MD, FACC, FHRS, *Guest Editors*

ISSUES OF RELATED INTEREST

Cardiology Clinics February 2010 (Vol. 28, No. 1)
Advanced Applied Interventional Cardiology
Samin K. Sharma, MD, FACC, and
Annapoorna S. Kini, MD, MRCP, FACC, *Guest Editors*
Available at: http://www.cardiology.theclinics.com/

Heart Failure Clinics July 2009 (Vol. 5, No. 3)
Cardiovascular Magnetic Resonance in Heart Failure
Raymond J. Kim, MD, and Dudley J. Pennell, MD, FRCP, FACC, *Guest Editors*
Available at: http://www.heartfailure.theclinics.com/

Foreword

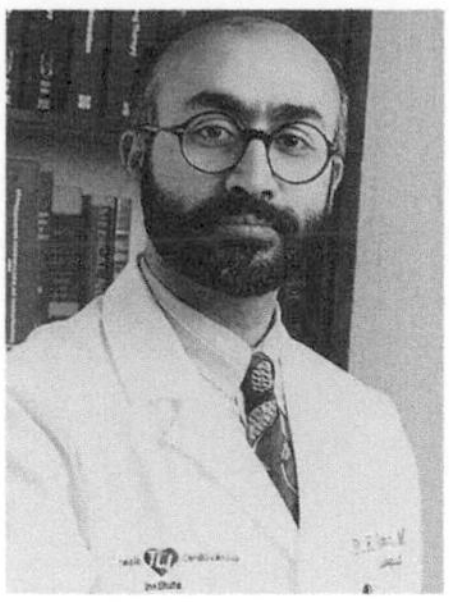

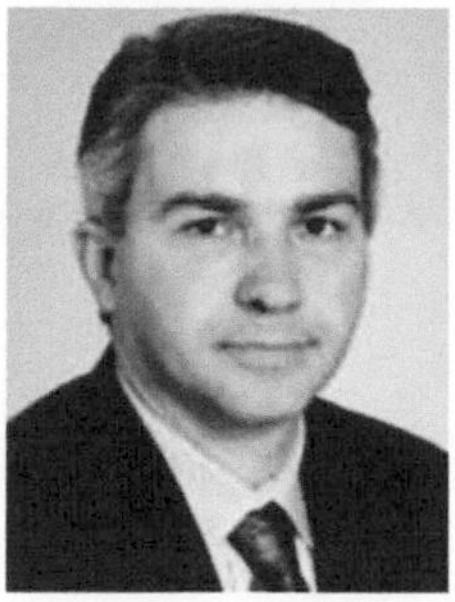

Ranjan K. Thakur, MD, MPH, FHRS Andrea Natale, MD, FACC, FHRS
Consulting Editors

We are pleased to introduce the second issue of *Cardiac Electrophysiology Clinics*. This publication was launched with the idea of providing comprehensive reviews on topics of interest to the clinical electrophysiology community. We set out to recruit eminent electrophysiologists who have expertise on a particular topic and have them assemble a table of contents and suitable contributors from all over the world to illuminate the issue at hand.

We are delighted that Dr Shivkumar and Dr Boyle have tackled epicardial interventions, which is becoming an ever more important approach for electrophysiologic interventions. They have done exactly what we had hoped for.

Most practicing electrophysiologists do not perform epicardial interventions because "the pericardial space has long evoked a sense of trepidation." The situation is not unlike transseptal catheterization a decade ago. When ablation for atrial fibrillation came along, electrophysiologists learned to perform transseptal puncture, and tools were developed subsequently (eg, intracardiac echocardiograpy, radiofrequency needle) so that we could do it safely, minimizing complications. The same will occur with pericardial access and interventions. As Dr Mittal has outlined in his article, this is a technique that can be learned and one can "get on the curve."

Catheter ablation for ventricular tachycardia has had limited success. In the last 5 years we have learned, however, that a significant number of these patients have epicardial circuits, and thus the success rate of catheter ablation can be enhanced by epicardial mapping and ablation. Epicardial access may also prove useful in the future if left ventricular epicardial pacing (to achieve biventricular pacing) can be achieved without a thoracotomy.

We have enjoyed reading the reviews and learning from our colleagues. We are convinced that the readership will find this issue educational and feel sanguine that any interventional electrophysiologist can master this technique.

Ranjan K. Thakur, MD, MPH, FHRS
Thoracic and Cardiovascular Institute
405 West Greenlawn, Suite 400
Michigan State University
Lansing, MI 48910, USA

Andrea Natale, MD, FACC, FHRS
Texas Cardiac Arrhythmia Institute
Center for Atrial Fibrillation at
St David's Medical Center
1015 East 32nd Street, Suite 516
Austin, TX 78705, USA

E-mail addresses:
Thakur@msu.edu (R.K. Thakur)
Andrea.natale@stdavids.com (A. Natale)

Card Electrophysiol Clin 2 (2010) xiii
doi:10.1016/j.ccep.2009.11.015
1877-9182/10/$ – see front matter

Preface

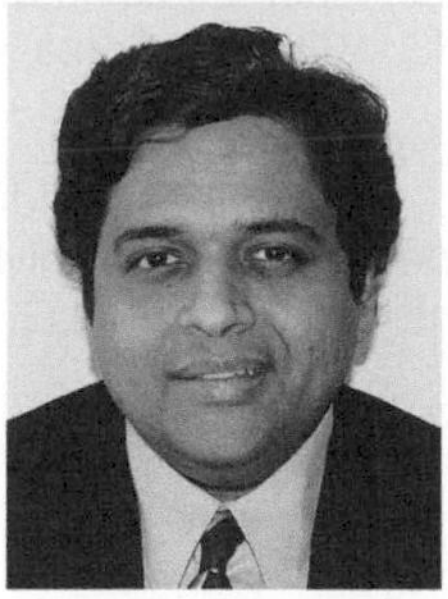

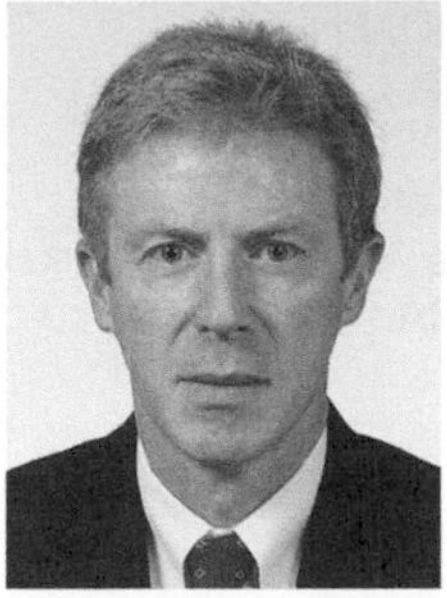

Kalyanam Shivkumar, MD, PhD, FHRS   Noel G. Boyle, MD, PhD, FHRS
Guest Editors

The pericardial space has long evoked a sense of trepidation for many cardiologists. Commonly associated with the pathologic pericardial effusion, it was rarely approached except when necessary to drain a chronic pericardial effusion or in the emergent setting of tamponade. The pioneering work of Sosa and colleagues, first reported in 1996 and described in the article by Drs Scanavacca and Sosa, opened up this new frontier to interventional cardiac electrophysiology and ablation.

This issue of *Cardiac Electrophysiology Clinics* focuses on the pericardial space, presents reviews from many leaders in the field of clinical cardiac electrophysiology, and outlines the latest advances in this area. Drs Ernst and Ho first present the anatomy of the pericardial space with its rediscovery in the setting of epicardial mapping and ablation, and Drs Syed, Asirvatham, and colleagues describe how a better understanding of the anatomy of the pericardial space and of radiology makes for safer access to pericardial space.

Drs Michowitz and Belhassen describe the electrocardiogram (EKG) recognition of epicardial arrhythmias, an important step in patient selection for the epicardial approach. Drs Garikipati, Paruchuri, and Mittal discuss how to learn the technique and how to set up a program for epicardial ablation. Drs Ghia and Haines provide a comprehensive description of the energy sources available for ablation with the epicardial approach.

Drs Scanavacca and Sosa describe their pioneering work in the field with the development of epicardial ventricular tachycardia (VT) ablation for the problem of VT in Chagas disease patients. Drs Tedrow and Stevenson discuss the epicardial ablation of scar-related VT, Drs Green and Wilber describe the method applied to idiopathic VT patients, and Drs Hutchinson and Marchlinski review the role of epicardial ablation in the setting of nonischemic cardiomyopathy–related VT. Dr Schweikert describes the application of the epicardial approach to supraventricular tachycardias, and Drs Buch, Nakahara and colleagues describe the potential for epicardial ablation of atrial fibrillation and important methods for protecting collateral structures.

The application of advances in remote navigation to epicardial ablation is discussed by Drs Burkhardt, Natale and associates, while Drs Yamada and Kay examine the important issue of procedure-related complications and how to prevent them. Drs Stanton, Friedman and coworkers conclude with a look at future prospects in the field.

The next decade will likely see major advances in the epicardial approach and wider use of the technique in ways analogous to how the first endocardial ablation procedure led to a revolution in the treatment of cardiac arrhythmias. These advances will come together with a new appreciation for the

Card Electrophysiol Clin 2 (2010) xv–xvi
doi:10.1016/j.ccep.2009.12.001

anatomy and physiology of the pericardial space and the development of new tools and therapeutics to make this procedure simpler and safer.

Kalyanam Shivkumar, MD, PhD, FHRS
UCLA Cardiac Arrhythmia Center
Ronald Reagan UCLA Medical Center
David Geffen School of Medicine at UCLA
A2-237 CHS, 10833 Le Conte Avenue
Los Angeles, CA 90095

Noel G. Boyle, MD, PhD, FHRS
UCLA Cardiac Arrhythmia Center
Ronald Reagan UCLA Medical Center
David Geffen School of Medicine at UCLA
A2-237 CHS, 10833 Le Conte Avenue
Los Angeles, CA 90095

E-mail addresses:
kshivkumar@mednet.ucla.edu (K. Shivkumar)
nboyle@mednet.ucla.edu (N.G. Boyle)

Anatomy of the Pericardial Space and Mediastinum: Relevance to Epicardial Mapping and Ablation

Sabine Ernst, MD, FESC[a,b],
Damian Sanchez-Quintana, MD, PhD[c],
Siew Yen Ho, PhD, FRCPath[d,e,*]

KEYWORDS

- Cardiac anatomy • Epicardial space
- Catheter ablation • Puncture technique
- Ventricular tachycardia • Atrial fibrillation

Catheter ablation for most arrhythmia substrates is performed frequently from within the cardiac chambers using an exclusively endocardial approach. Although epicardial ablations have been performed for many years; they have been from within the cardiac veins (mainly the coronary sinus) or from above the semilunar valves.[1,2] In most of these procedures, a fairly small area (eg, an accessory pathway or a focal origin of ventricular ectopy) was targeted, requiring only focal energy application. However, epicardial arrhythmias may require deployment of more complex lesions, such as linear lesions.

Because of the clinical need to manage ventricular tachycardia in patients with Chagas disease, the earliest experience of epicardial mapping and ablation using a subxiphoidal approach came from Brazil.[3] Although intraoperative mapping and subsequent arrhythmia surgery was commonly performed in the 1980s and 90s,[4] nowadays, arrhythmia surgery mostly concentrates on atrial fibrillation.[5,6] Arrhythmia surgery is mainly undertaken as an add-on or concomitant surgery, seldom as a stand-alone procedure. Because new tools have become available for an epicardial approach without the need to open the left atrium (LA), this procedure can be performed off-pump and in a purely thoracoscopic fashion.

Recently, reports on "sandwich" mapping and ablation for ischemic ventricular tachycardia have encouraged clinicians to widen their diagnostic and therapeutic window to this space (**Fig. 1**).[7–9] This article describes the anatomic background to the technical steps for the pericardial approach, which is an emerging clinical necessity and

Prof Ho's unit receives funding support from the Royal Brompton and Harefield Hospital Charitable Fund.
[a] Cardiology Department, Royal Brompton and Harefield Hospital, Sydney Street, London SW3 6NP, UK
[b] National Heart and Lung Institute, Imperial College London, London SW3 6LY, UK
[c] Departamento de Anatomía Humana, Facultad de Medicina, University of Extremadura, UEX, E-06071 Badajoz, Spain
[d] Cardiac Morphology Unit, Imperial College London, London SW3 6LY, UK
[e] Cardiac Morphology Unit, Royal Brompton and Harefield Hospital, Sydney Street, London SW3 6NP, UK
* Corresponding author. Cardiac Morphology Unit, Royal Brompton and Harefield Hospital, Sydney Street, London SW3 6NP, UK.
E-mail address: yen.ho@imperial.ac.uk (S.Y. Ho).

Card Electrophysiol Clin 2 (2010) 1–8
doi:10.1016/j.ccep.2009.11.003
1877-9182/10/$ – see front matter

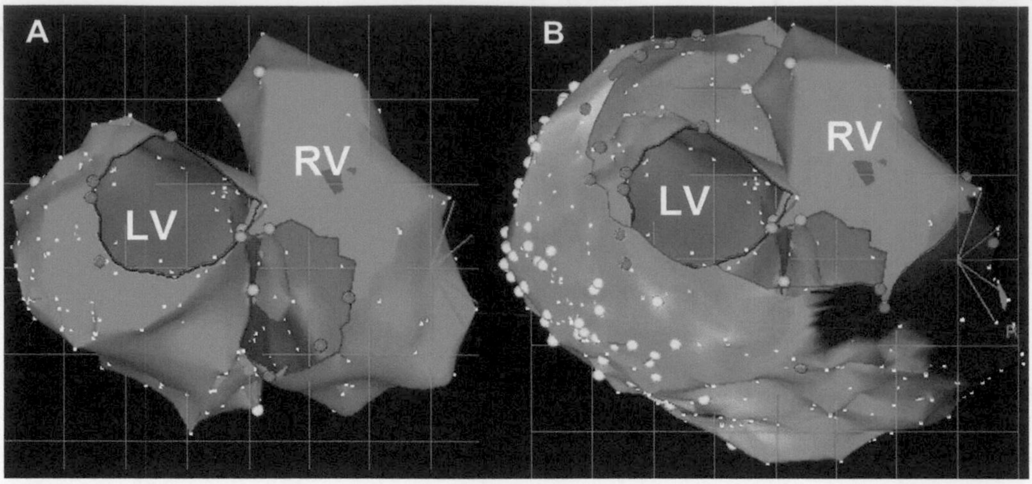

Fig. 1. (*A*) Three dimensional maps of the right (RV) and left ventricle (LV). (*B*) The additional epicardial map superimposed on the 2 ventricles.

increasingly important when dealing with complex arrhythmia.

THE ANATOMY OF THE PERICARDIAL SPACE

The heart and its adjoining great vessels are enclosed in a sac, the parietal (fibrous) pericardium. Superiorly, the fibrous pericardium is continuous with the adventitia of the great vessels, like cuffs attaching to the ascending aorta and pulmonary trunk and to the superior caval vein, several centimeters above the site of the sinus node. Anteriorly, it is attached to the posterior surface of the sternum by superior and inferior sternopericardial ligaments that are variably developed. Laterally are the pleural coverings of the mediastinal surface of the lungs. The esophagus, descending thoracic aorta, and posterior parts of the mediastinal surface of both lungs are related posteriorly. Inferiorly, the fibrous pericardium is attached to the central tendon of the diaphragm and a small muscular area to the left. The diaphragm separates the pericardium from the liver and fundus of the stomach. There is a small area behind the lower left half of the body of the sternum and the sternal ends of the left fourth and fifth costal cartilages where the fibrous pericardium is in direct contact with the thoracic wall. This area does allow the pericardial space to be accessed, but the operator should take care not to enter the right ventricle, which lies behind the space. Instead, most operators use a subxiphoid approach for the puncture (see later discussion).

Within the fibrous pericardium is a delicate double-layered membrane called the serous pericardium (**Fig. 2**A). One layer of the serous pericardium is fused to the inner surface of the fibrous pericardium, whereas the other layer lines the outer surface of the heart as the epicardium and continues over the surfaces of the vessels as the visceral pericardium. Over the great vessels, the junctions between the 2 layers are the pericardial reflections. The separation of the 2 layers of the serous pericardium creates a narrow space, the pericardial cavity. Under normal conditions, the pericardial cavity contains approximately 20 mL of fluid, which is a plasma ultrafiltrate. This pericardial fluid serves to lubricate the moving surfaces where the beating heart makes contact with fixed structures.

The pericardial cavity has 2 sinuses and several recesses. These are not complete compartments but represent extensions of the cavity. The transverse sinus is delineated anteriorly by the posterior surface of the ascending aorta and pulmonary trunk bifurcation and posteriorly by the anterior surface of the atria. The oblique sinus, a large cul-de-sac behind the left atrium (**Fig. 2**B), is formed by the continuity between the reflections along the pulmonary veins and caval veins. The right and left pulmonary venous recesses are at the back of the left atrium between the upper and lower pulmonary veins on each side, indenting the side walls of the oblique sinus to a greater or lesser extent. The pericardial reflections at the veins, particularly the pulmonary veins, are varied and they can restrict access around the veins.[10] The inferior and superior aortic recesses are extensions from the transverse sinus. The superior recess lies between the ascending aorta and the

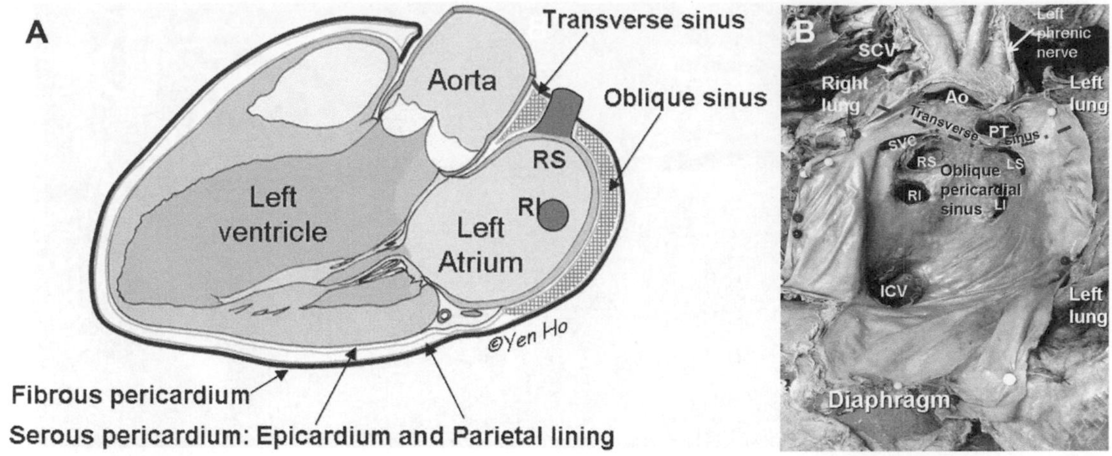

Fig. 2. (*A*) The layers of the pericardium and the transverse and oblique sinuses. (*B*) This dissection of a cadaver viewed from the front shows the sinuses following removal of the heart. Ao, aorta; ICV, inferior caval vein; SCV, superior caval vein; PT, pulmonary trunk; LI, left inferior; LS, left superior; RI, right inferior; and RS, right superior pulmonary veins.

right atrium, whereas the inferior recess between the aorta and the left atrium extends to the level of the aortic valve.

ACCESS TO THE EPICARDIUM (AS AN ELECTIVE PROCEDURE)

True epicardial approach is still a rarity and therefore requires expert skills and clear justification.[11] Subxiphoid puncture in the emergency of a tamponade in a hemodynamically unstable patient is an extremely stressfully situation. However, it can be performed successfully because the enlarged pericardial cavity (stretched by the blood accumulating) has the advantage of distancing the fibrous pericardium from the heart, reducing the risk of injury to the right ventricle.[12] By contrast, a "dry" puncture with only a few milliliters of pericardial fluid carries a significantly higher risk of unintentional injury to the ventricular myocardium; therefore, careful preparation and detailed knowledge of the underlying anatomy is the key.

Step-by-Step Approach

Most commonly, the epicardial space is accessed from the subxiphoidal space, aiming toward the left midclavicle (**Fig. 3**).[3,13] A long needle is advanced under fluoroscopic guidance at an angle of 20% to 30%, aiming at the heart shadow. Puncturing below the rib's cartilage usually does not encounter strong resistance until the stronger resistance of the diaphragm is felt. The cardiac contraction can be felt through the needle itself. Crossing this relatively thin zone that is directly attached to the strong texture of the fibrous pericardium should be performed under constant negative pressure. When entering the epicardial space, a small volume (2–3 mL) of clear yellowish fluid, the pericardial fluid, can be aspirated. Subsequently, injection of ca 3–5 mL of contrast agent results in it accumulating in a crescent-shaped outline of the pericardial space. In the event of an unintentional puncture of the apex of the right ventricle, the contrast agent moves with the blood flow upwards and becomes diluted, thus disappearing nearly instantly. To facilitate the depiction of the contrast properly, high resolution acquisition rather than fluoroscopy only should be performed to avoid missing the incorrect disappearance of the contrast. Once the pericardial space is outlined, injecting several more milliliters of saline allows widening of the pericardial space. Subsequently, a long J-tipped wire, when introduced under fluoroscopy, should wrap itself around the heart. Exiting the cardiac silhouette is definite evidence of unintentional ventricular puncture. The guidewire and needle need to be carefully withdrawn several millimeters, before the wire can be advanced again. Once a sufficient length of the guidewire is positioned in place, a long sheath (eg, 9 F) will be advanced in an over-the-wire fashion. Especially when crossing the diaphragm/fibrous pericardium, the resistance is rather high in some instances, and predilatation might be necessary. Choosing a sheath diameter of 1 F+ allows aspiration of excessive pericardial fluid, which might result from the use of an irrigated-tip mapping and ablation catheter in the later stages of the procedure. Pericardial

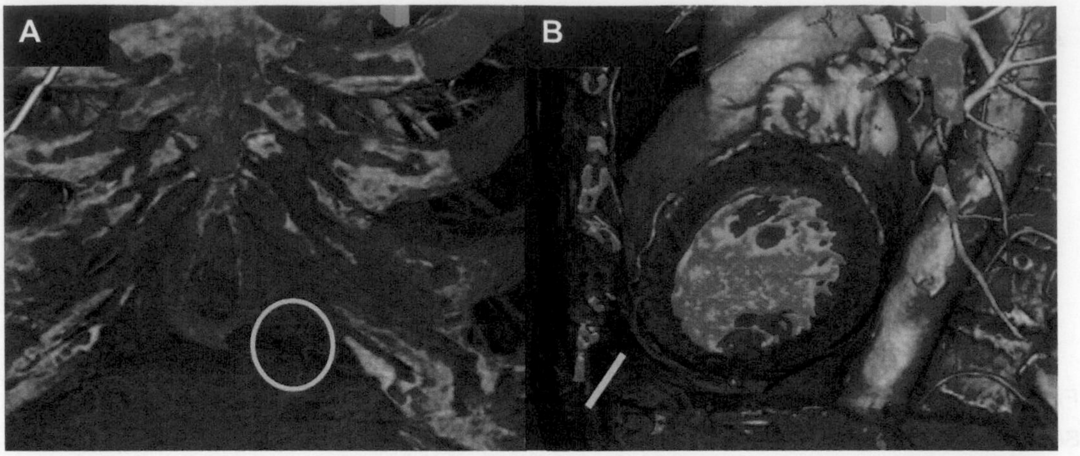

Fig. 3. Computed tomographic scans to demonstrate percutaneous access: (*A*) An anteroposterior projection with the green circle depicting the puncture site. (*B*) The left lateral projection demonstrates the angle that is necessary to target the anterior aspect of the pericardium.

adhesions that may be the result of a previous cardiac operation or any other pericardial inflammation process might limit the accessibility within the epicardial space. Detailed knowledge of the folds and reflections of the pericardium and frequent variations allows advance planning of the pericardial puncture.

To facilitate the puncture process itself, several technical improvements to the needle and assisting technologies have been introduced recently.[14,15] Advanced imaging, for example, by transgastric echo to directly visualize the perforating needle has been proposed, but there are no reports of large patient cohorts that underwent this procedure.

Especially after previous cardiac surgery (eg, for bypass grafting), the desired epicardial region might not be reachable by the conventional epicardial access. In these special cases, a surgically created minimal access to the epicardium has been reported.[8]

Also reported is an unusual technique, where despite several unsuccessful attempts to relieve a cardiac tamponade by conventional techniques, the operators finally perforated the left ventricular wall to relieve the effusion through a transseptal sheath.

The short-term follow-up was reported to be uneventful and the later surgical repair was uncomplicated.[16]

How to Exit the Pericardium?

Effusion, sterile pericarditis, hemopericardium, and retamponade are recognized frequent consequences after pericardial mapping and ablation. Therefore, the patients should be monitored carefully in an intensive care unit, with regular checks of vital signs and repeated transthoracic echocardiograms. It is recommended that a pigtail catheter be kept inside the pericardium for several hours (4–24 hours). The catheter should be flushed initially with heparinized saline to prevent clotting. Several investigators have recommended giving simultaneous antibiotic cover and recently, a group has published its experience with steroid installations to avoid sterile pericarditis.[13]

THE NEIGHBORHOOD: IMPORTANT CARDIAC STRUCTURES

Coronary Arteries

Detailed knowledge of the individual distribution of the coronary vessels is an obvious prerequisite of any epicardial mapping and ablation attempt (**Fig. 4**). However, using only the standard interventional fluoroscopic projections might make it difficult to understand the 3-dimensional (3D) anatomy. Because nowadays, most of these complex electrophysiologic procedures are performed using 3D mapping systems allowing merging of the endocardial volume reconstructions, a 3D registered image of the coronary arteries can also be used.[17] Nevertheless, if the final ablation site is close to any coronary artery, then a selective angiogram needs to be performed in at least 2 projections to establish the distance between the target site and the nearest vessel.

FAT PADS AND INNERVATION

The intrinsic cardiac nerves have been studied in detail by Armour and colleagues[18] and Pauza and colleagues[19] in the last decade, but gained

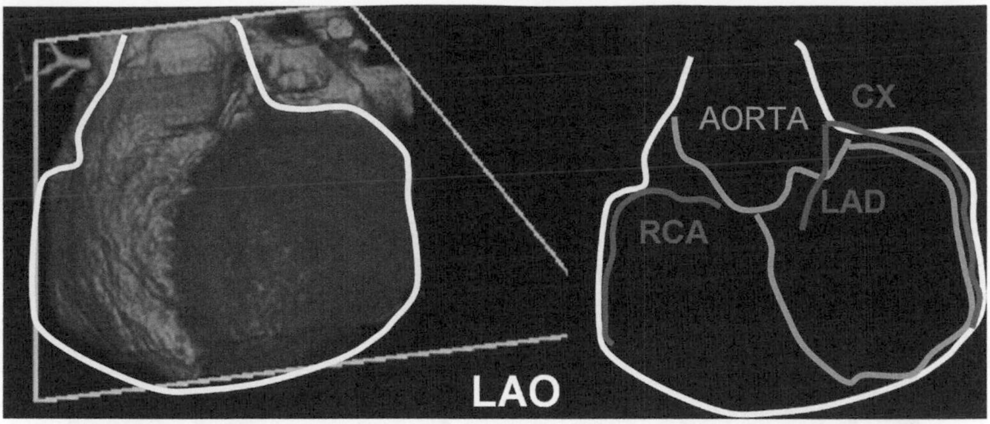

Fig. 4. Coronary arteries in epicardial space displayed in left anterior oblique (LAO) projection on a cardiac computed tomographic scan.

attention in recent years from electrophysiologists investigating their role in the initiation and maintenance of atrial fibrillation.[20,21] The ganglionated plexi predominantly occupy the epicardial fat pads. Five fat pads are recognized on the atria and there are 2 to 5 pads on the ventricles (**Fig. 5**).[18,19] Adrenergic and cholinergic nerves are distributed in the junctional areas between pulmonary veins and left atrium.[22] Transmurally, there are more nerves on the epicardial half than the endocardial half.[23]

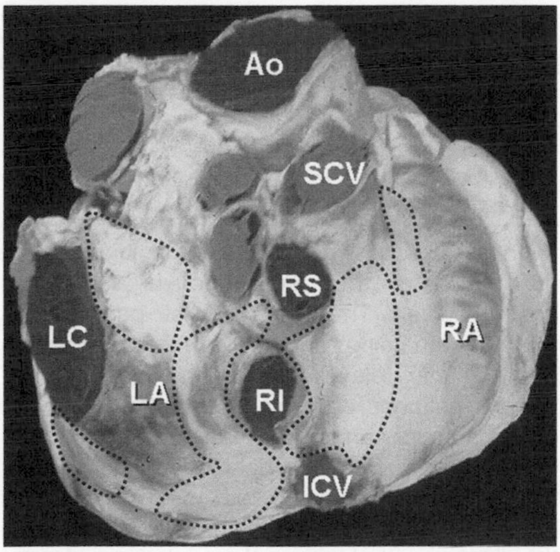

Fig. 5. This view of a heart from the right posterior aspect shows the areas of epicardial fat over the atrial chambers. Usually, 5 epicardial fat pads are recognized (*dotted lines*). LA, left atrium; RA, right atrium; LCC, left common pulmonary vein. Other abbreviations are as for **Fig. 2**.

THE NEIGHBORHOOD: IMPORTANT EXTRACARDIAC STRUCTURES

Phrenic Nerves

The importance of the phrenic nerves is often under-recognized. Accompanied by the pericardiophrenic vessels, the phrenic nerves descend bilaterally onto the fibrous pericardium. The right phrenic nerve descends almost vertically, first along the right brachiocephalic vein, then along the right anterolateral surface of the superior caval vein, and it continues its descent immediately in front of the right pulmonary veins in the lung hilum before reaching the diaphragm (**Fig. 6**A). Measurements made in cadavers show the right phrenic nerve has a close relationship with the superior caval vein (minimal distance 0.3 $\pm$ 0.5 mm) and the right superior pulmonary vein (PV, minimal distance 2.1 $\pm$ 0.4 mm) in its descent.

The left phrenic nerve descends behind the left brachiocephalic vein, continues over the aortic arch and pulmonary trunk onto the pericardium overlying the left atrial appendage, and then descends either anteriorly or anterolaterally over the area of the left ventricle to insert into the diaphragm behind the cardiac apex (**Fig. 6**B).[24,25] The course of the left phrenic nerve on the fibrous pericardium has 3 variants relating to various cardiac surfaces: (1) anteriorly across the anterior surface of the heart related to the high part of the right ventricular outflow tract and the high anterior left ventricular wall, (2) leftward over the tip of the left atrial appendage and obtuse margin of the left ventricle, and (3) posteriorly over the neck of the left atrial appendage and toward the inferior surface of the left ventricle, to be related to the epicardial surface of the high inferolateral left ventricular wall and the inferior left ventricular

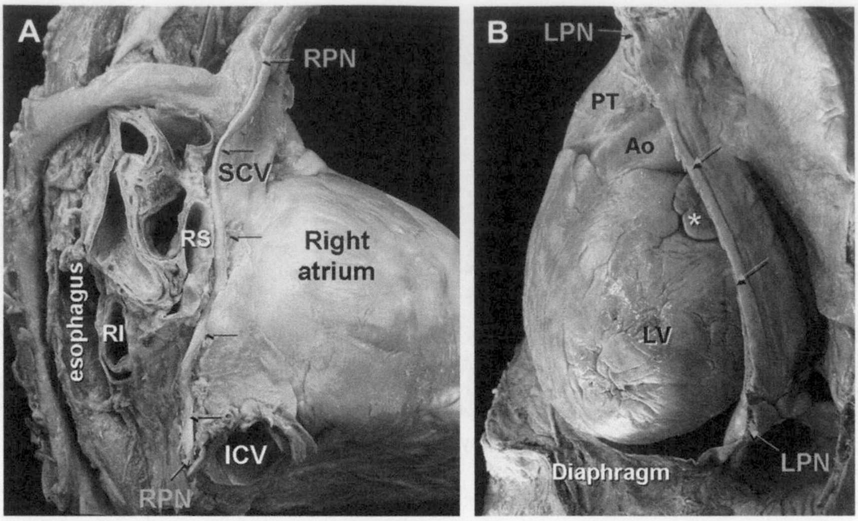

Fig. 6. (*A*) This dissection of a cadaver viewed from the right side shows the course of the right phrenic nerve (RPN) and its particularly close relationship to the superior caval vein and the right superior pulmonary vein. (*B*) This dissection of the left phrenic nerve (LPN) descending along the fibrous pericardium shows its course over the left atrial appendage (*) and relationship to the lateral wall of the left ventricle (LV).

vein.[25] The left phrenic nerve passes at a distance of less than 3 mm from the left marginal vein in 43% of postmortem heart specimens.

Although the damage of the right phrenic nerve has been described as a frequent complication of balloon PV isolation,[26,27] the left phrenic nerve is frequently encountered unknowingly during left ventricular lead placement in cardiac resynchronization therapy.[28] High-output stimulation from the tip of the mapping catheter can readily identify the location of the phrenic nerve on the corresponding side. Slow pacing in close proximity to the nerve results in involuntary diaphragmatic contractions (hiccups); these sites can then be marked using colored tags on the 3D mapping system.

The Esophagus

The esophagus descends through the mediastinum, related to the fibrous pericardium behind the posterior and inferior walls of the left atrium and the junctional areas of the atrium with the pulmonary veins. Because of its flexible position behind the heart, it serves as an excellent portal for transesophageal echocardiography. The proximity of the left atrium is obvious, and echocardiographers take advantage of this to measure flow and velocities in the left atrial appendage and the pulmonary veins.[29] During swallowing, the musculature of the esophagus relaxes sequentially to allow forward propulsion of food and saliva toward the stomach. However, there is also variable sideward movement, because the more posterior structures are relatively fixed in their position (aorta and spine; see earlier discussion). Swallowing occurs in different intervals depending on the amount of stimulation of the gastrointestinal nerve system. Therefore, the esophagus has the potential, at least, to be an irregularly "moving target," which makes static imaging alone a useless endeavor. A mere tube or 3D geometry confirming the retrocardiac position of the esophagus should be replaced by a dynamic imaging modality. Alternatively, operators should act always as if they were in close proximity to the esophagus when ablating at the posterior wall of the left atrium, using low RF energy settings and avoiding excessive contact force.

Periesophageal Nerve Plexus

Even less well known to electrophysiologists is the distribution of the periesophageal vagal and gastric nerves. The vagus nerves pass behind the root of the lungs and form right and left posterior pulmonary plexuses. From the caudal part of the left pulmonary plexus, 2 branches descend on the anterior surface of the esophagus forming, with a branch from the right pulmonary plexus, the anterior esophageal plexus. The posterior and anterior esophageal plexuses reunite beneath the diaphragm to become the posterior and anterior vagal trunks that innervate the stomach and pyloric canal and the digestive tract as far as the proximal part of the colon.[30] Damage of these nerves results in new gastric symptoms, like bloating and prolonged emptying.[31] Ultimately, it can result in pyloric spasms, which may necessitate dilatation or botulinum injections.[32]

The Diaphragm

The pericardium rests on an almost flat area of the diaphragm called the cardiac plateau, which extends more to the left than the right. The profile of the diaphragm rises on either side of the cardiac plateau to a smooth convex dome that is higher and slightly broader on the right than on the left. Most of the inferior surface of the diaphragm is covered by the peritoneum. The right side is molded over the convex surface of the right lobe of the liver, the right kidney, and the right suprarenal gland. The left side conforms to the left lobe of the liver, the fundus of the stomach, the spleen, the left kidney, and the left suprarenal gland.

SUMMARY

Detailed anatomic knowledge of the pericardial space and the neighboring structures inside the mediastinum is the key to entering this novel space. Accurate imaging and understanding of the 3D relationship should avoid causing unintentional "collateral damage" by catheter ablation.

REFERENCES

1. Ouyang F, Fotuhi P, Ho SY, et al. Repetitive monomorphic ventricular tachycardia originating from the aortic sinus cusp: electrocardiographic characterization for guiding catheter ablation. J Am Coll Cardiol 2002;39(3):500–8.
2. Sun Y, Arruda M, Otomo K, et al. Coronary sinus-ventricular accessory connections producing posteroseptal and left posterior accessory pathways: incidence and electrophysiological identification. Circulation 2002;106(11):1362–7.
3. Sosa E, Scanavacca M, d'Avila A, et al. A new technique to perform epicardial mapping in the electrophysiology laboratory. J Cardiovasc Electrophysiol 1996;7(6):531–6.
4. Waxman HL, Buxton AE, Marchlinski FE, et al. Medical versus surgical treatment of tachydysrhythmias. Eur Heart J 1984;5(Suppl B):103–8.
5. Cui YQ, Sun LB, Li Y, et al. Intraoperative modified Cox mini-maze procedure for long-standing persistent atrial fibrillation. Ann Thorac Surg 2008;85(4): 1283–9.
6. McClelland JH, Duke D, Reddy R. Preliminary results of a limited thoracotomy: new approach to treat atrial fibrillation. J Cardiovasc Electrophysiol 2007;18(12):1289–95.
7. Schweikert RA, Saliba WI, Tomassoni G, et al. Percutaneous pericardial instrumentation for endo-epicardial mapping of previously failed ablations. Circulation 2003;108(11):1329–35.
8. Soejima K, Stevenson WG, Sapp JL, et al. Endocardial and epicardial radiofrequency ablation of ventricular tachycardia associated with dilated cardiomyopathy: the importance of low-voltage scars. J Am Coll Cardiol 2004;43(10):1834–42.
9. Garcia FC, Bazan V, Zado ES, et al. Epicardial substrate and outcome with epicardial ablation of ventricular tachycardia in arrhythmogenic right ventricular cardiomyopathy/dysplasia. Circulation 2009;120(5):366–75.
10. D'Avila A, Scanavacca M, Sosa E, et al. Pericardial anatomy for the interventional electrophysiologist. J Cardiovasc Electrophysiol 2003;14(4):422–30.
11. Cappato R. NICE guidance on catheter ablation of atrial fibrillation using an epicardial (non-thorascoscopic) approach. Heart 2009;95:1956–7.
12. Tsang TS, Freeman WK, Barnes ME, et al. Rescue echocardiographically guided pericardiocentesis for cardiac perforation complicating catheter-based procedures. The Mayo Clinic experience. J Am Coll Cardiol 1998;32(5):1345–50.
13. Grimard C, Lacotte J, Hidden-Lucet F, et al. Percutaneous epicardial radiofrequency ablation of ventricular arrhythmias after failure of endocardial approach: a 9-year experience. J Cardiovasc Electrophysiol 2009. [Epub ahead of print].
14. d'Avila A, Scanavacca M, Sosa E. Transthoracic epicardial catheter ablation of ventricular tachycardia. Heart Rhythm 2006;3(9):1110–1.
15. Hou D, March KL. A novel percutaneous technique for accessing the normal pericardium: a single-center successful experience of 53 porcine procedures. J Invasive Cardiol 2003;15(1):13–7.
16. Hsu LF, Scavee C, Jais P, et al. Transcardiac pericardiocentesis: an emergency life-saving technique for cardiac tamponade. J Cardiovasc Electrophysiol 2003;14(9):1001–3.
17. Zeppenfeld K, Tops LF, Bax JJ, et al. Images in cardiovascular medicine. Epicardial radiofrequency catheter ablation of ventricular tachycardia in the vicinity of coronary arteries is facilitated by fusion of 3-dimensional electroanatomical mapping with multislice computed tomography. Circulation 2006; 114(3):e51–2.
18. Armour JA, Murphy DA, Yuan BX, et al. Gross and microscopic anatomy of the human intrinsic cardiac nervous system. Anat Rec 1997;247(2):289–98.
19. Pauza DH, Skripka V, Pauziene N, et al. Morphology, distribution, and variability of the epicardiac neural ganglionated subplexuses in the human heart. Anat Rec 2000;259(4):353–82.
20. Hou Y, Scherlag BJ, Lin J, et al. Interactive atrial neural network: determining the connections between ganglionated plexi. Heart Rhythm 2007; 4(1):56–63.

21. Scanavacca M, Pisani CF, Hachul D, et al. Selective atrial vagal denervation guided by evoked vagal reflex to treat patients with paroxysmal atrial fibrillation. Circulation 2006;114(9):876–85.
22. Tan AY, Li H, Wachsmann-Hogiu S, et al. Autonomic innervation and segmental muscular disconnections at the human pulmonary vein-atrial junction: implications for catheter ablation of atrial-pulmonary vein junction. J Am Coll Cardiol 2006;48(1):132–43.
23. Tan AY, Chen PS, Chen LS, et al. Autonomic nerves in pulmonary veins. Heart Rhythm 2007;4(Suppl 3): S57–60.
24. Sánchez-Quintana D, Cabrera JA, Climent V, et al. How close are the phrenic nerves to cardiac structures? Implications for cardiac interventionalists. J Cardiovasc Electrophysiol 2005;16(3):309–13.
25. Sánchez-Quintana D, Ho SY, Climent V, et al. Anatomic evaluation of the left phrenic nerve relevant to epicardial and endocardial catheter ablation: implications for phrenic nerve injury. Heart Rhythm 2009;6(6):764–8.
26. Chun KR, Schmidt B, Metzner A, et al. The 'single big cryoballoon' technique for acute pulmonary vein isolation in patients with paroxysmal atrial fibrillation: a prospective observational single centre study. Eur Heart J 2009;30(6):699–709.
27. Neumann T, Vogt J, Schumacher B, et al. Circumferential pulmonary vein isolation with the cryoballoon technique results from a prospective 3-center study. J Am Coll Cardiol 2008;52(4):273–8.
28. Leclercq C, Gadler F, Kranig W, et al. A randomized comparison of triple-site versus dual-site ventricular stimulation in patients with congestive heart failure. J Am Coll Cardiol 2008;51(15):1455–62.
29. Schneider C, Ernst S, Malisius R, et al. Transesophageal echocardiography: a follow-up tool after catheter ablation of atrial fibrillation and interventional therapy of pulmonary vein stenosis and occlusion. J Interv Card Electrophysiol 2007;18(2): 195–205.
30. Ho SY, Cabrera JA, Sánchez-Quintana D. Vagaries of the vagus nerve: relevance to ablationists. J Cardiovasc Electrophysiol 2006;17(3):330–1.
31. Shah D, Dumonceau JM, Burri H, et al. Acute pyloric spasm and gastric hypomotility: an extracardiac adverse effect of percutaneous radiofrequency ablation for atrial fibrillation. J Am Coll Cardiol 2005;46(2):327–30.
32. Pisani CF, Hachul D, Sosa E, et al. Gastric hypomotility following epicardial vagal denervation ablation to treat atrial fibrillation. J Cardiovasc Electrophysiol 2008;19(2):211–3.

The Pericardial Space: Obtaining Access and an Approach to Fluoroscopic Anatomy

Faisal Syed, MBChB[a], Nirusha Lachman, PhD[b], Kevin Christensen, BA[c], Jennifer A. Mears, BS[d], Traci Buescher, RN[d], Yong-Mei Cha, MD[d], Paul A. Friedman, MD, FHRS, FACC[d], Thomas M. Munger, MD[d], Samuel J. Asirvatham, MD, FHRS[d,e,*]

KEYWORDS

• Pericardium • Access • Fluoroscopy • Anatomy • Ablation

Percutaneous access to the pericardium is now a well-established means for catheter ablation of ventricular tachycardia (VT) in selected patients.[1–5] The principle has since been extended to atrial fibrillation ablation.[6] Here specific advantages, in addition to targeting epicardial circuits, are the potential for introducing devices to protect the esophagus and phrenic nerves as well as allowing access to the vein of Marshall and ganglionic plexi.[7] Some accessory pathways may be better ablated epicardially.[8] The approach may be used to apply epicardial left ventricular (LV) pacing leads.[9] Preclinical studies have demonstrated its feasibility in targeted myocardial stem cell and gene vector delivery,[10,11] and localized pharmaceutical therapy to myocardial tissue and coronary vasculature.[12–18] A more recent utility is in the percutaneous closure of the left atrial appendage (LAA).[19] The discovery that the pericardium is itself a source of myocardial stem cells may lead to further extension of this technique for stem cell harvesting.[20–23]

An intimate understanding of fluoroscopic anatomy is integral to performing any of these procedures. Although there is growing utility of electroanatomic mapping and intracardiac ultrasound,[24,25] fluoroscopy remains the most robust method currently available for the accurate real-time imaging of catheters in an interventional setting.

OUTLINE OF THIS ARTICLE

The first part of this article deals with the practicalities of obtaining access to the pericardial space with a focus on technique, complications to avoid, and navigation within the space. The subsequent broader section is an approach to fluoroscopic anatomy. Each section introduces the need to be familiar with the fluoroscopic anatomy in that region; a brief review of the relevant anatomy is then followed by examples of fluoroscopic images, with explanations to develop an approach to understanding the fluoroscopic anatomy of the pericardial space in general.

[a] Department of Internal Medicine, Mayo Clinic, 200 1st Street, SW, Rochester, MN 55905, USA
[b] Department of Anatomy, Mayo Clinic, 200 1st Street, SW, Rochester, MN 55905, USA
[c] Mayo Medical School, Mayo Clinic, 200 1st Street, SW, Rochester, MN 55905, USA
[d] Division of Cardiovascular Diseases and Internal Medicine, Mayo Clinic College of Medicine, 200 1st Street, SW, Rochester, MN 55905, USA
[e] Division of Pediatric Cardiology, Department of Pediatrics and Adolescent Medicine, Mayo Clinic College of Medicine, 200 1st Street, SW, Rochester, MN 55905, USA
* Corresponding author. Division of Cardiovascular Diseases and Internal Medicine, Mayo Clinic College of Medicine, 200 1st Street, SW, Rochester, MN 55905.
E-mail address: asirvatham.samuel@mayo.edu (S.J. Asirvatham).

Card Electrophysiol Clin 2 (2010) 9–23
doi:10.1016/j.ccep.2009.11.001
1877-9182/10/$ – see front matter

ANATOMY OF THE PERICARDIUM

The pericardial cavity (**Figs. 1** and **2**) is a potential space between the parietal and visceral layers of the serous pericardium. This space is continuous with the epicardium and reflects around the roots of the great vessels and onto the visceral surface of the fibrous pericardium.

The fibrous pericardium is continuous with the adventitia of the great vessels superiorly and is related posteriorly to the bronchi, esophagus, descending thoracic aorta, and mediastinal surface of each lung. The phrenic nerves descend between it and the mediastinal pleural layers that adhere to its lateral sides.

The oblique sinus, a recess located behind the left atrium, is formed as the pericardium envelops the pulmonary veins and vena cava. Within it rests the vein of Marshall, connected by the fetal remnant of the duct of Couvier to the highest left intercostal vein, draining into the coronary sinus. The transverse sinus is located superior to the heart between the arterial mesocardium, which envelops the ascending aorta and pulmonary trunk anteriorly, and the venous mesocardium, which covers the superior vena cava (SVC), left atrium, and pulmonary veins posteriorly and inferiorly.

OBTAINING ACCESS TO THE PERICARDIAL SPACE

Subxiphoid Access

Percutaneous subxiphoid access to the pericardium was traditionally reserved for the management of pericardial effusion[26] until Sosa and colleagues[27] first described a technique for safely accessing the normal space using a modification of the traditional method. The subxiphoid approach holds the advantage of allowing free access to the entire ventricular surfaces, the right atrium, and the majority of the left atrium.

The patient is positioned horizontally and prepared surgically. Generous sedation is required, and at times general anesthesia is used. For ablation procedures, it is best to first position the intracardiac catheters as these act dually as anatomic landmarks of the right ventricular (RV) apex anteriorly and coronary sinus posteriorly (see **Figs. 1** and **2**). After the delivery of local anesthesia, skin entry is approximately 2 cm below the subxiphoid process (see **Figs. 1** and **2**). A blunt-tipped 18-gauge Tuohy epidural needle with a soft-tipped wire is used. The needle is directed posteriorly toward the left shoulder. Unlike in pericardiocentesis when a 30° angle to skin is preferred, the angle of entry is adjusted according to whether an anterior or posterior approach is preferred. Fluoroscopic guidance is used in the right anterior oblique (RAO) projection if the needle is directed anteriorly, or the left anterior oblique (LAO) projection if posteriorly. When the needle approaches the cardiac border, small volumes of contrast are injected using a 5-mL syringe attached to the needle. The fluid is seen to pool in the extrapericardial tissue until the needle enters the potential pericardial space, when further injection of contrast outlines the pericardium as a thin film surrounding the cardiac silhouette. Tenting of the pericardium is usually seen fluoroscopically before puncture (see **Figs. 1** and **2**), and the transmitted cardiac impulse can be felt at the needle tip. Lack of blood on aspiration at this stage confirms that the ventricle has not been breached, although this is usually identified on contrast injection. Once in the pericardial space, the needle is stabilized with one hand while the syringe is removed and the wire advanced through the bevel. Guidewire placement is monitored fluoroscopically to ensure that inadvertent entry into the RV or the extrapericardial space has not occurred. Pericardial placement is confirmed by the wire wrapping around the cardiac silhouette, traversing chamber boundaries as it traverses both right and left cardiac borders (see **Figs. 1** and **2**). Some authorities advocate the LAO view here, as in RAO or anteroposterior (AP) projections, the wire can puncture the RV and travel into the right atrium or pulmonary artery and still appear to be in the pericardium.[5] It is important to ensure pericardial wire placement before the needle is withdrawn over the wire and the sheath introduced. An 8-French sheath with a sidearm is useful for most procedures. Once placed, the wire is withdrawn and any blood is aspirated from the side hole; bleeding is usually limited to 30 mL. Two sheaths can allow for simultaneous mapping and ablation,[28] and this can be achieved either with a separate puncture or by using the first sheath to introduce 2 wires and sheathing each in turn.

Possible Complications and How to Avoid Them

There is potential damage to several important surrounding structures, including the myocardium itself, great vessels, coronary arteries, lungs, mediastinum, esophagus, liver, diaphragmatic vessels, and phrenic nerves. However, with careful understanding of fluoroscopic anatomy serious complications are rare, the most frequent reported complications of epicardial ablation being pericarditis and hemopericardium.[1–3,5] The former can be treated with systemic and intrapericardial anti-inflammatory agents. Pericardial hemorrhage is

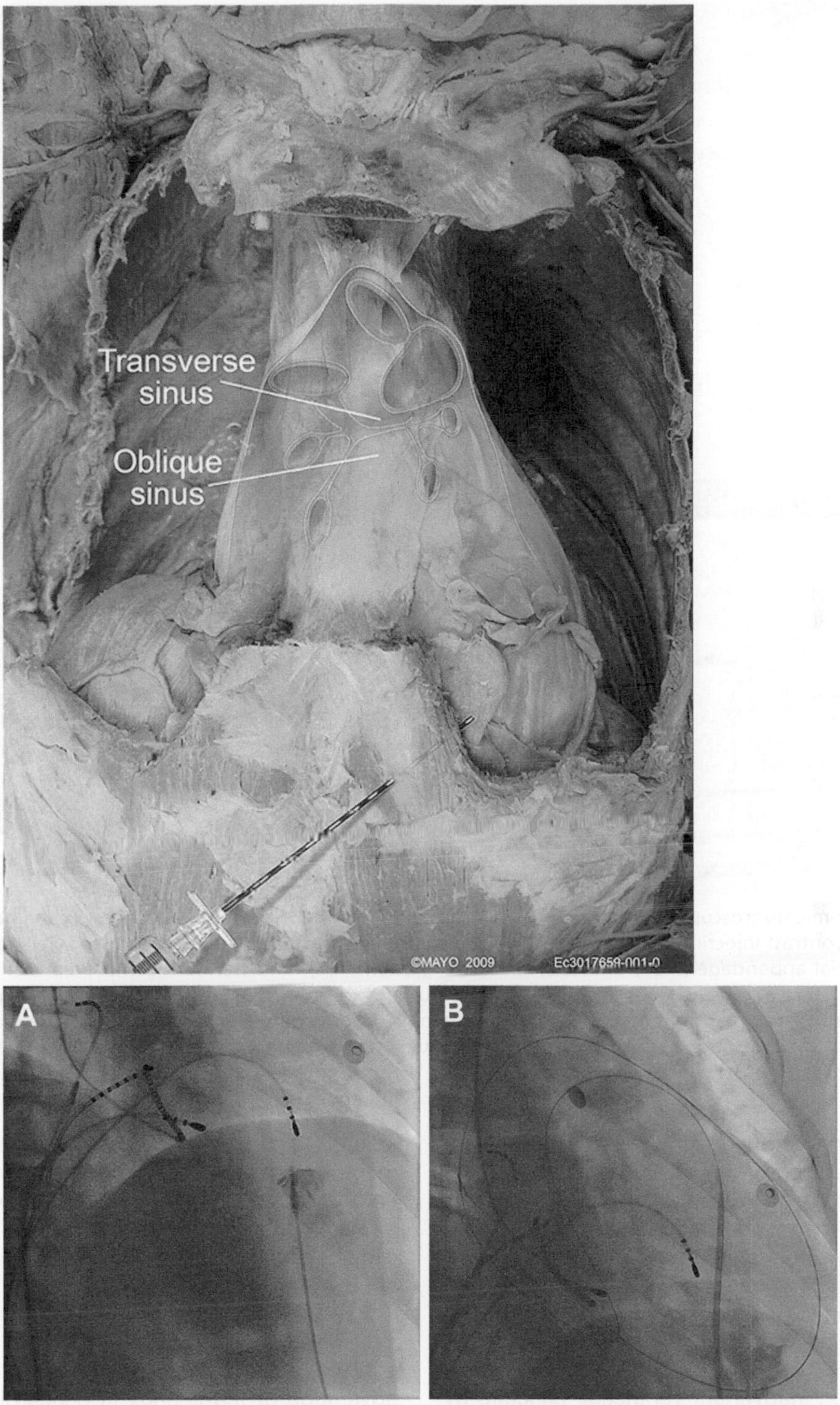

Fig. 1. Pericardial access and orientation to fluoroscopic anatomy. The dissection shows the site of needle puncture, and the transposed diagram of the pericardium outlines the primary pericardial space and the posteriorly located oblique and transverse sinuses and their boundaries. The point of pericardial entry is shown in (*A*), with tenting of the pericardium at the needle tip and pooling of injected contrast in the extrapericardial tissue. In (*B*), a wire lies in the pericardial space; the needle has been withdrawn and a sheath introduced. (*Image A courtesy of* Mayo Clinic Foundation; with permission.)

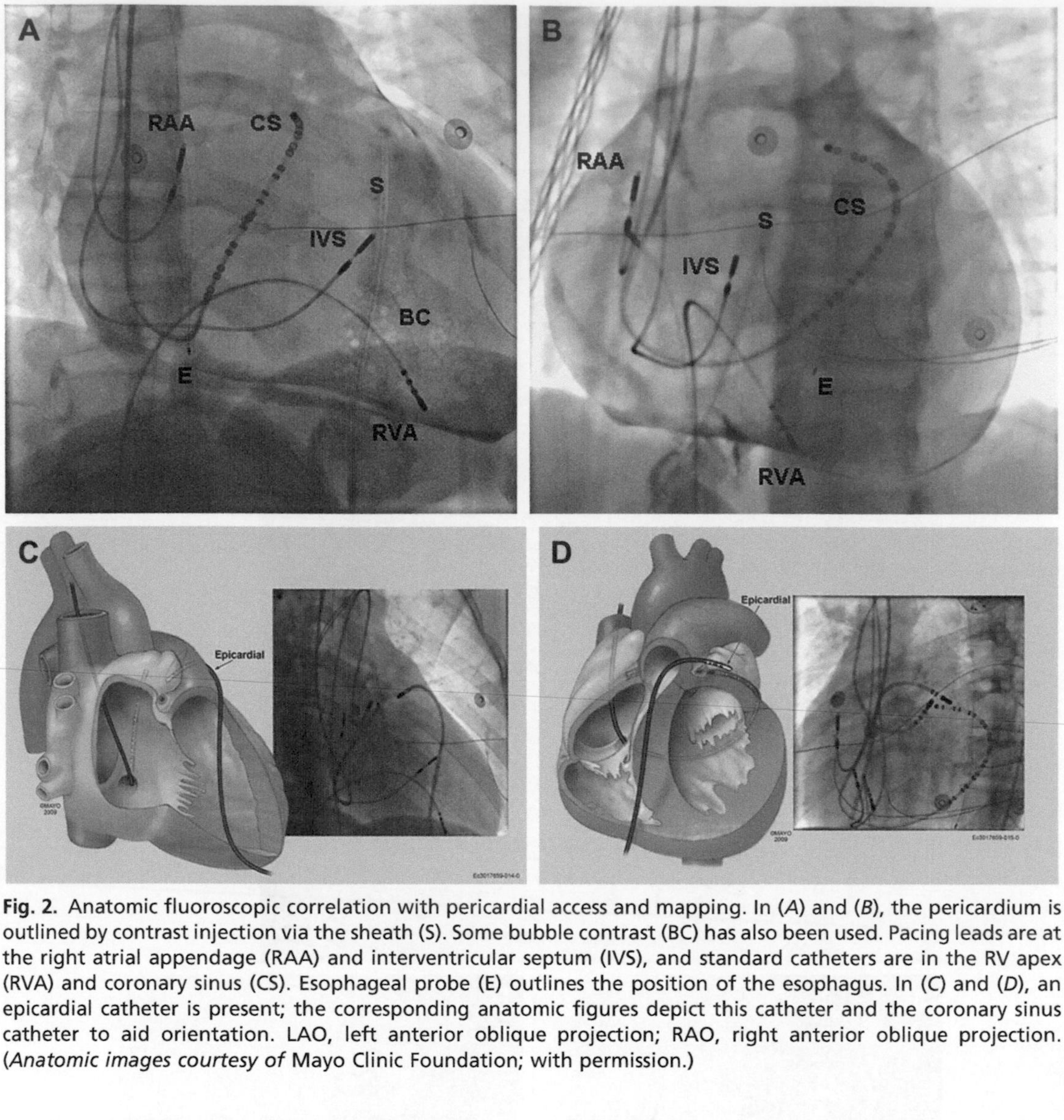

Fig. 2. Anatomic fluoroscopic correlation with pericardial access and mapping. In (*A*) and (*B*), the pericardium is outlined by contrast injection via the sheath (S). Some bubble contrast (BC) has also been used. Pacing leads are at the right atrial appendage (RAA) and interventricular septum (IVS), and standard catheters are in the RV apex (RVA) and coronary sinus (CS). Esophageal probe (E) outlines the position of the esophagus. In (*C*) and (*D*), an epicardial catheter is present; the corresponding anatomic figures depict this catheter and the coronary sinus catheter to aid orientation. LAO, left anterior oblique projection; RAO, right anterior oblique projection. (*Anatomic images courtesy of* Mayo Clinic Foundation; with permission.)

usually seen at the start of the procedure, and an important practice is to aspirate immediately on sheath placement to empty the pericardium. It is considered normal to aspirate up to 30 mL of blood; rarely there may be more (up to 300 mL),[1] but any bleeding is usually self limited. A related complication is myocardial puncture; this can be dry in the case of partial puncture or result in the aspiration of blood if the needle reaches the chamber. Inadvertent ventricular puncture by the needle alone is tolerated: the needle can be gently withdrawn with negative syringe suction until cessation of bloody return and the procedure continued. Certain steps can be taken to minimize the risk of this occurring. Fluoroscopy is used to determine proximity to the cardiac border and determine an oblique entry into the pericardial space. As the needle contacts the myocardium there is tactile feedback, and there may also be ectopics as the needle tip irritates the ventricle. Monitoring for a current of injury from a crocodile clip attached to the shaft of the needle can identify entry into myocardium.

Devices have been developed to try and minimize the risk of complications from pericardial entry. A novel device under development takes advantage of the change in pericardial pressure during the cardiac cycle, identifying pericardial entry from the frequency of pressure changes at the needle tip as it traverses the thoracic cavity into the pericardial space.[29] There is some reported clinical experience from the PerDUCER device (Comedicus Inc, Columbia Heights, MN), which houses a 21-gauge needle in a 12-French metal tube. The device is percutaneously inserted into the anterior mediastinal space until it contacts the anterior pericardium when suction is applied to capture a bleb of pericardium, which is then pierced with the needle allowing for guidewire entry into the pericardial space.[30,31] There is also a device that delivers a continuous positive pressure of 20 to 30 mm Hg using a continuous saline infusion through the advancing needle, which is designed to push the right ventricle away from the needle tip as it enters the pericardium.[32] Finally, the Cooper retractor, designed for transcervical thymectomy, has been described as facilitating subxiphoid pericardiotomy in a case report.[33]

Another related complication is wire entry into the extrapericardial space; if there is a concern for this, one technique involves monitoring for a current of injury from the needle to identify partial myocardium entry and advancing the wire on subsequent partial withdrawal of the needle. In the case when a sheath is already in place and the second puncture is attempted, injection of 120 mL of air to create a pneumopericardium has been described as a method of reducing the risk of myocardial or coronary artery laceration on the second puncture.[28]

Coronary vascular damage during needle entry is rare, and can be minimized by directing the needle away from the ventricular septum. Coronary damage is of greater concern during ablation, with a higher risk near the base of the heart or the septum. Here, the fluoroscopic identification of anatomic landmarks can be supplemented by intracardiac catheters including retrograde placement at the aortic root, but when there is doubt this should prompt performing coronary angiography.

Liver laceration during needle entry can be avoided in most cases by pushing the liver gently out of the way with one hand as the other advances the needle, and maintaining the course of the needle once the subcutaneous tissues are traversed. Finally, diaphragmatic vessel injury with hemoperitoneum has been reported. Although rare, it may require blood transfusion and surgery.[1,5]

Other Routes of Pericardial Access

The clinical utility of transesophageal puncture for pericardiocentesis in 2 cases and biopsy of a left atrial mass in 1 case has been reported, supplemented by experimental experience in 8 pigs.[34] Transbronchial pericardiocentesis has also been described in 3 patients, with puncture through the anterior wall of the left lower lobe bronchus into the pericardial space of the left atrium or through the second intercartilage space of the distal trachea to reach the aortic pericardial recess.[35] Neither method has shown demonstrable clinical utility for obtaining access to the normal pericardial space or epicardial ablation. Entry through the anterior mediastinum has been described as safe in a study of 10 pigs.[36] A 21-gauge, 2-part trocar needle inserted subcutaneously below the xiphoid process is advanced at 10° to 15° to the abdominal wall, first along the posterior surface of the sternum into the anterior mediastinal space and then toward the heart apex. On pericardial entry, the needle hub is seen to move with the heartbeat, whereupon trocar withdrawal and guidewire entry into the pericardial space allows insertion of the sheath. The right atrial appendage has also been reported as a point of entry into the pericardium, but again the experience is so far limited to preclinical studies. The first report was in 6 dogs and 13 pigs that tolerated introduction of a 4-French sheath into the pericardial space.[37] A subsequent study in 8 pigs reported right atrial and terminal anterior SVC access as a feasible modality for placing pacing leads through a 9-French sheath, though at the time of the procedure a hemodynamically significant pericardial effusion developed in half the cases.[38] There seems to be potential for clinical utility in these latter approaches for pericardial ablation.

NAVIGATING THE PERICARDIAL SPACE

Once within the pericardial space, the catheter usually moves around without difficulty. However, in patients with previous insult to the pericardium such as with previous cardiac surgery or myopericarditis, adhesions may limit intrapericardial mobility and access to the likely target region. In the case of prior cardiac surgery, these adhesions are usually more restrictive anteriorly, and approaching the inferior wall of the LV has been reported to allow ablation of the inferolateral LV.[39] The catheter can be used to try and gently lyse adhesions manually, by vibration, or by application of radiofrequency. A subxiphoid pericardiotomy with local adhesiolysis and placement of a pericardial sheath under direct vision has been described in a series of 6 patients with prior cardiac surgery and difficult access, with reported subsequent catheter access to the diaphragmatic border in all and the anterior and lateral surfaces for 4 of 6 patients.[40] Open-chested ablation in the operating room has also been described, but with limited direct mapping and ablation.[5,41]

Novel Aids to Intrapericardial Navigation

Fiberoptic endoscopy using the 7-mm flexible necked FLEXview system (Boston Scientific

Cardiac Surgery, Santa Clara, CA) has been used to facilitate electroanatomic mapping, although introduction in this case report was via surgical subxiphoid pericardiotomy under general anesthesia.[42] In a study in pigs, the 5.3-mm EB-1530T3 steerable bronchoscope (Pentax, Montvale, NJ) was introduced through an 18-Frech subxiphoid sheath, with clear visualization of intrapericardial structures such as coronary vessels, LAA, and pulmonary veins, and catheter ablation under direct vision.[43] The ingenious HeartLander (The Robotics Institute, Pittsburgh, PA) is a miniature robotic device that is introduced through the subxiphoid approach and can navigate on the epicardial surface to deliver semiautonomous epicardial injections.[44] There are also reports of using intracardiac ultrasound probes in the pericardial space,[45] and a novel 9-French catheter combing ultrasound and ablation capability has been developed.[46]

Phrenic Nerve Injury

Phrenic nerve injury is a well-recognized complication of radiofrequency ablation even when radiofrequency energy is delivered endocardially, with the most common sites of injury being at the ostium of the SVC, within the right upper pulmonary vein (RUPV), the left atrium, and the lateral LV wall.[47,48] The intimate relation of these nerves to the pericardium warn of the potential for this complication in epicardial procedures.[49] Within the thorax, the phrenic nerve passes downward and in front of the hilum of the lung between the fibrous pericardium and mediastinal pleura. However, it must be noted that there is interindividual variation in its course.[49,50] On the right, the nerve descends along the right anterolateral border of the SVC and becomes separated from it at the right atrial junction by pericardium as it curves posteriorly; here it lies briefly between the RUPV (being particularly closely related to mid and distal portions of this vein) and the SVC before continuing its downward descent along the right atrial wall. On the left, the phrenic nerve descends over the aortic arch, pulmonary trunk, and the pericardium overlying the lateral wall of the LAA and the high LV free wall. Damage to the phrenic nerve results in diaphragmatic paralysis, and there are 4 general methods used to prevent this.[49] Fluoroscopic screening for diaphragmatic stimulation by pacing the site before ablating identifies proximity to the nerve. Electroanatomic mapping extends this principle by combining it with electrical mapping techniques. Cryomapping makes use of the early reversible effects of freezing as diaphragmatic movement is visualized under fluoroscopic screening, and is a means of successfully ablating despite nerve proximity.[51] The fourth method involves protecting the nerve if ablation must be at a site of proximity; here the infusion of air and saline together has been reported to be superior to infusion of air or saline alone or insertion of balloons to create distance between the catheter and the nerve.[52]

Esophageal Injury

The esophagus is vulnerable to thermal injury when ablating the left atrium posteriorly. If this occurs, the patient presents some weeks later with an esophageal-atrial fistula, a serious condition with high mortality.[53] To avoid this, it is the authors' practice to place an esophageal temperature probe routinely to monitor for thermal injury and act as a fluoroscopic anatomic marker (see **Figs. 1** and **2**). Cooling with a water-irrigated balloon placed in the esophagus has also been described.[54]

RADIOGRAPHIC ANATOMY

The standard fluoroscopic projections of the heart are in the RAO and LAO positions (see **Figs. 1** and **2**). These positions allow a view of the heart in its anatomic sagittal and coronal planes such that in RAO the left and right sides are superimposed but there is good atrioventricular differentiation, whereas the LAO looks at the heart from apex to base and allows left-right differentiation, but the atria and ventricles are superimposed. The coronary sinus catheter marks the mitral valve annulus from the interatrial septum medially.

The Primary Pericardial Space and Ventricular Arrhythmia Ablation

Once a catheter is inserted into the pericardial space, it can be moved freely laterally, anteriorly, and inferiorly. Various parts of the ventricle ranging from the right ventricular outflow tract (RVOT) to the posterior crux can be mapped and ablation performed without difficulty. On the anterior surface of the heart, the catheter can be readily moved to the RVOT. The RV free wall, LV free wall, and the posterior LV can be mapped and ablation performed without difficulty (**Fig. 3**). However, the left ventricular outflow tract (LVOT) cannot be reached using this approach.

The Ventricular Outflow Tracts

As with other portions of the ventricle, the RVOT and LVOT may have arrhythmia origin on the epicardial surface. The anatomy of the outflow tract region is complex. The RVOT lies anterior to

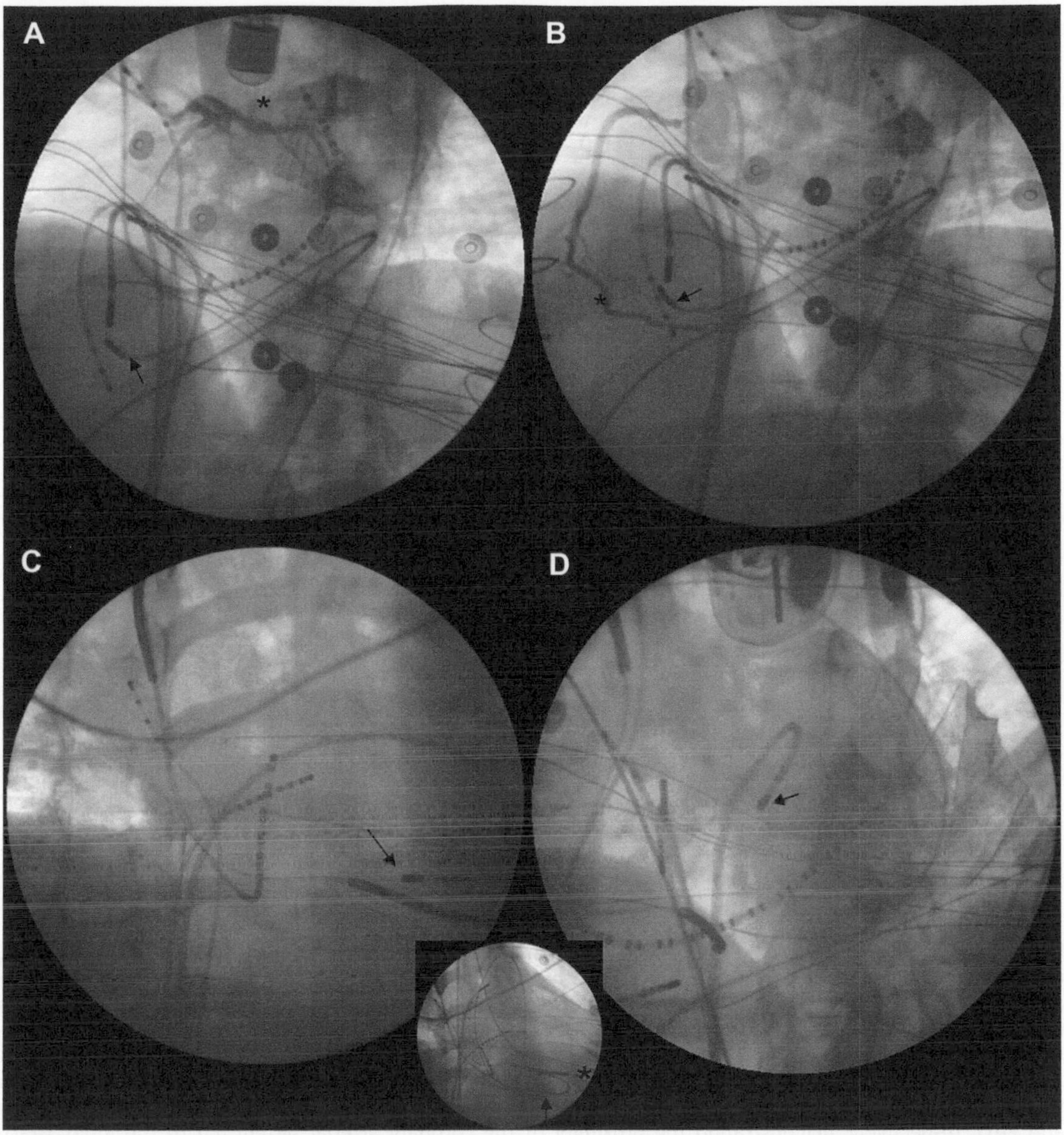

Fig. 3. (*A, B*) Left anterior oblique (LAO) projection of epicardial ablation of the RV free wall. Left and right coronary injections (*star*) are shown in (*A*) and (*B*), respectively, demonstrating the proximity of the coronary artery to the ablation catheter (*arrow*). (*C, D*) Epicardial ablation at the LV free wall. The epicardial catheter (*arrow*) has been maneuvered from an anterior position. Inset (right anterior oblique [RAO]) shows the maneuver of wrapping around the heart to maintain catheter stability in the face of free wall mobility. (*Courtesy of* Mayo Clinic Foundation; with permission.)

the LVOT, but as the conus tapers to the level of the pulmonary valve, the RVOT is to the left of the LVOT. The pulmonary artery continues leftward and slightly posterior at the point of its bifurcation to the ascending aorta as it becomes the arch.[55] The central anatomic location of the aortic valve and the LVOT means that the epicardial portion of the anterior wall of the LVOT is actually the posterior wall of the RVOT, while posteriorly the LVOT, especially the supravalvar portion, lies in relationship to the mitral valve or the left atrium. Thus, the epicardial route is rarely relevant to ablating aortic root tachycardia as an example.[56] **Fig. 4** demonstrates this anatomic relationship. The proximal coronary arteries and distal coronary veins are closely related to the RVOT, with the left main lying adjacent and posterior to the RVOT, the left anterior descending artery coursing down

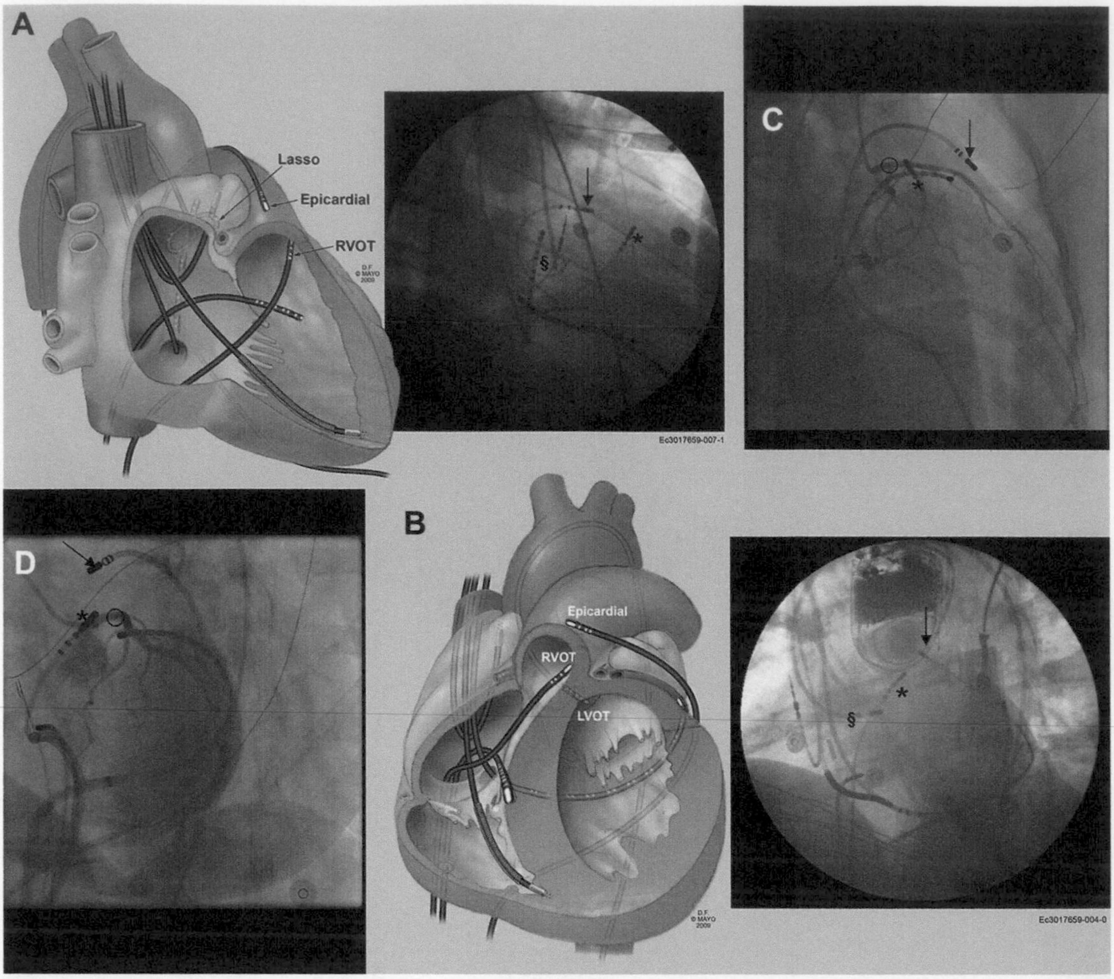

Fig. 4. (*A, B*) RAO and LAO projections, respectively, demonstrating the epicardial catheter (*arrow*) at the RVOT, and corresponding diagrammatic representation. Catheters positioned in the RVOT (*star*), and retrogradely in the aortic root (*section sign*), mark the ventricular outflow tracts intraluminally. A standard catheter in (*B*) has replaced the retrograde aortic root lasso in (*A*). The RVOT lies anterior to the LVOT. The coronary sinus (CS) catheter can be seen posterior to the LVOT as it wraps around the mitral annulus. The epicardial catheter has been advanced inferoposteriorly along the LV to reach the RVOT. The true distance of the epicardial catheter from the LVOT is more easily appreciated in LAO (*B*), and is taken up by the RVOT and epicardial fat. (*C, D*) RAO and LAO, respectively, demonstrating the proximity of the coronary arterial system (O) to the RVOT (*star*). (*Anatomic images courtesy of* Mayo Clinic Foundation; with permission.)

the lateral aspect of the muscular portion of the RVOT, and the right coronary artery lying in the region of the superior proximal RVOT close to the tricuspid annulus (see **Fig. 4**).[55]

Oblique Sinus

The oblique sinus has gained importance in contemporary ablation practice of atrial arrhythmias because of its unique anatomic location behind the pulmonary venous atrium and the posterior left atrial wall. Within it rests the vein of Marshall, which can itself be a source of arrhythmia amenable to ablation.[57] Immediately posterior rests the esophagus, which confers its sensitivity to thermal damage and formation of atrio-esophageal fistula (see **Figs. 1** and **2**).[58–61]

The oblique sinus lies in the region of the 4 pulmonary veins and can be reached by a finger passed superiorly behind the heart, its opening being bounded by the 2 inferior pulmonary veins (see **Figs. 1** and **2**). The oblique sinus is of variable shape, averaging 4.1 cm at its opening and 3.1 cm in its extension superiorly.[62] The right boundary is formed by the SVC and the left by the pericardial reflection connecting the 2 pulmonary veins, while superiorly it is bounded by a pericardial reflection connecting the right and left superior pulmonary veins. Beyond this superior margin rests the transverse sinus. **Fig. 5** demonstrates fluoroscopic visualization of a catheter in the oblique sinus.

Transverse Sinus

The transverse sinus is of functional importance because a catheter placed at this site may ablate the roof of the left atrium or Bachmann's bundle and important sites for certain atrial arrhythmias.[63] The transverse sinus also allows access to the anterior LVOT. The fluoroscopic anatomy is depicted in **Fig. 6**. The transverse sinus lies superior to the oblique sinus, its inferior border being formed by the pericardial reflection between the right and left superior pulmonary veins, and which separates it from the oblique sinus below (see **Figs. 1** and **2**). The roof of the left atrium also forms part of the floor of the sinus and allows access to Bachmann's bundle. Anteriorly lie the posterior wall of the ascending aorta, part of the main pulmonary trunk, and the dome of the left atrium. The anterior wall of the descending aorta forms its posterior border, and the roof is formed in parts by the arch of the aorta, the floor of the right pulmonary artery, and a part of the main pulmonary artery. The sinus houses the right pulmonary artery as it protrudes into it. This sinus communicates with the epicardial aspect of the noncoronary and right coronary aortic cusps via the inferior aortic recess (see **Figs. 1** and **2**). It also communicates with the vena cava by way of the aortocaval sinus, a small virtual space between the SVC and the ascending aorta that in some individuals is large enough to bypass with a catheter and reach the right heart border (see **Fig. 6**).[55] In the vicinity are 3 parasympathetic ganglia that can be found within epicardial fat pads: at the junction of the right atrium and the right superior pulmonary vein, at the junction of the IVC and LA, and at the aortocaval recess.[56,64] To reach the transverse sinus, the catheter is passed around the lateral wall of the LV and left atrium, and then under the pulmonary arteries.

The Left Atrial Appendage

When navigating in the pericardial space, the first atrial structure to be encountered when a catheter is advanced laterally and cranially is the LAA. The expected and characteristic change in electrograms while moving the catheter cranially can be used to identify this structure (**Fig. 7**).[19] The LAA lies completely within the pericardial space and originates from the superior portion of the left atrium body to cross posterolaterally to the pulmonary trunk origin, draping over the left-sided portion of the RVOT (see **Fig. 7**). At the junction of the LAA to the RVOT, the proximal left anterior descending and the anterior interventricular vein are seen. When a posterior lobe of the LAA is present (secondary lobe), it is often invaginated between the pulmonary annulus and the region of the left

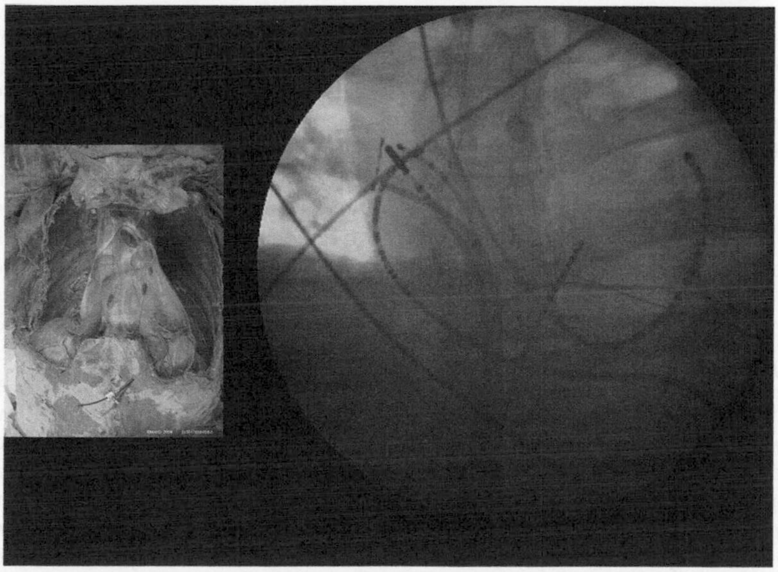

Fig. 5. Epicardial catheter in the oblique sinus. LAO projection. (*Dissection image courtesy of* Mayo Clinic Foundation; with permission.)

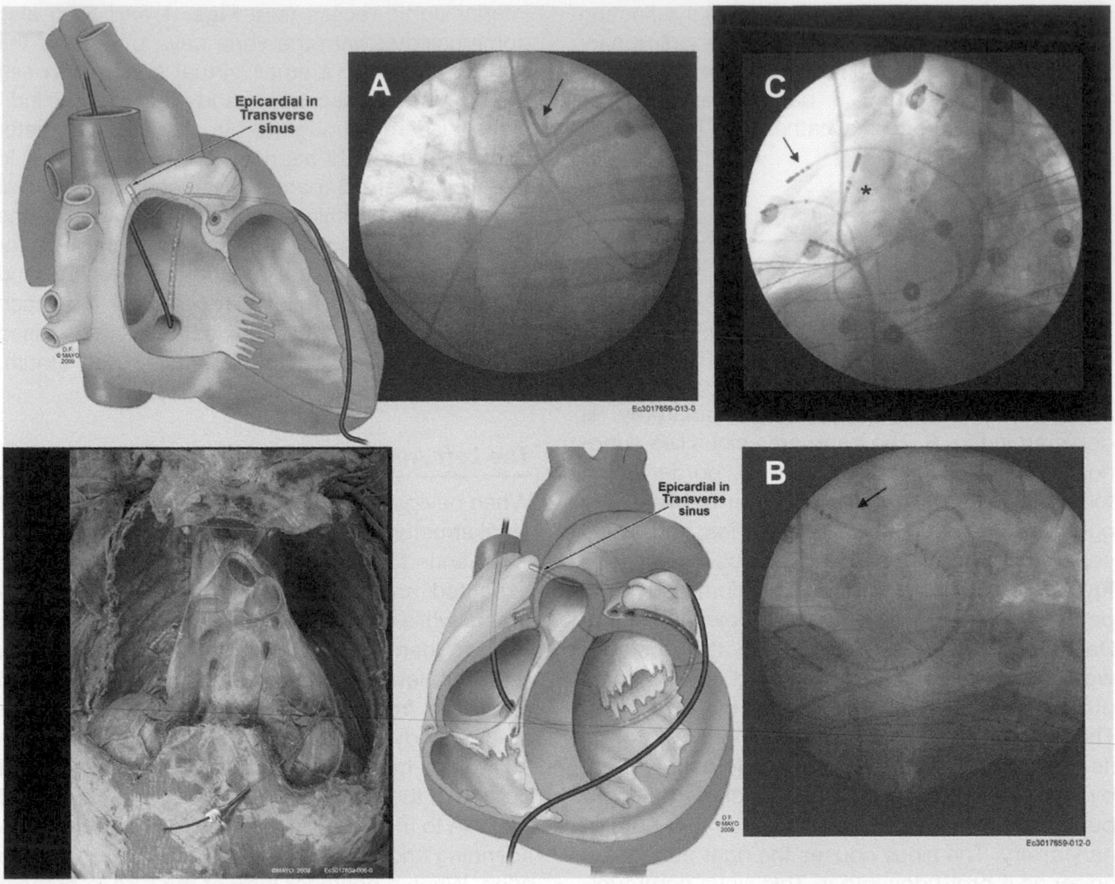

Fig. 6. (*A, B*) RAO and LAO images, respectively, and their diagrammatic representations, showing the epicardial catheter (*arrow*) in the transverse sinus. In (*C*) the epicardial catheter has traversed the transverse sinus to reach the vena cavae and right heart border via the aortocaval sinus, and there is an endoluminal ablation catheter at the RVOT (*star*). (*Anatomic images and dissection image courtesy of* Mayo Clinic Foundation; with permission.)

coronary cusp of the aorta.[55] Understanding the fluoroscopic anatomy of this structure is important for ablationists because of its close proximity to the RVOT and the proximal coronary arterial system. Catheter-based epicardial approaches for nonablation reasons such as snaring of the appendage or epicardial atrial pacing have further increased the reason for accurate regional and fluoroscopic anatomic knowledge of this structure.

Tricuspid and Mitral Annulus

Epicardial ablation along the annulus is occasionally required for accessory pathways that could not otherwise be ablated with an endocardial or intravenous approach. The mitral and tricuspid annuli are intimately related to the major arteries and veins of the heart. In general, the veins lie atrial and superficial to the arterial system such that the coronary sinus lies atrial to the distal circumflex artery; however, the great cardiac vein overlaps the artery and the anterior intraventricular vein lies ventricular to the proximal left anterior descending artery and circumflex coronary artery. Ablation within the coronary veins or with high energy along the annulus can damage the circumflex artery. This damage is particularly more likely to occur with epicardial ablation either via the pericardial space from within the coronary venous system, or when ablating on the left atrial tissue as it "overhangs" the mitral annulus rather than on the mitral annulus itself.

The major coronary vessels are typically cushioned in a layer of epicardial fat, which tends also to be concentrated along the atrioventricular and interventricular grooves, the acute margin, and the RV free wall.[64,65] Knowledge of the distribution of the epicardial fat along the annulus, the exact course of the coronary vessels, and the extensions of the vessels and fat along the main intraventricular grooves is essential to correlate with

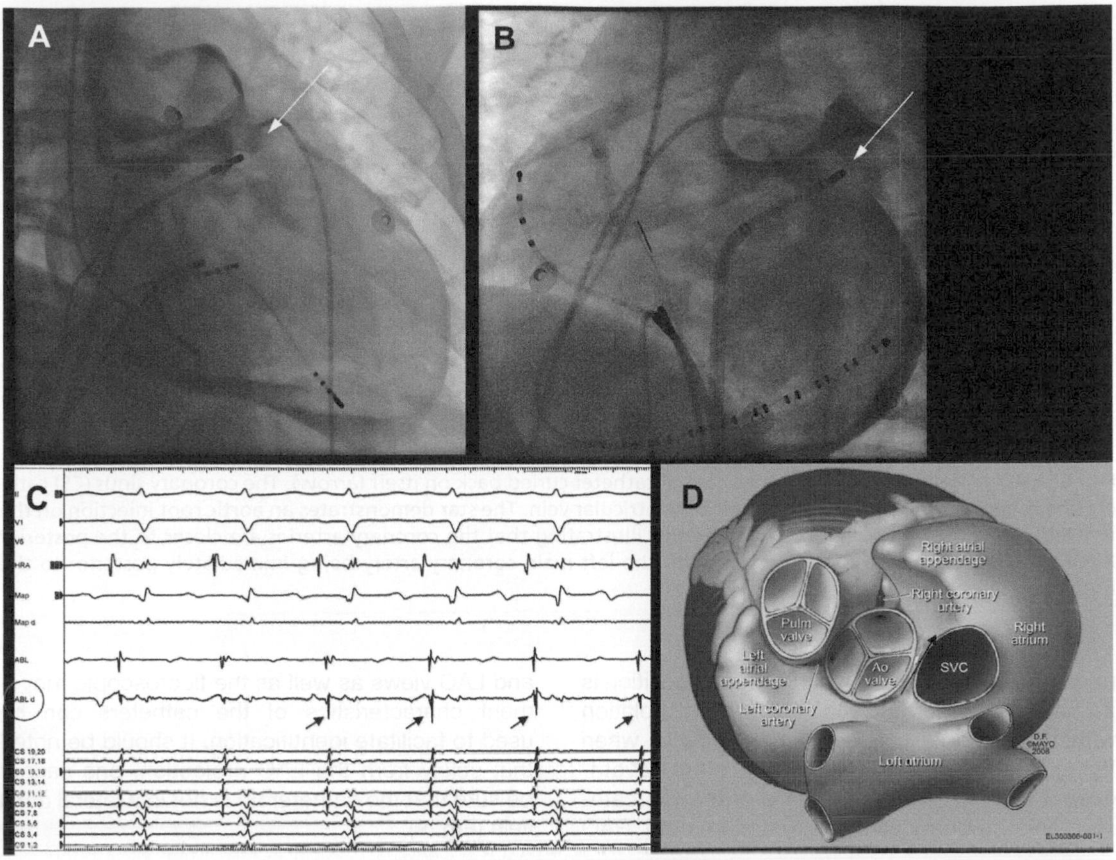

Fig. 7. (*A, B*) The left atrial appendage (*arrow*) in RAO and LAO, respectively. Radiocontrast has been introduced into the pericardium, outlining the appendage. (*C*) Electrocardiographic changes used to identify the left atrial appendage. The atrial signal on the pericardial catheter (ABL d, *red circle*) characteristically becomes more prominent after the third complex on this tracing (*arrows*), coincident with it crossing over the appendage. (*D*) Cranial view of the base of the heart, illustrating the important relationship of the left atrial appendage to the right ventricular outflow tract and the proximal coronary arteries. The left main coronary artery is just posterior to the pulmonary valve, closely related to the overlying left atrial appendage base. Note also the variable amount of epicardial fat between the right atrial appendage, aortic valve, and around the right coronary artery. The aortocaval sinus (*arrow*) between the aorta and SVC allows passage to the right venous chambers as discussed in the text. (*Image D courtesy of* Mayo Clinic Foundation; with permission.)

fluoroscopy and electrograms being recorded from the catheters placed in the epicardial space.

The mitral annulus is outlined by the coronary sinus catheter and the tricuspid annulus identified by the endoluminal RV catheter. The septum is defined fluoroscopically by the His catheter. **Fig. 8** demonstrates catheter positioning in the venous system.

Cardiac Veins and Epicardial Ablation

The epicardial surface of the heart can be reached with catheters for mapping and ablation via the venous system. The fluoroscopic anatomy for epicardial ablation via the veins is important because true epicardial and venous-based epicardial approaches may be complementary, with some areas better reached by one modality than another. The coronary veins, specifically the anterior interventricular vein, course on the interventricular septum. Near the base, they move close to the epicardial surface of the leftward portion of the RVOT. Smaller tributaries may occasionally drain the tissue between the RVOT and LVOT, and these veins can be used to map or ablate foci in this region.

Fluoroscopic differentiation of veins can sometimes be difficult, such as with distinguishing catheters in the middle cardiac vein from other closely separated veins or from a position on the interventricular septum parallel to the middle cardiac vein. The distinction between middle cardiac vein

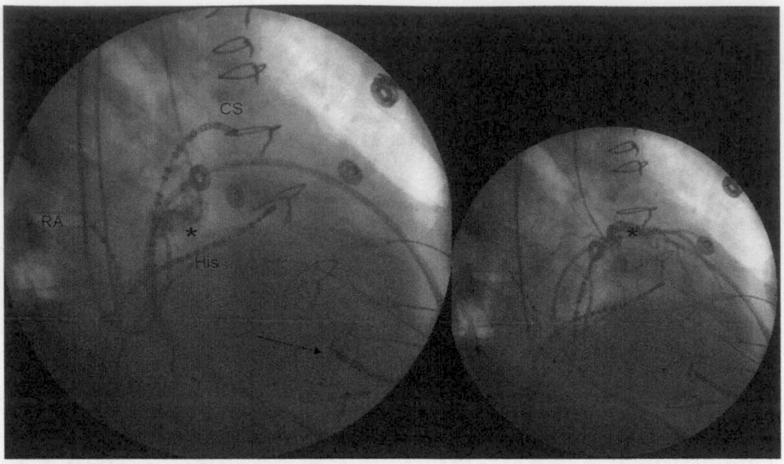

Fig. 8. RAO projection showing the epicardial catheter curled back on itself (*arrow*). The coronary sinus (CS) catheter has been advanced to the anterior interventricular vein. The star demonstrates an aortic root injection on the left and a left coronary injection on the right, illustrating that the coronary arteries are closer to the posterior RVOT than they are to the aortic cusps, with the left main coronary artery being immediately posterior to the RVOT and pulmonary valve.

position and right interventricular septal position is particularly important, as inadvertent ablation within the middle cardiac vein may occur when trying to ablate the slow pathway or the cavotricuspid isthmus. Careful analysis of the His catheter and coronary sinus catheter in both RAO and LAO views as well as the fluoroscopic movement characteristics of the catheters can be used to facilitate identification. It should be noted that solely from the LAO projection, one cannot be sure that the catheter tip is not in a lateral atrial vein (**Fig. 9**).

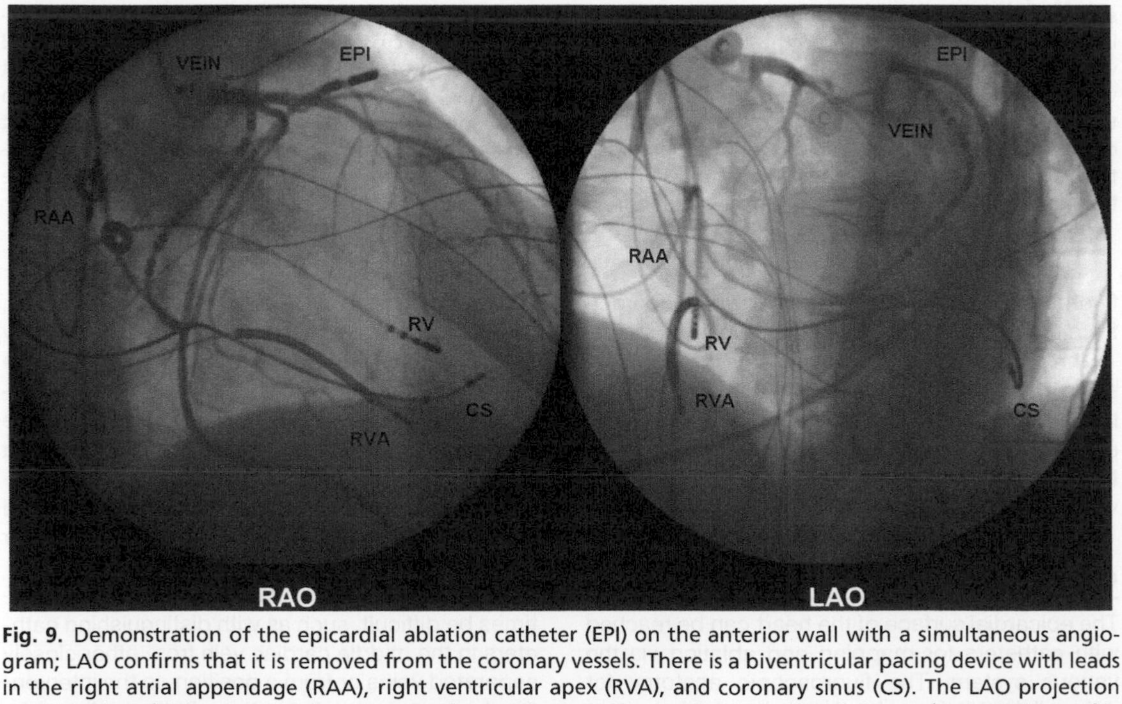

Fig. 9. Demonstration of the epicardial ablation catheter (EPI) on the anterior wall with a simultaneous angiogram; LAO confirms that it is removed from the coronary vessels. There is a biventricular pacing device with leads in the right atrial appendage (RAA), right ventricular apex (RVA), and coronary sinus (CS). The LAO projection suggests that the location of the coronary sinus catheter is in a cardiac vein (VEIN), but only on RAO can this be seen to be in a lateral atrial vein.

Table 1
Summary of fluoroscopy correlations for arrhythmia ablation

Arrhythmia	Anatomic Target	Fluoroscopic Pericardial Anatomy	Vulnerable Structures
Atrial fibrillation	Left atrial appendage	Primary pericardial space	Coronary arteries Left phrenic nerve
	Posterior left atrial wall Vein of Marshall Parasympathetic plexi	Oblique sinus	Esophagus Inferior pulmonary veins
	Left atrial roof Bachmann's bundle Parasympathetic plexi	Transverse sinus	Aorta Pulmonary arteries Superior pulmonary veins
Atrial tachycardia	As above		
	Right atrium	Aortocaval sinus via transverse sinus	Right phrenic nerve
AV reentry tachycardia	Epicardial accessory pathway	Mitral and tricuspid annulus Middle cardiac vein Posterior vein Coronary sinus	Coronary arteries
Ventricular tachycardia	LVOT	Left sinus of Valsalva Great cardiac vein Transverse sinus	
	RVOT	Primary pericardial space	Coronary arteries
	LV	Primary pericardial space	Left phrenic nerve
	RV	Primary pericardial space	

SUMMARY

Table 1 focuses the concepts discussed toward the various arrhythmias amenable to ablation. Understanding the orientation and anatomic relations of the cardiac chambers, great vessels, and epicardial structures is critical in realizing how the folds, sinuses, and recesses of the pericardial space can be taken advantage of. Fluoroscopy remains the technique of choice, and a working knowledge of fluoroscopic anatomy of the pericardium and cardiac veins equips the interventionist to safely and effectively engage in epicardial intervention.

REFERENCES

1. d'Avila A. Epicardial catheter ablation of ventricular tachycardia. Heart Rhythm 2008;5(Suppl 6):S73–5.
2. Hammill SC. Epicardial ablation: reducing the risks. J Cardiovasc Electrophysiol 2006;17(5):550–2.
3. Sosa E, Scanavacca M. Epicardial mapping and ablation techniques to control ventricular tachycardia. J Cardiovasc Electrophysiol 2005;16(4):449–52.
4. Sosa E, Scanavacca M, D'Avila A, et al. Endocardial and epicardial ablation guided by nonsurgical transthoracic epicardial mapping to treat recurrent ventricular tachycardia. J Cardiovasc Electrophysiol 1998;9(3):229–39.
5. Tedrow U, Stevenson WG. Strategies for epicardial mapping and ablation of ventricular tachycardia. J Cardiovasc Electrophysiol 2009;20(6):710–3.
6. Pak HN, Hwang C, Lim HE, et al. Hybrid epicardial and endocardial ablation of persistent or permanent atrial fibrillation: a new approach for difficult cases. J Cardiovasc Electrophysiol 2007;18(9):917–23.
7. Buch E, Shivkumar K. Epicardial catheter ablation of atrial fibrillation. Minerva Med 2009;100(2):151–7.
8. Valderrabano M, Cesario DA, Ji S, et al. Percutaneous epicardial mapping during ablation of difficult accessory pathways as an alternative to cardiac surgery. Heart Rhythm 2004;1(3):311–6.
9. Zenati MA, Bonanomi G, Chin AK, et al. Left heart pacing lead implantation using subxiphoid videopericardioscopy. J Cardiovasc Electrophysiol 2003;14(9):949–53.
10. March KL, Woody M, Mehdi K, et al. Efficient in vivo catheter-based pericardial gene transfer mediated by adenoviral vectors. Clin Cardiol 1999;22(1 Suppl 1):I23–9.

11. Hamdi H, Furuta A, Bellamy V, et al. Cell delivery: intramyocardial injections or epicardial deposition? A head-to-head comparison. Ann Thorac Surg 2009; 87(4):1196–203.
12. Stoll HP, Carlson K, Keefer LK, et al. Pharmacokinetics and consistency of pericardial delivery directed to coronary arteries: direct comparison with endoluminal delivery. Clin Cardiol 1999; 22(1 Suppl 1):I10–6.
13. Waxman S, Moreno R, Rowe KA, et al. Persistent primary coronary dilation induced by transatrial delivery of nitroglycerin into the pericardial space: a novel approach for local cardiac drug delivery. J Am Coll Cardiol 1999;33(7):2073–7.
14. Laham RJ, Post M, Sellke FW, et al. Therapeutic angiogenesis using local perivascular and pericardial delivery. Curr Interv Cardiol Rep 2000;2(3): 213–7.
15. Ujhelyi MR, Hadsall KZ, Euler DE, et al. Intrapericardial therapeutics: a pharmacodynamic and pharmacokinetic comparison between pericardial and intravenous procainamide delivery. J Cardiovasc Electrophysiol 2002;13(6):605–11.
16. Gleason JD, Nguyen KP, Kissinger KV, et al. Myocardial drug distribution pattern following intrapericardial delivery: an MRI analysis. J Cardiovasc Magn Reson 2002;4(3):311–6.
17. Matthews KG, Devlin GP, Stuart SP, et al. Intrapericardial IGF-I improves cardiac function in an ovine model of chronic heart failure. Heart Lung Circ 2005;14(2):98–103.
18. van Brakel TJ, Hermans JJ, Accord RE, et al. Effects of intrapericardial sotalol and flecainide on transmural atrial electrophysiology and atrial fibrillation. J Cardiovasc Electrophysiol 2009;20(2):207–15.
19. Friedman PA, Asirvatham SJ, Dalegrave C, et al. Percutaneous epicardial left atrial appendage closure: preliminary results of an electrogram guided approach. J Cardiovasc Electrophysiol 2009;20(8): 908–15.
20. Wessels A, Perez-Pomares JM. The epicardium and epicardially derived cells (EPDCs) as cardiac stem cells. Anat Rec A Discov Mol Cell Evol Biol 2004; 276(1):43–57.
21. Ota T, Patronik NA, Schwartzman D, et al. Minimally invasive epicardial injections using a novel semiautonomous robotic device. Circulation 2008; 118(Suppl 14):S115–20.
22. Zhou B, Ma Q, Rajagopal S, et al. Epicardial progenitors contribute to the cardiomyocyte lineage in the developing heart. Nature 2008;454(7200):109–13.
23. Smart N, Riley PR. Derivation of epicardium-derived progenitor cells (EPDCs) from adult epicardium. Curr Protoc Stem Cell Biol 2009; Chapter 2:unit2C.2.
24. Packer DL, Johnson SB, Kolasa MW, et al. New generation of electro-anatomic mapping: full intracardiac ultrasound image integration. Europace 2008;10(Suppl 3):iii35–41.
25. Sra J. Cardiac image integration implications for atrial fibrillation ablation. J Interv Card Electrophysiol 2008;22(2):145–54.
26. Krikorian JG, Hancock EW. Pericardiocentesis. Am J Med 1978;65(5):808–14.
27. Sosa E, Scanavacca M, d'Avila A, et al. A new technique to perform epicardial mapping in the electrophysiology laboratory. J Cardiovasc Electrophysiol 1996;7(6):531–6.
28. Nault I, Nguyen BL, Wright M, et al. Double pericardial access facilitated by iatrogenic pneumopericardium. J Cardiovasc Electrophysiol 2009;20(9):1068–9.
29. Tucker-Schwartz JM, Gillies GT, Scanavacca M, et al. Pressure-frequency sensing subxiphoid access system for use in percutaneous cardiac electrophysiology: prototype design and pilot study results. IEEE Trans Biomed Eng 2009;56(4):1160–8.
30. Macris MP, Igo SR. Minimally invasive access of the normal pericardium: initial clinical experience with a novel device. Clin Cardiol 1999;22(1 Suppl 1): I36–9.
31. Seferovic PM, Ristic AD, Maksimovic R, et al. Initial clinical experience with PerDUCER device: promising new tool in the diagnosis and treatment of pericardial disease. Clin Cardiol 1999;1(Suppl 1):I30–5.
32. Laham RJ, Simons M, Hung D. Subxyphoid access of the normal pericardium: a novel drug delivery technique. Catheter Cardiovasc Interv 1999;47(1): 109–11.
33. Temeck BK, Pass HI. A method to facilitate subxiphoid pericardiotomy. Ann Thorac Surg 1994; 57(4):1015–7.
34. Fritscher-Ravens A, Ganbari A, Mosse CA, et al. Transesophageal endoscopic ultrasound-guided access to the heart. Endoscopy 2007;39(5):385–9.
35. Ceron L, Manzato M, Mazzaro F, et al. A new diagnostic and therapeutic approach to pericardial effusion: transbronchial needle aspiration. Chest 2003; 123(5):1753–8.
36. Sun F, Sanchez FM, Crisostomo V, et al. Subxiphoid access to normal pericardium with micropuncture set: technical feasibility study in pigs. Radiology 2006;238(2):719–24.
37. Verrier RL, Waxman S, Lovett EG, et al. Transatrial access to the normal pericardial space: a novel approach for diagnostic sampling, pericardiocentesis, and therapeutic interventions. Circulation 1998; 98(21):2331–3.
38. Mickelsen SR, Ashikaga H, DeSilva R, et al. Transvenous access to the pericardial space: an approach to epicardial lead implantation for cardiac resynchronization therapy. Pacing Clin Electrophysiol 2005; 28(10):1018–24.
39. Sosa E, Scanavacca M, D'Avila A, et al. Nonsurgical transthoracic epicardial approach in patients with

ventricular tachycardia and previous cardiac surgery. J Interv Card Electrophysiol 2004;10(3): 281–8.

40. Soejima K, Couper G, Cooper JM, et al. Subxiphoid surgical approach for epicardial catheter-based mapping and ablation in patients with prior cardiac surgery or difficult pericardial access. Circulation 2004;110(10):1197–201.
41. Maury P, Marcheix B, Duparc A, et al. Surgical catheter ablation of ventricular tachycardia using left thoracotomy in a patient with hindered access to the left ventricle. Pacing Clin Electrophysiol 2009; 32(4):556–60.
42. Zenati MA, Shalaby A, Eisenman G, et al. Epicardial left ventricular mapping using subxiphoid video pericardioscopy. Ann Thorac Surg 2007;84(6): 2106–7.
43. Nazarian S, Kantsevoy SV, Zviman MM, et al. Feasibility of endoscopic guidance for nonsurgical transthoracic atrial and ventricular epicardial ablation. Heart Rhythm 2008;5(8):1115–9.
44. Ota T, Degani A, Schwartzman D, et al. A novel highly articulated robotic surgical system for epicardial ablation. Conf Proc IEEE Eng Med Biol Soc 2008;2008:250–3.
45. Horowitz BN, Vaseghi M, Mahajan A, et al. Percutaneous intrapericardial echocardiography during catheter ablation: a feasibility study. Heart Rhythm 2006;3(11):1275–82.
46. Stephens DN, O'Donnell M, Thomenius K, et al. Experimental studies with a 9F forward-looking intracardiac imaging and ablation catheter. J Ultrasound Med 2009;28(2):207–15.
47. Sacher F, Monahan KH, Thomas SP, et al. Phrenic nerve injury after atrial fibrillation catheter ablation: characterization and outcome in a multicenter study. J Am Coll Cardiol 2006;47(12):2498–503.
48. Fan R, Cano O, Ho SY, et al. Characterization of the phrenic nerve course within the epicardial substrate of patients with nonischemic cardiomyopathy and ventricular tachycardia. Heart Rhythm 2009;6(1):59–64.
49. Mears JA, Lachman N, Christensen K, et al. The phrenic nerve and atrial fibrillation ablation procedures. J Atr Fibrillation 2009;1(7):430–46.
50. Sanchez-Quintana D, Cabrera JA, Climent V, et al. How close are the phrenic nerves to cardiac structures? Implications for cardiac interventionalists. J Cardiovasc Electrophysiol 2005;16(3):309–13.
51. Dib C, Kapa S, Powell BD, et al. Successful use of "cryo-mapping" to avoid phrenic nerve damage during ostial superior vena caval ablation despite nerve proximity. J Interv Card Electrophysiol 2008; 22(1):23–30.
52. Di Biase L, Burkhardt JD, Pelargonio G, et al. Prevention of phrenic nerve injury during epicardial ablation: comparison of methods for separating the phrenic nerve from the epicardial surface. Heart Rhythm 2009;6(7):957–61.
53. Crandall MA, Bradley DJ, Packer DL, et al. Contemporary management of atrial fibrillation: update on anticoagulation and invasive management strategies. Mayo Clin Proc 2009;84(7):643–62.
54. Tsuchiya T, Ashikaga K, Nakagawa S, et al. Atrial fibrillation ablation with esophageal cooling with a cooled water-irrigated intraesophageal balloon: a pilot study. J Cardiovasc Electrophysiol 2007; 18(2):145–50.
55. Asirvatham SJ. Correlative anatomy for the invasive electrophysiologist: outflow tract and supravalvar arrhythmia. J Cardiovasc Electrophysiol 2009; 20(8):955–68.
56. Suleiman M, Asirvatham SJ. Ablation above the semilunar valves: when, why, and how? Part I. Heart Rhythm 2008;5(10):1485–92.
57. Olson TM, Alekseev AE, Moreau C, et al. KATP channel mutation confers risk for vein of Marshall adrenergic atrial fibrillation. Nat Clin Pract Cardiovasc Med 2007;4(2):110–6.
58. Gillinov AM, Pettersson G, Rice TW. Esophageal injury during radiofrequency ablation for atrial fibrillation. J Thorac Cardiovasc Surg 2001;122(6): 1239–40.
59. Mohr FW, Fabricius AM, Falk V, et al. Curative treatment of atrial fibrillation with intraoperative radiofrequency ablation: short-term and midterm results. J Thorac Cardiovasc Surg 2002;123(5): 919–27.
60. Sonmez B, Demirsoy E, Yagan N, et al. A fatal complication due to radiofrequency ablation for atrial fibrillation: atrio-esophageal fistula. Ann Thorac Surg 2003;76(1):281–3.
61. Pappone C, Oral H, Santinelli V, et al. Atrio-esophageal fistula as a complication of percutaneous transcatheter ablation of atrial fibrillation. Circulation 2004;109(22):2724–6.
62. Chaffanjon P, Brichon PY, Faure C, et al. Pericardial reflection around the venous aspect of the heart. Surg Radiol Anat 1997;19(1):17–21.
63. Cabrera JA, Ho SY, Climent V, et al. The architecture of the left lateral atrial wall: a particular anatomic region with implications for ablation of atrial fibrillation. Eur Heart J 2008;29(3):356–62.
64. D'Avila A, Scanavacca M, Sosa E, et al. Pericardial anatomy for the interventional electrophysiologist. J Cardiovasc Electrophysiol 2003; 14(4):422–30.
65. Abbara S, Desai JC, Cury RC, et al. Mapping epicardial fat with multi-detector computed tomography to facilitate percutaneous transepicardial arrhythmia ablation. Eur J Radiol 2006;57(3):417–22.

Electrocardiographic Recognition of Epicardial Arrhythmias

Yoav Michowitz, MD[a,b,*], Bernard Belhassen, MD[a]

KEYWORDS

- Epicardial ablation • Epicardial origin
- Ventricular arrhythmias • Atrial tachycardias

In the current electrophysiologic practice, ablation of most cardiac arrhythmias is performed, with high success rates, using an endocardial approach. However, in some cases, endocardial mapping techniques fail to identify the origin of a focal tachyarrhythmia or the critical site of a reentrant circuit and an epicardial origin is suspected.[1] Although successful ablation will depend ultimately on the results of detailed intracardiac mapping, early suspicion of the epicardial origin of an arrhythmia by standard 12-lead ECG is very useful.

Epicardial ventricular tachyarrhythmias are more common in certain patient populations with structural heart disease such as chagasic heart disease, nonischemic dilated cardiomyopathy and arrhythmogenic right ventricular dysplasia.[1–3] However, they may also occur in patients with ischemic cardiomyopathy—most frequently after inferior myocardial infarction.[4] In patients with structurally normal heart, an epicardial origin has been described in the outflow tract (OT) region, sometimes in proximity to perivascular sites and in the crux of the heart.[5,6]

Most cases of epicardial ablation have involved ventricular tachyarrhythmias, as the thickness of the ventricular myocardium makes it more difficult for endocardial ablation lesions to penetrate through the wall and reach an epicardial site. There are also some reports of epicardial radiofrequency ablation of atrial arrhythmias in the left atrial appendage area where the thick cords of pectinate muscle may preclude endocardial ablation success.[1,7–9] Also, epicardial accessory atrioventricular pathways have been described in the area of the right atrial appendage and coronary sinus (CS) tributaries.[10–14] The term epicardial origin is used indifferently throughout this article regardless of the mechanism of the arrhythmia (reentry vs focal). Since this term only refers to the arrhythmia exit site, it is not excluded that some reentrant mechanisms exhibiting an epicardial exit site actually may have critical components (Isthmus, entrance site) located at an endocardial site.

VENTRICULAR ARRHYTHMIAS

Several criteria have been proposed to differentiate epicardial from endocardial origin of ventricular tachycardia (VT). These include general criteria,[5,15] and site-specific criteria.[16,17] The general criteria are related to the morphology of the QRS. They are all based on the presumed slower conduction during the initial part of the QRS as the wave of depolarization traverses slowly from the epicardium to the endocardium and then spreads faster using the endocardial Purkinje fibers.

[a] The Department of Cardiology, Tel Aviv Sourasky Medical Center and the Sackler Faculty of Medicine, Tel Aviv University, 6 Weizman Street, Tel Aviv 64239, Israel
[b] UCLA Cardiac Arrhythmia Center, Ronald Reagan UCLA Medical Center, David Geffen School of Medicine at UCLA, A2-237 CHS, 10833 Le Conte Avenue, Los Angeles, CA 90095, USA
* Corresponding author. UCLA Cardiac Arrhythmia Center, Ronald Reagan UCLA Medical Center, David Geffen School of Medicine at UCLA, A2-237 CHS, 10833 Le Conte Avenue, Los Angeles, CA 90095.
E-mail address: ymichowitz@gmail.com (Y. Michowitz).

Card Electrophysiol Clin 2 (2010) 25–33
doi:10.1016/j.ccep.2009.11.008
1877-9182/10/$ – see front matter

GENERAL CRITERIA

Pseudodelta Wave

Pseudodelta wave is defined as the interval from the earliest QRS activation to the earliest fast deflection in the precordial leads (**Fig. 1**). Berruezo and colleagues[15] studied patients with VT and a right bundle branch block (RBBB) morphology associated with ischemic or dilated cardiomyopathy. They analyzed the ECG pattern in VTs successfully ablated from the epicardium after a failed endocardial approach and in VTs successfully ablated from the endocardium. They demonstrated that a pseudodelta wave cut-off greater than or equal to 34 msec has a sensitivity and specificity of 83% and 95%, respectively, in predicting an epicardial origin. Bazan and colleagues[16] tested this parameter in a group of 15 patients (9 with structural heart disease, but no history of myocardial infarction, and 6 patients without heart disease) with refractory ventricular arrhythmias. They compared the QRS morphology during pace-mapping from multiple endocardial and epicardial left ventricular (LV) sites. They found that (1) the pseudodelta wave was significantly longer from the epicardium compared with the endocardium and (2) the reported cut-off value of greater than or equal to 34msec was overall very sensitive (96%) but not specific (29%) in predicting an epicardial LV-VT origin. Berruezo and colleagues[15] mentioned that measuring the duration of pseudodelta wave may be difficult.

Intrinsicoid Deflection Time

Intrinsicoid deflection (ID) time is defined as the interval from the earliest ventricular activation to the peak of the R wave in lead V2 (see **Fig. 1**). A cut-off of greater than or equal to 85 ms was found to have a sensitivity and specificity of 87% and 90%, respectively, in predicting epicardial origin.[15] When this parameter was tested by Bazan and colleagues,[16] a longer ID time was confirmed during epicardial pacing as compared with endocardial pacing. However, the 85 msec cut-off

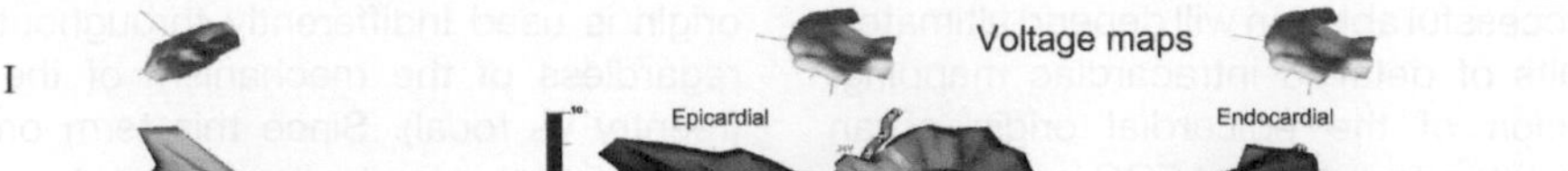

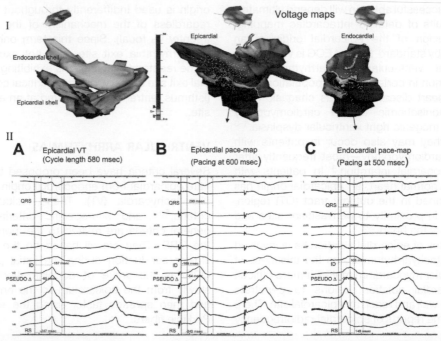

Fig. 1. Panel I. Endocardial and epicardial left ventricular shells (*left*) and voltage maps (*right*) in a patient with nonischemic cardiomyopathy undergoing VT ablation. A scar is demonstrated at the base of the heart in proximity to the mitral valve. The CS catheter is shown in blue. Panel II (same patient). (*A*) Twelve-lead ECG of an epicardial VT (cycle length 580 ms). (*B*) Epicardial pace-map during pacing at a cycle length of 600 ms. (*C*) Endocardial pace-map during pacing at a cycle length of 500 ms. All recordings at a paper speed of 100 mm/s. The VT originated from the base of the heart as manifested by positive concordance of the precordial leads. Pacing was performed from the scar border zone on the epicardial and endocardial sides (pacing site is marked on the voltage maps). Measurements of the ID time pseudodelta wave (PSEUDO Δ) and the shortest RS complex (RS) during VT (*A*) and during both pace-maps (*B, C*) are consistent with an epicardial origin. The similarity in morphology and measurements between the epicardial pace-map and the VT supports an epicardial origin.

reached sensitivity and specificity of only 39% and 24%, respectively.[16]

Shortest Precordial Complex

Shortest RS complex is measured from the earliest ventricular activation to the nadir of the first S wave in any precordial lead (see **Fig. 1**).

A cutoff of greater than or equal to 121 ms yielded specificity and sensitivity of 76% and 85%, respectively, by Berruezo and colleagues[15]; and lower values of 53% and 79%, respectively, by Bazan and colleagues.[16]

QRS-Complex Duration

The QRS complex duration is defined as the interval measured from the earliest ventricular activation (from the stimulation artifact in paced patients) to the offset of QRS in the precordial leads. The QRS duration is longer when pacing is performed from the epicardium, as compared with endocardial pacing at a similar LV site[16] (due to the presence of pseudodelta wave). However, due to considerable overlap in QRS duration during VT, an exact cut-off value for QRS width could not be identified to differentiate between epicardial and endocardial VTs.[16]

Precordial Maximum Deflection Index

Maximum deflection index (MDI) is defined as the time from the beginning of the QRS to the earliest maximal deflection (largest amplitude deflection either above or below the baseline) in any of the precordial leads divided by the maximal QRS duration.[5] A cut-off value of 0.55 had high sensitivity and specificity to predict epicardial VT origin in patients with idiopathic left VTs arising close to the aortic sinus of Valsalva[5] and near the crux of the heart.[6] MDI was not tested systematically in patients with structural heart disease.

Precordial Pattern Break

Another finding that may point to an epicardial origin is the pattern break or R wave regression or progression sign (Marchlinski, 2nd annual VT symposium, Philadelphia, PA, unpublished data, 2007) manifested as an abrupt loss of R wave in V2 with resumption in V3-V6.[18] According to Haqqani and colleagues,[18] this criterion was not tested in patients with structural heart disease although it is likely to be helpful in this patient group as well.

SITE-SPECIFIC CRITERIA

Several articles have examined region-specific ECG features of epicardial ventricular arrhythmia, including the LV,[16] right ventricle (RV),[17] the OT area[5,17,19] and the crux of the heart.[6] The difference between epicardial and endocardial electrograms may be related to two factors: slowed initial conduction in the epicardial layer and differences in propagation of the depolarizing wave. QRS morphology in leads reflecting initial activation will manifest as a Q wave (activation moving away from the electrode) when the origin is epicardial. However, when the origin is endocardial it will manifest as an rS complex as part of the activation (endocardial to epicardial) moves toward the recording electrode.

LV

Bazan and colleagues[16] divided the LV into five parts: basal superior, basal inferior, apical superior, apical inferior, and LV apex.

Basal LV area

VT originating from the base of the heart can be recognized by positive concordance in the precordial leads.[20] The presence of a Q wave in lead I and the absence of Q in leads II, III, and AVF are good predictors of an epicardial origin for the basal superior LV region.[16] Conversely, the presence of Q wave in inferior leads is a good predictor of an epicardial origin in the basal inferior LV area.[16]

Apical LV area

Apical superior VT will have a negative concordance in the precordial leads and right inferior axis.[20] The presence of Q wave in lead I supports an epicardial location at the superior area, while the presence of Q wave in inferior leads (as opposed to rS pattern) supports an epicardial location at the inferior part.[16]

LV apex

VT arising from the LV apex suggested by negative precordial concordance and QS pattern from V4-V6.[20] An initial Q wave in lead V2 was significantly associated with epicardial sites but this finding was not confirmed in the matched pace-mapping analysis.[16]

These site-specific criteria were developed in patients without myocardial infarction; obviously, infarct-related Q waves will likely affect the ability of this criterion to differentiate epicardial from endocardial foci.

RV

A region-specific study with RV epicardial and endocardial pace-mapping demonstrated several findings[17]: pacing from the epicardial anterior RV is more likely to manifest Q or QS complex in lead I and V2, whereas inferior wall epicardial pacing will manifest Q wave in inferior leads.

Cut-off values for the general criteria described for the LV (pseudodelta, ID time, shortest precordial RS complex, and QRS duration) were not applicable to the RV, though some significant differences between epicardial and endocardial pacing were observed.

These findings were explained by two factors[17]: the thinner RV wall and the less abundant Purkinje network over the RV free wall making difference in conduction velocity between epicardial and endocardial pacing less robust. As this study included only two patients with ischemic heart disease, the results cannot be extrapolated to this patient subgroup. In addition, there are no studies in patients with RV hypertrophy.

OT

VT arising from the OT typically has a left bundle branch block (LBBB) pattern and an inferior axis. Criteria for differentiating right- from left-sided origin have been described.[21–23] No pathognomonic differences in ECG morphology were noted between epicardial and endocardial pacing in the RVOT region.[17]

Daniels and colleagues[5] described a series of patients with epicardial tachycardia originating from LV sites close to the coronary vessels. Tachycardias from the anterior interventricular vein (AIV) region exhibit a LBBB pattern in V1 with precordial transition beyond V2.[24] As the AIV or great cardiac vein (GCV) junction lies immediately lateral to the left coronary cusp (LCC),[25] VTs from this location have a pattern similar to those originating from the aortic sinus of Valsalva (ie, R/S amplitude index >0.5 and R wave duration index >0.3 in V1 or V2). Whether it has M or W pattern in V1 like LCC VT has not been described. VTs originating more distally in the AIV had narrower QRS complex and were similar to RVOT VTs.

Obel and colleagues[19] described a series of five patients with epicardial VTs originating in the distal GCV region, all patients had slurring of the precordial R wave, four or five had RBBB pattern in V1 and 1 had transition in V3.

MDI, which was first introduced by Daniels and colleagues,[5] had a sensitivity of 100% and specificity of 98.7% in identifying epicardial VTs. Ito and colleagues[22] developed an algorithm to locate origin of OT VT. In patients with ECG compatible with LVOT VTs, an aVL to aVR Q ratio greater than 1.4, or an S wave in V1 greater than 1.2 mV differentiated epicardial from endocardial origin. Another study from the same group[26] reported findings of ECGs from 10 patients with LVOT perivascular epicardial VTs. Using either their algorithm or MDI they could correctly identify 6 out of 10 ECG with each method separately. However, using both they could identify 9 out of 10 ECGs.

Crux of the Heart

Another recent study described epicardial VTs originating from the crux of the heart[6] (which corresponds to the junction between the CS and middle cardiac vein). All four patients had MDI greater than or equal to 55 (pseudodelta $\geq$34 and ID $\geq$85). However, only one had shortest RS less than 121. These VTs had left superior axis and demonstrated an abrupt precordial transition in V2. Their main differential diagnosis is VT from the posterior mitral annulus. Deep negative deltoid wave in the inferior leads with very positive V2 and MDI greater than or equal to 55 can be helpful in differentiating the two sites.

SUMMARY ALGORITHM

An algorithm summarizing the current evidence and approach to ECG recognition of epicardial VT is presented in **Tables 1** and **2**. None of the criteria is absolute and all were tested in a limited number of patients. In addition, the effect of slowed conduction by antiarrhythmic drugs on surface ECG characteristics was not tested. Representative ECG of presumed epicardial VT in a patient with structural heart disease is presented in **Fig. 1**. An example of OT epicardial VT is presented in **Fig. 2**.

ACCESSORY PATHWAYS

Epicardial accessory pathways have been described mainly in two anatomic locations: (1) in the CS tributaries and (2) the area between the atrial appendages and ventricular myocardium, mainly on the right side.[10–13]

The CS has extensive electrical connections with the left and right atria. It may have a connection to the ventricles along the middle cardiac vein and posterior cardiac vein (related to CS diverticulum in 30%) creating the substrate for an accessory pathway between the ventricles and the atria.[12] These connections manifest electrocardiographically as posteroseptal or left posterior pathways. Their distinguishing features are an immediately negative delta wave in lead II,[12,13] a steep positive delta wave in aVR and a deep S wave in lead V6 (R wave $\leq$ S wave). According to Takahashi and colleagues,[13] an immediate negative delta wave in lead II has the highest sensitivity (found in 70%–87% of cases). However, steep positive delta wave in aVR has the highest specificity (98%) and positive predictive value

Table 1
An algorithm summarizing the current evidence and approach to ECG recognition of epicardial VTs in patients with structural heart disease

Ischemic Heart Disease (RBBB VT)	Dilated Cardiomyopathy (RBBB VT)	Arrhythmogenic Right Ventricular Dysplasia[d] (LBBB VT)
General criteria • Pseudo $\Delta \geq 34$ ms • ID ≥ 85 ms • RS ≥ 121 ms • MDI $\geq 55\%$[a] • Precordial pattern break[a]	General criteria • Pseudo $\Delta \geq 34$ms[b] • ID ≥ 85ms[b] • RS ≥ 121ms[b] • MDI $\geq 55\%$[a] • Precordial pattern break[a]	General criteria • Pseudo Δ, ID, RS—may be higher from epi pacing[c] • MDI—not tested
Site specific criteria • In case of non Q MI,[a] Q-wave in leads reflecting the VT exit region may favor an epicardial exit • Differential epi- or endo-pacing Compare QRS duration and morphology to the clinical VT	Site specific criteria • Q in inferior leads for inferior VT • Q in lead I in basal superior or apical superior VT • Absence of Q in inferior leads in basal superior VT • Differential epi- or endo-pacing Compare QRS duration and morphology to the clinical VT	Site specific criteria • Q in leads that reflect local activation • Differential epi- or endo-pacing • QRS duration—not helpful

If any of the above criteria is found, an epicardial VT is suggested.

Abbreviations: AIV, anterior interventricular vein; ARVD, arrhythmogenic right ventricular dysplasia; CMP, cardiomyopathy; GCV, great cardiac vein; HD, heart disease; ID, intrinsicoid deflection time; LBBB, left bundle branch block; LV, left ventricle; LVOT, left ventricular outflow tract; MDI, maximal deflection index; Pseudo Δ, pseudodelta wave; RBBB, right bundle branch block; RV, right ventricle; RVOT, right ventricular outflow tract; SHD, structural heart disease.

[a] Not tested in this patient subgroup.
[b] Sensitivity and specificity vary in different articles.
[c] Cutoff reported for LV VT are not applicable to RV V.
[d] Or other structural heart disease patient with RV VT.

Table 2
An algorithm summarizing the current evidence and approach to ECG recognition of epicardial VTs in patients with structurally normal heart

RVOT	LVOT[a]	CRUX
(VT with inferior axis and precordial R/S transition beyond V3)	(VT with inferior axis and early precordial R/S transition)	(VT with left superior axis and abrupt precordial transition in V2)
Possible epicardial location: distal AIV	Possible epicardial location: AIV/GCV Junction-precordial R transition beyond V2 Distal GCV—RBBB pattern in V1	
• MDI ≥ 55% • No pathognomonic differences between epicardial and endocardial pacing • Pseudo Δ, ID, RS—may be higher from epicardial pacing[b]	• MDI ≥ 55% • aVL/aVR Q ratio >1.4 or an S wave in V1 ≥1.2 mV • Pseudo Δ, ID, RS—Not tested in this group, may prove useful	• MDI ≥ 55% • Pseudo Δ ≥ 34 • ID ≥ 85 • RS—not useful

If any of the above criteria is found, an epicardial VT is suggested.

Abbreviations: AIV, anterior interventricular vein; ARVD, arrhythmogenic right ventricular dysplasia; CMP, cardiomyopathy; GCV, great cardiac vein; HD, heart disease; ID, intrinsicoid deflection time; LBBB, left bundle branch block; LV, left ventricle; LVOT, left ventricular outflow tract; MDI, maximal deflection index; Pseudo Δ, pseudodelta wave; RBBB, right bundle branch block; RV, right ventricle; RVOT, right ventricular outflow tract; SHD, structural heart disease.

[a] Other ECG Criteria for LVOT VT include: R-wave duration index ≥50% and R/S-wave amplitude ratio ≥30% in V1 or V2.[18]

[b] Cutoffs reported for LV VT are not applicable to RV VT.

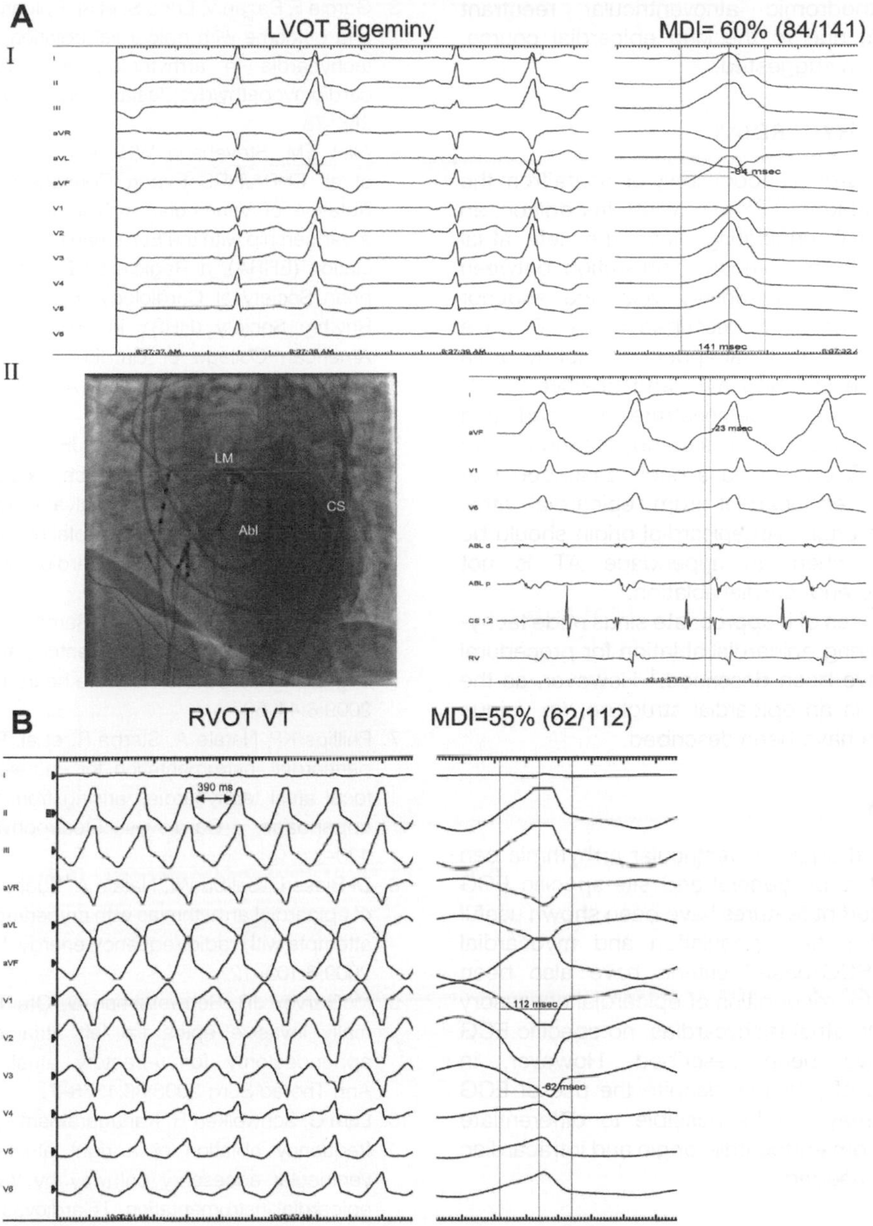

Fig. 2. (*A*) OT ventricular arrhythmias. Panel I. A patient with ventricular premature complex resembling left OT VT (paper speed 50 mm/s). Endocardial ablation failed to ablate the arrhythmia. MDI above 55% supports an epicardial origin (paper speed of 200 mm/s). Panel II. Earliest ventricular activation during the tachycardia was recorded in the distal CS (23 ms before the surface QRS), which supports an origin in the GCV area. On the left, catheter position during recordings and contrast injection to the left main (LM) coronary artery. The endocardial ablation catheter was located endocardially in the LVOT through retrograde aortic approach and the CS catheter was pushed deep into the coronary sinus. (*B*) ECG of a patient with RVOT VT ablated from epicardial approach. An MDI of 55% suggests an epicardial location.

especially when combined with deep S wave in lead V6.

Epicardial connections between the right atrial appendage and the RV have been described. They can be located 10 mm away from the annulus. Surface ECG features of these accessory pathways correspond to the anatomic location of appendage and thus may be similar to those of right anterior or anterolateral accessory pathways. A relatively long ventriculoatrial conduction time during orthodromic atrioventricular reentrant tachycardia, due to the long epicardial course, has also been suggested.

ATRIAL TACHYCARDIAS

Atrial tachycardias uncommonly originate from the atrial appendages,[27–29] mainly left. In addition, an epicardial AT originating near the left atrial appendage from a venous connection between the left superior pulmonary vein and superior vena cava has been described.[30] The P wave morphology of left atrial appendage tachycardia was negative in I and aVL, and positive in V1. The inferior leads demonstrate a broad and notched P wave due to superior location.[27] No specific ECG criteria have been described that differentiate endocardial from epicardial atrial tachycardia origin. An epicardial origin should be considered when an appendage AT is not amenable to endocardial ablation.

Finally, cases of inappropriate sinus node tachycardia requiring epicardial ablation for procedural success have been described.[1] However, as the sinus node is an epicardial structure, no unique ECG criteria have been described.

SUMMARY

An epicardial origin of ventricular arrhythmia can be suggested by general and site-specific ECG criteria. Different features have been shown useful in different patient population and myocardial locations. ECG-based criteria have also been developed for recognition of epicardial accessory pathways. In atrial tachycardias, no specific ECG criteria have been described. However, in a subgroup of patients, despite the use of ECG criteria, it may not be possible to differentiate epicardial from endocardial origin and intracardiac mapping is needed.

ACKNOWLEDGMENTS

The authors thank Dr Roderick Tung for his help in preparing the figures.

REFERENCES

1. Schweikert RA, Saliba WI, Tomassoni G, et al. Percutaneous pericardial instrumentation for endo-epicardial mapping of previously failed ablations. Circulation 2003;108:1329–35.
2. Cesario DA, Vaseghi M, Boyle NG, et al. Value of high-density endocardial and epicardial mapping for catheter ablation of hemodynamically unstable ventricular tachycardia. Heart Rhythm 2006;3:1–10.
3. Garcia F, Bazan V, Erica S, et al. Epicardial substrate and outcome with epicardial ablation of ventricular tachycardia in arrhythmogenic right ventricular cardiomyopathy/dysplasia. Circulation 2009;120: 366–75.
4. Aliot EM, Stevenson WG, Almendral-Garrote JM, et al. EHRA/HRS Expert Consensus on Catheter Ablation of Ventricular Arrhythmias: developed in a partnership with the European Heart Rhythm Association (EHRA), a Registered Branch of the European Society of Cardiology (ESC), and the Heart Rhythm Society (HRS); in collaboration with the American College of Cardiology (ACC) and the American Heart Association (AHA). Heart Rhythm 2009;6:886–933.
5. Daniels DV, Lu YY, Morton JB, et al. Idiopathic epicardial left ventricular tachycardia originating remote from the sinus of Valsalva: electrophysiological characteristics, catheter ablation, and identification from the 12-lead electrocardiogram. Circulation 2006;113:1659–66.
6. Doppalapudi H, Yamada T, Ramaswamy K, et al. Idiopathic focal epicardial ventricular tachycardia originating from the crux of the heart. Heart Rhythm 2009;6:44–50.
7. Phillips KP, Natale A, Sterba R, et al. Percutaneous pericardial instrumentation for catheter ablation of focal atrial tachycardias arising from the left atrial appendage. J Cardiovasc Electrophysiol 2008;19: 430–3.
8. Di Biase L, Saliba WI, Natale A. Successful ablation of epicardial arrhythmias with cryoenergy after failed attempts with radiofrequency energy. Heart Rhythm 2009;6:109–12.
9. McGarvey JR, Schwartzman D, Ota T, et al. Minimally invasive epicardial left atrial ablation and appendectomy for refractory atrial tachycardia. Ann Thorac Surg 2008;86:1375–7.
10. Lam C, Schweikert R, Kanagaratnam L, et al. Radiofrequency ablation of a right atrial appendage-ventricular accessory pathway by transcutaneous epicardial instrumentation. J Cardiovasc Electrophysiol 2000;11:1170–3.
11. Haghjoo M, Mahmoodi E, Fazelifar AF, et al. Electrocardiographic and electrophysiologic predictors of successful ablation site in patients with manifest posteroseptal accessory pathway. Pacing Clin Electrophysiol 2008;3:103–11.
12. Sun Y, Arruda M, Otomo K, et al. Coronary sinus-ventricular accessory connections producing posteroseptal and left posterior accessory pathways: incidence and electrophysiological identification. Circulation 2002;106:1362–7.
13. Takahashi A, Shah DC, Jais P, et al. Specific electrocardiographic features of manifest coronary vein posteroseptal accessory pathways. J Cardiovasc Electrophysiol 1998;9:1015–25.

14. Valderrabano M, Cesario DA, Ji S, et al. Percutaneous epicardial mapping during ablation of difficult accessory pathways as an alternative to cardiac surgery. Heart Rhythm 2004;1:311–6.
15. Berruezo A, Mont L, Nava S, et al. Electrocardiographic recognition of the epicardial origin of ventricular tachycardias. Circulation 2004;109: 1842–7.
16. Bazan V, Gerstenfeld EP, Garcia FC, et al. Site-specific twelve-lead ECG features to identify an epicardial origin for left ventricular tachycardia in the absence of myocardial infarction. Heart Rhythm 2007;4:1403–10.
17. Bazan V, Bala R, Garcia FC, et al. Twelve-lead ECG features to identify ventricular tachycardia arising from the epicardial right ventricle. Heart Rhythm 2006;3:1132–9.
18. Haqqani HM, Morton JB, Kalman JM. Using the 12-lead ECG to localize the origin of atrial and ventricular tachycardias: part 2—ventricular tachycardia. J Cardiovasc Electrophysiol 2009;20:825–32.
19. Obel OA, d'Avila A, Neuzil P, et al. Ablation of left ventricular epicardial outflow tract tachycardia from the distal great cardiac vein. J Am Coll Cardiol 2006;48:1813–7.
20. Josephson ME, Callans DJ. Using the twelve-lead electrocardiogram to localize the site of origin of ventricular tachycardia. Heart Rhythm 2005;2: 443–6.
21. Ouyang F, Fotuhi P, Ho SY, et al. Repetitive monomorphic ventricular tachycardia originating from the aortic sinus cusp: electrocardiographic characterization for guiding catheter ablation. J Am Coll Cardiol 2002;39:500–8.
22. Ito S, Tada H, Naito S, et al. Development and validation of an ECG algorithm for identifying the optimal ablation site for idiopathic ventricular outflow tract tachycardia. J Cardiovasc Electrophysiol 2003; 14:1280–6.
23. Yang Y, Saenz LC, Varosy PD, et al. Using the initial vector from surface electrocardiogram to distinguish the site of outflow tract tachycardia. Pacing Clin Electrophysiol 2007;30:891–8.
24. Hirasawa Y, Miyauchi Y, Iwasaki YK, et al. Successful radiofrequency catheter ablation of epicardial left ventricular outflow tract tachycardia from the anterior interventricular coronary vein. J Cardiovasc Electrophysiol 2005;16:1378–80.
25. Asirvatham SJ. Correlative anatomy for the invasive electrophysiologist: outflow tract and supravalvar arrhythmia. J Cardiovasc Electrophysiol 2009;20: 955–68.
26. Kaseno K, Tada H, Tanaka S, et al. Successful catheter ablation of left ventricular epicardial tachycardia originating from the great cardiac vein: a case report and review of the literature. Circ J 2007;71:1983–8.
27. Teh AW, Kistler PM, Kalman JM. Using the 12-lead ECG to localize the origin of ventricular and atrial tachycardias: Part 1. Focal atrial tachycardia. J Cardiovasc Electrophysiol 2009;20:706–9.
28. Lesh MD, Van Hare GF, Epstein LM, et al. Radiofrequency catheter ablation of atrial arrhythmias. Results and mechanisms. Circulation 1994;89: 1074–89.
29. Hillock RJ, Singarayar S, Kalman JM, et al. Tale of two tails: the tip of the atrial appendages is an unusual site for focal atrial tachycardia. Heart Rhythm 2006;3:467–9.
30. Tse HF, Lau CP, Lee KL, et al. Atrial tachycardia arising from an epicardial site with venous connection between the left superior pulmonary vein and superior vena cava. J Cardiovasc Electrophysiol 2003;14:540–3.

How to Learn Epicardial Intervention Techniques in Electrophysiology

Naga Vamsi Garikipati, MD, MPH[a],
Vijayapraveena Paruchuri, MD[a], Suneet Mittal, MD[b,*]

KEYWORDS

• Pericardial space • Catheter ablation • Ventricle

During the past 20 years, catheter ablation of ventricular tachycardia (VT) has emerged as an important therapeutic modality. Conventionally, the endocardium of the right and left ventricles is accessed through a percutaneous femoral approach. However, an endocardial approach fails in a significant proportion of patients because of the presence of epicardial circuits. These epicardial circuits are observed in up to 15% of patients with prior myocardial infarction and in up to 40% of patients with Chagas disease.[1–4]

Access to the epicardium without resorting to open heart surgery has historically been challenging. Initial attempts sought to use the coronary vasculature to access epicardial circuits[5,6]; however, the challenge of reaching epicardial circuits that are remote from the vasculature remained. Today, there is great interest in percutaneous access to the epicardium. Franz Schuh pioneered the first blind percutaneous pericardial puncture in 1840; a subxiphoid approach was then described by Marfan in 1911.[7] Building on this technique, Sosa and colleagues[5] in 1996 pioneered a nonsurgical access to the pericardium by using a percutaneous approach. Initial attempts involved only mapping; subsequently, Sosa refined the technique to guide endocardial VT ablation and to perform epicardial VT ablation[1] in patients with Chagas disease. This innovation heralded the era of percutaneous epicardial ablation in the electrophysiology laboratory.

INDICATIONS

With time, the indications for epicardial ablation have gradually expanded to include various conditions. For example, epicardial VT ablation is necessary in patients in whom endocardial ablation cannot be performed. This situation occurs in patients with severe peripheral vascular disease, in patients in whom transseptal access is contraindicated or difficult (eg, previously placed interatrial septal occlusion devices), in patients with an existing thrombus with the left ventricular cavity,[8] and in patients with mechanical aortic and mitral valves.[9] More importantly,

Conflict of interest disclosures: N.V.G.: none; V.P.: none; S.M.: consultant (Bard, Biotronik, Boston Scientific, Johnson & Johnson, Lifewatch, Medtronic, St Jude Medical, Transoma Medical); fellowship support (Biotronik, Boston Scientific, Medtronic, St Jude Medical); research grants (Transoma Medical).

[a] Clinical Electrophysiology, The Al-Sabah Arrhythmia Institute, The St Luke's and Roosevelt Hospitals Center, Columbia University College of Physicians & Surgeons, 1111 Amsterdam Avenue, New York, NY 10025, USA
[b] Electrophysiology Laboratory, The Al-Sabah Arrhythmia Institute, The St Luke's and Roosevelt Hospitals Center, Columbia University College of Physicians & Surgeons, 1111 Amsterdam Avenue, New York, NY 10025, USA
* Corresponding author. Division of Cardiology, The St Luke's and Roosevelt Hospitals Center, 1111 Amsterdam Avenue, New York, NY 10025.
E-mail address: smittal@chpnet.org (S. Mittal).

Card Electrophysiol Clin 2 (2010) 35–43
doi:10.1016/j.ccep.2009.11.009

epicardial ablation is necessary in patients with prior failed endocardial ablations[10] as has been observed in patients with Chagas disease[1,11]; cardiac sarcoidosis[12]; and ischemic,[13] idiopathic dilated,[6,14] and right ventricular cardiomyopathy.[15] Epicardial mapping is increasingly being performed concomitantly with endocardial mapping in an attempt to identify the optimal sites for ablation. More recently, investigators have applied the technique to manage supraventricular arrhythmias, including inappropriate sinus tachycardia, atrial tachycardia arising from the left atrial appendage, accessory pathways,[10,16] and atrial fibrillation.[8,17–19] Therefore, there has been an increased interest for the practicing electrophysiologist to learn the skills that are necessary to perform successful epicardial ablation. This article outlines an approach to begin an epicardial ablation program in the electrophysiology laboratory.

INITIATING THE PROGRAM

Because epicardial ablation is a relative newcomer to electrophysiology, most electrophysiologists interested in the procedure were either trained before the procedure was available or trained at an institution that did not offer the procedure. Therefore, there are some logistical hurdles in getting an epicardial ablation program up and running. Nothing is more important as an initial step than visiting a center performing a high number of these procedures and observing several procedures being performed, thus providing a good opportunity to review the indications, the risks that are inherent in the procedure, and the infrastructure necessary in the electrophysiology laboratory and institution to perform the procedure safely and effectively. Ideally, this observership is followed by direct proctorship of the first few cases by an experienced operator.

INDIVIDUAL CASES

In the beginning, it may be best to consider an epicardial approach in patients with VT (1) who have not had prior cardiac surgery, (2) who have failed to respond to medical therapy (including those patients who have received frequent implantable cardioverter-defibrillator shocks), and (3) who have failed a prior attempt at endocardial ablation. With initial experience in this patient group and adequate skill and comfort level with the procedure, it is reasonable to expand the program to include patients in whom endocardial ablation is not possible (see the earlier discussion) and who have had prior cardiac surgery and as part of a concomitant endocardial and epicardial ablation procedure.

Preprocedure Considerations

Before scheduling the procedure, attention has to be directed toward managing antiplatelet and anticoagulant medications. The authors continue the administration of aspirin but discontinue (whenever possible) clopidogrel at least 5 days in advance of the procedure. For patients taking anticoagulants, the authors discontinue warfarin 5 days in advance of the procedure to allow the international normalized ratio to normalize. If necessary, the patients are administered low-molecular-weight heparin for 2 to 3 days before the procedure as a bridging therapy and discontinue it at least 12 hours before the procedure. In all cases the authors "type and crossmatch" the patient for 2 units of packed red blood cells on the morning of the procedure and ensure that the platelet count is greater than 100,000/µL.

Anesthesia Considerations

For epicardial ablations, it is important that an anesthesiologist be present for the procedure. The patient can be deeply sedated using intravenous fentanyl and midazolam with spontaneous ventilation[5,20] or placed under intravenous general anesthesia. The latter is preferred because these procedures can be lengthy and because ablation in the epicardial space can often be painful. General anesthesia also guards against patient movement, which can adversely affect 3-dimensional mapping data (see later discussion). In addition, an arterial catheter is placed for continuous blood pressure monitoring, and a Foley catheter is placed to monitor urinary output.

Procedural Considerations

It is preferred that these procedures be performed in a laboratory that is equipped with biplane fluoroscopy. Standard femoral arterial and venous access is obtained. A coronary sinus catheter is placed via a transfemoral approach in all patients; this helps to define the posteroseptal space (**Fig. 1**). In addition, a standard quadripolar catheter is placed into the right ventricle. There are limited dedicated tools or catheters for epicardial procedures to assist electrophysiologists working in the pericardial space. Most of the tools currently used were developed for standard electrophysiology procedures. The authors obtain epicardial access (see the next section) and perform epicardial mapping before endocardial mapping to minimize the period of anticoagulation. A

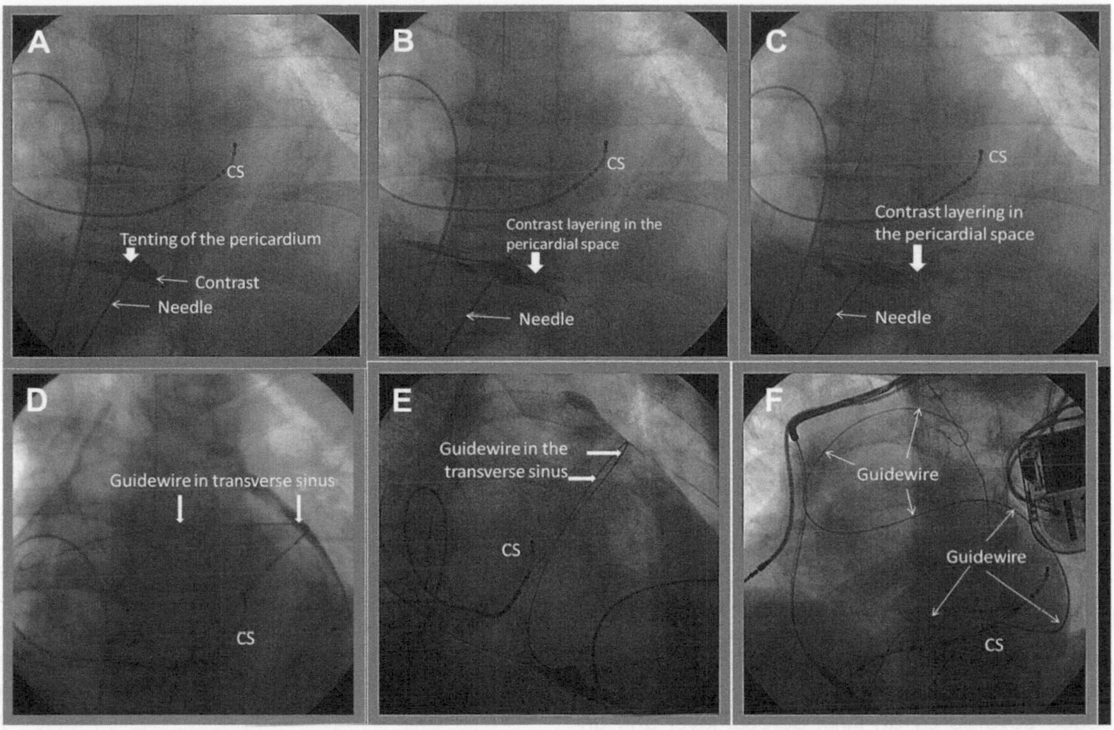

Fig. 1. Sequential fluoroscopic images of an epicardial access procedure. A decapolar catheter has been placed into the coronary sinus (CS) through a femoral venous approach. (*A*) Left anterior oblique (LAO) image. Contrast injection through the Tuohy needle demonstrates tenting of the pericardium before puncture. (*B, C*) LAO image. As the needle is advanced, additional contrast is injected. Layering of contrast in the pericardial space confirms successful entry into the desired space. (*D*) LAO image. A guidewire is present in the pericardial space and traverses the transverse sinus. Note that the guidewire abuts the outer fluoroscopic border of the heart, thereby confirming its location in the proper space. (*E*) Right anterior oblique image. The guidewire remains within the transverse sinus. (*F*) LAO image of a different patient showing the position of the guidewire.

3-dimensional mapping system is essential for these types of procedures.

Epicardial Access

The authors routinely administer prophylactic antibiotics (cefazolin 1 g or vancomycin 1 g intravenously) before starting the procedure. The subxiphoid area is shaved, cleansed, and prepared in an aseptic fashion. The skin overlying the subxiphoid region is anesthetized with 1% lidocaine. Commercially available epidural needles designed to perform lumbar puncture (Tuohy needle) are used for the procedure. These needles come in different lengths; the choice of length is based on the size of the thorax. Either a 17 Ga × 3-7/8-in or a 17 Ga × 5-in Tuohy needle with centimeter markings (Arrow International Inc, Reading, PA, USA) is most commonly used.

The skin is punctured at the angle between the left border of the subxiphoid process and the lower left rib. The spatial orientation of the needle determines the portion of the ventricle reached. The needle should always point to the left shoulder of the patient; it is introduced more horizontally to access the anterior portion of the ventricles and more vertically to access the diaphragmatic portion. Fluoroscopy is used to guide the needle after the skin puncture. In the left anterior oblique view (35°–40°), the needle is guided toward the cardiac silhouette until the heart movement can be detected by the operator. At this point, the needle should reach the mid portion between the base and apex of the heart. The location can be verified in the right anterior oblique view (35°–40°). Radiocontrast (approximately 1 mL) is then injected to verify the location of the needle (see **Fig. 1**A). If the needle has not reached the pericardial sac and is below the diaphragm, contrast is visualized under the diaphragm. When the needle reaches the pericardial sac, the injected contrast outlines the cardiac silhouette (see **Fig. 1**B, C). A soft, floppy-tipped guidewire is then passed into the hollow of the needle (see **Fig. 1**D, E).

It is absolutely critical that the guidewire is confirmed to be in the pericardial space. Toward that end, it is ensured that in the left anterior oblique view the guidewire follows the outer border of the heart; in addition, whenever possible, the authors try to pass the guidewire into the transverse sinus as added confirmation of entry into the pericardial space (see **Fig. 1**D, E). The dilator from a 5F sheath is introduced into the pericardial space, the guidewire is removed, and a pericardiogram is obtained by injecting 20 mL radiocontrast material (**Fig. 2**). The guidewire is then replaced back in the pericardial space, and a sheath is introduced. A bidirectional steerable sheath specifically for use in this setting has recently become available (Agilis Steerable Introducer; St Jude Medical, St Paul, MN, USA). The mapping and ablation catheters can now be introduced to begin the epicardial aspect of the procedure (**Fig. 3**).

UNDERSTANDING PERICARDIAL ANATOMY

Before embarking on an epicardial ablation program, it is essential to have a thorough understanding of the anatomy of the pericardial space. The pericardial cavity is a flask-shaped virtual space covered by an inner serosal layer and an outer fibrous layer. The cavity separates the heart from its surrounding mediastinal structures, thus allowing free movement of the heart (within this cavity). The serosal layer is further divided into a parietal layer fixed to the outer fibrous layer and the visceral layer known as the epicardium. Unlike a flask, the pericardial cavity is not a continuous space. The pericardium forms reflections around the great vessels and the heart (on the posterior aspect), breaking it down into a series of sinuses and recesses. These reflections can assist by forming landmarks against which the catheters can be placed. At the same time, they can become anatomic obstacles for electrophysiologic procedures. For example, the pericardial reflections that separate the superior and the inferior pulmonary veins form pulmonary venous recesses, which preclude the ability to completely encircle a single pulmonary vein during epicardial ablation.[4]

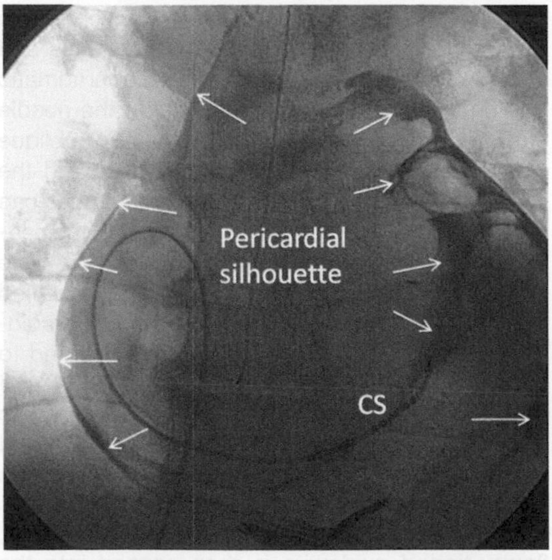

Fig. 2. Pericardiogram. After obtaining epicardial access, a pericardiogram is obtained after injecting 20 mL radiocontrast material via a 5F dilator. CS, coronary sinus.

The 2 pericardial space sinuses that can be accessed in electrophysiology procedures are the transverse and oblique sinuses. The transverse sinus is bound anteriorly by the left atrium and inferiorly by the pericardial reflection connecting the right and left pulmonary veins. The sinus contains the right pulmonary artery and inferior aortic recess. By exploring the transverse sinus, one can gain access to the left atrium and the pulmonary veins for atrial fibrillation ablation and to the noncoronary and right coronary aortic cusps in the aortic recess for epicardial ablation. In contrast, the oblique sinus is bound anteriorly by the atria, to the right by a reflection extending from the right pulmonary veins to the inferior vena cava and to the left by a reflection between the left pulmonary veins. The oblique sinus allows for extensive mapping of the ventricles.

SPECIAL SITUATIONS

Adhesions

Dense adhesions form on the surface of the heart in patients who have previously undergone cardiac surgery. A similar problem has been observed in some patients with prior myocarditis or myocardial infarction, likely secondary to associated pericarditis. Sosa and colleagues[21] reported adhesions on the right and left ventricular lateral walls along the anterior surface of the heart in postsurgical patients. These investigators were able to access the pericardial space in these patients and insert ablation catheters but were unable to manipulate the catheters within the pericardial space. In such patients, the puncture needs to be directed toward the inferior wall of the heart. The electrophysiologist can gently separate the pericardial adhesions by blunt dissection (making use of the ablation catheter) to progressively enlarge the epicardial surface available for mapping and ablation.

Soejima and colleagues[22] have described the use of a direct surgical subxiphoid approach in patients in whom dense adhesions are also present along the inferior wall. In a patient who is

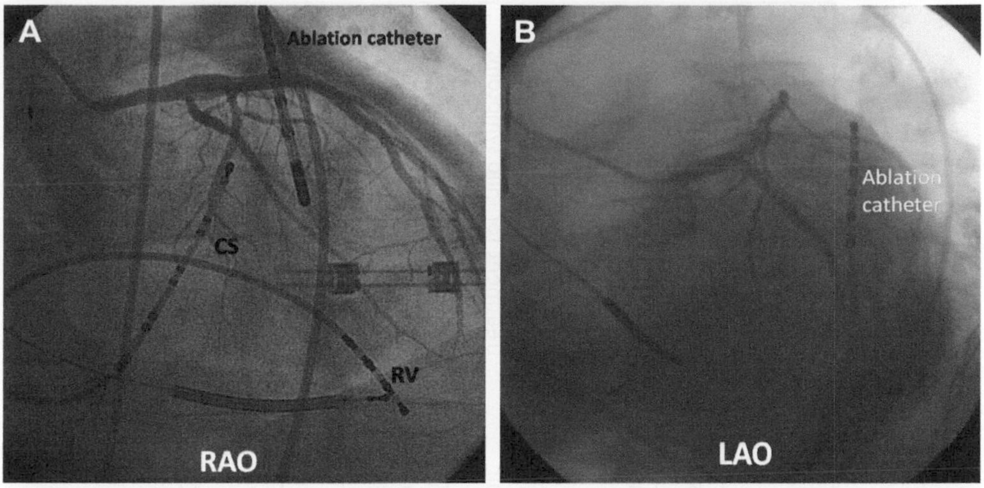

Fig. 3. Coronary angiography performed in RAO (*A*) and LAO (*B*) projections. Before ablation, coronary angiography is performed to assess the location of the ablation catheter to the major epicardial coronary arteries. CS, coronary sinus catheter; LAO, left anterior oblique; RAO, right anterior oblique; RV, right ventricular quadripolar catheter.

endotracheally intubated and is under general anesthesia, the cardiothoracic surgeon makes a 3-in midepigastric incision. The abdominal fascia is opened along the linea alba to the left of the xiphoid process. The pericardium is then exposed and opened horizontally, parallel to the diaphragmatic reflection. The pericardiotomy is then extended to visualize the ventricles, and blunt dissection of the adhesions is done to expose the diaphragmatic and posterior epicardium. A sheath can then be placed for further introduction of mapping and ablation catheters. After ablation, the pericardial sheath is removed and the surgical incision is closed. A Jackson-Pratt drain is placed in the pericardial space and left to drain overnight.

Epicardial Fat

The presence of epicardial fat is an important procedural consideration. Epicardial fat covers 80% of the heart surface and constitutes 20% of the total heart weight.[23,24] The thickness of the epicardial fat layer increases from age 20 to 40 years and is independent of age afterward. Women tend to have a thicker epicardial fat layer than men (1.65:1).[25] Epicardial fat embeds the coronary arteries and their main branches, and is concentrated along the coronary sulcus and the interventricular groove. On the right ventricle, the greatest amount of epicardial fat is located over the basal aspect of the lateral wall.[25,26] Less is known about the distribution of epicardial fat on the left ventricle. However, it seems that epicardial fat over the left ventricle is only a third to a quarter of that found over the right ventricle.[23]

Epicardial fat between the ablation catheter and the target site can act as an insulator, resulting in the failure of epicardial ablation lesions. Furthermore, epicardial fat more than 5 mm in thickness alters the amplitude/duration of the recorded electrogram, making it difficult to differentiate fat from scar. The fat layer also alters the ventricular stimulation threshold, which can further affect one's ability to differentiate epicardial fat from true scar.[27]

TECHNIQUES IN DEVELOPMENT

Pressure-Frequency Sensing Needle

At present, access to the pericardial space is done blindly, which can lead to certain complications as outlined later in this article. Because the pericardial space is not visible under fluoroscopy, it is difficult to distinguish whether the needle is in the thoracic cavity, the pericardial space, or the ventricles. The mean pressures in the thorax and the pericardial space are the same. Hence, a pressure sensing needle would not differentiate between the two; however, the parietal pericardium moves at a frequency close to the respiratory rate, and the visceral pericardium moves at a frequency of that of the heart rate. Mahapatra and colleagues[28] have designed, built, and tested an early prototype of an epicardial needle that connects to a computer via a pressure transducer and displays the changes of pressure and frequency during pericardial access. Such a needle may provide additional information and assist the operator in localizing the tip of the needle, thereby reducing the complications inherent in obtaining epicardial access.

Table 1
Major complications associated with epicardial procedures

Complication	Mechanism of Injury	Possible Precautions	Treatment
Intra-abdominal bleeding[6]	Diaphragmatic vessel rupture	Needle tip localization by contrast injection	Blood transfusion, laparotomy
Gastroparesis[33]	Damage to the esophageal plexus of the vagus nerve	Real-time esophageal position and esophageal temperature monitoring	Motility-enhancing drugs, endoscopic botulinum injection, pyloric endoscopic dilatation, surgery
Diaphragmatic paralysis[34,35,a]	Phrenic nerve injury	Phrenic nerve mapping, controlled progressive balloon inflation (air and saline filled) of the pericardium[36–38]	Bronchodilators, conservative treatment for mild symptoms
Coronary occlusion[6]	Ablation-induced injury to the coronary arteries	Concomitant coronary angiography, monitoring endocardial ventricular potential[39]	Medical or surgical intervention
Elevated defibrillation threshold[40]	Residual air in the pericardial space	Removal of air after procedure	Lateral placement of sternal defibrillation pad
Cardiac tamponade and perforation	Puncture of the right ventricle	Injecting contrast to localize the needle[27]; using pressure sensing needles for access[28]	Emergent pericardiocentesis or a pericardial window

[a] Diaphragmatic paralysis has not been reported in epicardial procedures.

Intrapericardial Echocardiography

The feasibility of an intrapericardial echocardiography in patients undergoing epicardial ablation was recently evaluated by Horowitz and colleagues.[29] After obtaining epicardial access, 2 sheaths (8F and 10.5F) were introduced into the pericardial space. A 10F intracardiac echocardiography catheter was then introduced into the pericardial space via the 10.5F sheath, and imaging performed at a setting of either 6 or 7 MHz. It was possible to localize endocardial and epicardial catheters without the need for fluoroscopy.

Fiberoptic Endoscopy

Nazarian and colleagues[30] have reported on the feasibility of fiberoptic endoscopy for direct visualization within the pericardial space. After accessing the pericardial space, 2 large bore sheaths (14F and 18F) are introduced. A flexible endoscope is advanced through the 18F sheath under endoscopic and fluoroscopic guidance. The endoscope is retroflexed to identify the distal end of the 14F sheath through which epicardial mapping and ablation catheters are introduced under endoscopic guidance. Endocardial electrophysiology catheters are placed in the coronary sinus and the pulmonary veins. These endocardial catheters are then used as fluoroscopic markers to confirm the location of the endoscope. Air is insufflated through the endoscope for better visualization of the target sites. If visualization is poor despite air insufflation, an inflatable balloon is inserted through the remaining 14F sheath, positioned next to the target site, and expanded with saline; this improves the ability to visualize pericardial structures. The major coronary vessels, coronary sinus, left atrial appendage, lateral aspect of all pulmonary veins, and right ventricular outflow tract were well visualized using this procedure. Ablation of targeted sites was then achieved under endoscopic guidance. Direct visual identification of pericardial structures might enhance the safety of the procedure and reduce fluoroscopy and procedure times.

Transesophageal Epicardial Access

Sumiyama and colleagues[31] have evaluated the feasibility of accessing the epicardium via the esophagus during gastrointestinal endoscopy. This method is known as the submucosal endoscopy with mucosal flap safety valve (SEMF) technique, and belongs within the emerging field of natural orifice transluminal endoscopic surgery. In this procedure, gastrointestinal endoscopy is performed under mechanically ventilated general anesthesia. Esophageal lavage is performed with povidone-iodine solution. A saline bleb is created 15 cm proximal to the gastroesophageal junction to confirm access to the submucosa. Subsequently, a burst of high-pressure CO_2 is insufflated through the injection needle. A 10-cm long submucosal tunnel is created in the distal esophagus. A few milliliters of methylcellulose compound are injected to act as a sealant to prevent CO_2 leakage. Using the injection needle and a balloon dilator, the muscularis layer of the submucosal tunnel is separated. The gastroscope is then inserted into the posterior mediastinum through myotomy. The endoscope is then retroflexed at the level of esophageal entry, and the pleura opened and entered with the scope. Pericardial puncture is done after visual identification of the heart. Subsequently, a 3-cm pericardial window is made with a needle knife and the pericardial space is accessed. On completion, the pleura and submucosa are decompressed, and the submucosal entry site is closed with mucosal clips. This SEMF technique promises to be an alternative method for accessing the epicardial space, and could find potential uses when transcutaneous access is not feasible or contraindicated.

COMPLICATIONS

Both major and minor complications can ensue from epicardial procedures (**Table 1**). Notable major complications include hemopericardium, which is observed in up to 30% of cases, with the amount of blood drained from the pericardial space ranging from 20 to 300 mL. "Dry" puncture of right ventricle is observed in 10% to 20% of patients. Coronary arterial injury occurs in less than 1% of patients. Routine coronary angiography is performed before the delivery of lesions, especially when the target sites are located along the base of the heart (see **Fig. 3**). Minor complications involve transient chest discomfort from procedural related pericarditis; this can be prevented with intrapericardial instillation of anti-inflammatory or steroid medications, or treated with oral formulations of the same medications.[27,32]

SUMMARY

Epicardial mapping and ablation through percutaneous access to the pericardial space has emerged as an important therapeutic modality for patients with supraventricular and ventricular arrhythmias. This technique has opened a new window of opportunity for the successful management of some of these arrhythmias. Anatomic,

procedural, and technological limitations exist, which need to be addressed with continued clinical investigation and research.

REFERENCES

1. Sosa E, Scanavacca M, D'Avila A, et al. Endocardial and epicardial ablation guided by nonsurgical transthoracic epicardial mapping to treat recurrent ventricular tachycardia. J Cardiovasc Electrophysiol 1998;9(3):229–39.
2. Kaltenbrunner W, Cardinal R, Dubuc M, et al. Epicardial and endocardial mapping of ventricular tachycardia in patients with myocardial infarction. Is the origin of the tachycardia always subendocardially localized? Circulation 1991;84(3):1058–71.
3. Svenson RH, Littmann L, Gallagher JJ, et al. Termination of ventricular tachycardia with epicardial laser photocoagulation: a clinical comparison with patients undergoing successful endocardial photocoagulation alone. J Am Coll Cardiol 1990;15(1):163–70 [see comment].
4. D'Avila A, Scanavacca M, Sosa E, et al. Pericardial anatomy for the interventional electrophysiologist. J Cardiovasc Electrophysiol 2003;14(4):422–30.
5. Sosa E, Scanavacca M, d'Avila A, et al. A new technique to perform epicardial mapping in the electrophysiology laboratory. J Cardiovasc Electrophysiol 1996;7(6):531–6.
6. Sosa E, Scanavacca M. Epicardial mapping and ablation techniques to control ventricular tachycardia. J Cardiovasc Electrophysiol 2005;16(4):449–52.
7. Kilpatrick ZM, Chapman CB. On pericardiocentesis. Am J Cardiol 1965;16(5):722–8.
8. Shivkumar K. Percutaneous epicardial ablation of atrial fibrillation. Heart Rhythm 2008;5(1):152–4.
9. Anh DJ, Hsia HH, Reitz B, et al. Epicardial ablation of postinfarction ventricular tachycardia with an externally irrigated catheter in a patient with mechanical aortic and mitral valves. Heart Rhythm 2007;4(5):651–4.
10. Schweikert RA, Saliba WI, Tomassoni G, et al. Percutaneous pericardial instrumentation for endo-epicardial mapping of previously failed ablations. Circulation 2003;108(11):1329–35.
11. Sosa E, Scanavacca M, D'Avila A, et al. Radiofrequency catheter ablation of ventricular tachycardia guided by nonsurgical epicardial mapping in chronic Chagasic heart disease. Pacing Clin Electrophysiol 1999;22(1 Pt 1):128–30.
12. Koplan BA, Soejima K, Baughman K, et al. Refractory ventricular tachycardia secondary to cardiac sarcoid: electrophysiologic characteristics, mapping, and ablation. Heart Rhythm 2006;3(8):924–9.
13. Sosa E, Scanavacca M, D'Avila A, et al. Nonsurgical transthoracic epicardial catheter ablation to treat recurrent ventricular tachycardia occurring late after myocardial infarction. J Am Coll Cardiol 2000;35(6):1442–9.
14. Soejima K, Stevenson WG, Sapp JL, et al. Endocardial and epicardial radiofrequency ablation of ventricular tachycardia associated with dilated cardiomyopathy: the importance of low-voltage scars. J Am Coll Cardiol 2004;43(10):1834–42.
15. Garcia FC, Sussman JS, Bala R, et al. AB2-6: epicardial ablation to eliminate ventricular tachycardia associated with right ventricular cardiomyopathy: characterization of the substrate. Heart Rhythm 2006;3(5 Suppl 1):S4–5.
16. Phillips KP, Natale A, Sterba R, et al. Percutaneous pericardial instrumentation for catheter ablation of focal atrial tachycardias arising from the left atrial appendage. J Cardiovasc Electrophysiol 2008;19(4):430–3.
17. Pak HN, Hwang C, Lim HE, et al. Hybrid epicardial and endocardial ablation of persistent or permanent atrial fibrillation: a new approach for difficult cases. J Cardiovasc Electrophysiol 2007;18(9):917–23 [see comment].
18. Reddy VY, Neuzil P, D'Avila A, et al. Isolating the posterior left atrium and pulmonary veins with a "box" lesion set: use of epicardial ablation to complete electrical isolation. J Cardiovasc Electrophysiol 2008;19(3):326–9.
19. Scanavacca M, Pisani CF, Hachul D, et al. Selective atrial vagal denervation guided by evoked vagal reflex to treat patients with paroxysmal atrial fibrillation. Circulation 2006;114(9):876–85.
20. Brugada J, Berruezo A, Cuesta A, et al. Nonsurgical transthoracic epicardial radiofrequency ablation: an alternative in incessant ventricular tachycardia. J Am Coll Cardiol 2003;41(11):2036–43 [see comment].
21. Sosa E, Scanavacca M, D'Avila A, et al. Nonsurgical transthoracic epicardial approach in patients with ventricular tachycardia and previous cardiac surgery. J Interv Card Electrophysiol 2004;10(3):281–8.
22. Soejima K, Couper JM, Cooper JM, et al. Subxiphoid surgical approach for epicardial catheter-based mapping and ablation in patients with prior cardiac surgery or difficult pericardial access. Circulation 2004;110(10):1197–201.
23. Corradi D, Maestri R, Callegari S, et al. The ventricular epicardial fat is related to the myocardial mass in normal, ischemic and hypertrophic hearts. Cardiovasc Pathol 2004;13(6):313–6.
24. Rabkin SW. Epicardial fat: properties, function and relationship to obesity. Obes Rev 2007;8(3):253–61.
25. Schejbal V. [Epicardial fatty tissue of the right ventricle–morphology, morphometry and functional significance]. Pneumologie 1989;43(9):490–9 [in German].

26. Tansey DK, Aly Z, Sheppard MN. Fat in the right ventricle of the normal heart. Histopathology 2005; 46(1):98–104.
27. d'Avila A. Epicardial catheter ablation of ventricular tachycardia. Heart Rhythm 2008;5(6 Suppl 1):S73–5.
28. Mahapatra S, Jason Tucker-Schwartz M, Gillies GT, et al. Real-time analysis of needle tip pressure frequency allows for differentiation of pericardial from non-pericardial location during subxiphoid access for epicardial VT ablation. Heart Rhythm 2008;5(5S):124–5.
29. Horowitz BN, Vaseghi M, Mahajan A, et al. Percutaneous intrapericardial echocardiography during catheter ablation: a feasibility study. Heart Rhythm 2006;3(11):1275–82.
30. Nazarian S, Kantsevoy SV, Zviman MM, et al. Feasibility of endoscopic guidance for nonsurgical transthoracic atrial and ventricular epicardial ablation. Heart Rhythm 2008;5(8):1115–9.
31. Sumiyama K, Gostout CJ, Rajan E, et al. Pilot study of transesophageal endoscopic epicardial coagulation by submucosal endoscopy with the mucosal flap safety valve technique (with videos). Gastrointest Endosc 2008;67(3):497–501.
32. Sosa E, Scanavacca M, d'Avila A. Transthoracic epicardial catheter ablation to treat recurrent ventricular tachycardia. Curr Cardiol Rep 2001; 3(6):451–8.
33. Pisani CF, Hachul D, Sosa E, et al. Gastric hypomotility following epicardial vagal denervation ablation to treat atrial fibrillation. J Cardiovasc Electrophysiol 2008;19(2):211–3.
34. Rumbak MJ, Chokshi SK, Abel N, et al. Left phrenic nerve paresis complicating catheter radiofrequency ablation for Wolff-Parkinson-White syndrome. Am Heart J 1996;132(6):1281–5.
35. Sacher F, Monahan KH, Thomas SP, et al. Phrenic nerve injury after atrial fibrillation catheter ablation: characterization and outcome in a multicenter study. J Am Coll Cardiol 2006;47(12):2498–503.
36. Matsuo S, Jais P, Knecht S, et al. Images in cardiovascular medicine. Novel technique to prevent left phrenic nerve injury during epicardial catheter ablation. Circulation 2008;117(22):e471.
37. Di Biase L, Burkhardt JD, Perlargonio G, et al. Prevention of phrenic nerve injury during epicardial ablation: comparison of methods for separating the phrenic nerve from the epicardial surface. Heart Rhythm 2009;6(7):957–61.
38. Fan R, Cano O, Ho SY, et al. Characterization of the phrenic nerve course within the epicardial substrate of patients with nonischemic cardiomyopathy and ventricular tachycardia. Heart Rhythm 2009;6(1): 59–64.
39. Kawamura M, Kobayashi Y, Ito H, et al. Epicardial ablation with cooled tip catheter close to the coronary arteries is effective and safe in the porcine heart if the ventricular potential is being monitored in the epicardium and endocardium. Circ J 2006; 70(7):926–32.
40. Yamada T, McElderry HT, Platnov M, et al. Aspirated air in the pericardial space during epicardial catheterization may elevate the defibrillation threshold. Int J Cardiol 2009;135(1):e34–5.

Energy Sources for Ablation in the Pericardial Space

Kasturi K. Ghia, MD, David E. Haines, MD*

KEYWORDS

- Catheter ablation • Cardiac arrhythmias
- Epicardial ablation

Catheter ablation has been widely used for the management of cardiac arrhythmias. Transvenous endocardial catheter ablation has successfully eliminated or modified the critical substrate for most arrhythmias. Most arrhythmias can be eliminated with conventional endocardial mapping and radiofrequency energy delivery, but some critical arrhythmic substrates are not accessible endocardially. The experience with surgical ablation of scar-related ventricular tachycardia (VT) identified 23% of critical ablation sites as subepicardial rather than subendocardial in origin.[1] This led to epicardial mapping and ablation in addition to traditional endocardial mapping techniques. Other arrhythmias with subepicardial origin include many idiopathic left VTs, high-density premature ventricular complexes in which the focal site of origin is left ventricular, and some reentrant VTs in patients with nonischemic cardiomyopathy.[2] In addition, ablation of some arrhythmias such as atrial fibrillation may be accomplished more effectively with an epicardial approach. Because radiofrequency lesions are usually no deeper than 6 to 8 mm and do not penetrate scar well, it is difficult or impossible to ablate a subepicardial site from a subendocardial approach. Even if the endocardially delivered ablative lesion were extensive enough to incorporate the subepicardial target, a large volume of healthy subendocardial and midmyocardial tissue would need to be destroyed to reach the subepicardial sites. Thus, epicardial ablation is preferred in theses select cases.

The unique considerations required for epicardial ablation include catheter access to the epicardium and optimizing energy delivery. There are few vascular conduits to the epicardium and no easy access sites to the pericardial space. Catheterization of the coronary sinus can provide limited access to epicardial sites, but this is dependent on cardiac anatomy and is not useful when the site of origin is not close to the vessel. Once the ideal epicardial site has been mapped, conventional radiofrequency ablation may be ineffective. This article reviews current approaches to epicardial ablation and discusses the specialized tools that increase ablation efficacy and safety.

ENDOCARDIAL VERSUS EPICARDIAL ABLATION

Although the initial results have been promising, epicardial mapping and ablation pose a unique set of challenges. Specific anatomic targets can determine the type of ablation approach. The left ventricular surface is easily accessible for ablation of epicardial VT; however, sites along the septum and anterior portions of the right-sided pulmonary veins (PVs) are not accessible because of pericardial reflections of the oblique sinus. These sites are traditionally ablated from an endocardial approach. Epicardial ablation as an adjunctive treatment strategy to endocardial ablation for persistent atrial fibrillation has been reported with some early success.[3] Specific target sites in the left atrium such as the ligament of Marshall or the ridge between the left atrial (LA) appendage and superior PV may be challenging to ablate

Department of Cardiovascular Medicine, William Beaumont Hospital, Oakland University William Beaumont School of Medicine, 3601 West 13 Mile Road, Royal Oak, MI 48073, USA
* Corresponding author.
E-mail address: dhaines@beaumont.edu (D.E. Haines).

Card Electrophysiol Clin 2 (2010) 45–54
doi:10.1016/j.ccep.2009.11.011
1877-9182/10/$ – see front matter

from an endocardial approach but are more successful from an epicardial approach.

Whereas the endocardium is a uniform, muscular surface, the anatomy of the epicardium requires special consideration in catheter ablation. Epicardial fat is found in the coronary grooves and variably on the surface of the heart. It insulates the coronary arteries and myocardium from thermal damage during ablation. Older patients and obese patients (more commonly found in the population with heart disease) may have a greater quantity of epicardial fat. Epicardial fat thickness is variable and may interfere with catheter mapping. Saba and colleagues[4] measured left and right ventricular epicardial electrograms on 10 patients undergoing open heart surgery. Recordings were taken from regions of thick (>0.5 cm) and thin (<0.5 cm) epicardial fat. Electrogram amplitudes over thick fat with normal myocardium were found to measure less than 0.5 mV. This value traditionally represents scar; therefore, the presence of thick epicardial fat may mimic low-voltage scar. In addition, the presence of epicardial fat may lead to inaccurate activation times caused by recording of far-field signals. Reference values for endocardial substrate mapping exist; however, these reference values for epicardial electrogram voltage are currently being defined. Lower mapping resolution is sometimes met by use of ablation technologies that create larger lesions.

Coronary blood flow in epicardial coronary arteries results in a substantial heat-sink effect that helps protect the artery against injury but also makes it difficult to ablate contiguous tissue. Epicardial ablation over a perfused coronary artery has been studied in a rabbit model.[5] This study found that flow through small epicardial coronary arteries can prevent transmural lesion formation, arterial flow rate and vessel diameter were directly related to the volume of preserved myocardium, and high tissue temperatures (80°C) may overcome the protective effects of vascular perfusion.[5] The clinical implications of these findings are that the presence of epicardial arteries close to ablation targets can prevent lesion formation, resulting in incomplete ablation.

The most important feature differentiating endocardial from epicardial ablation is the presence of flowing blood and its associated convective cooling effects over the endocardium, and absence of this effect in the pericardial space (**Fig. 1**). With any hyperthermic ablation technology, a small volume of tissue is directly heated by the energy source. From this volume of heated tissue, the heat spreads to contiguous tissue by conduction. The combination of volume heating and conductive heating generates the temperature distribution through the tissue.[6] Heating the tissue to temperatures of 50°C or greater can induce irreversible thermal injury, thus destroying an arrhythmogenic focus.[7] The major factor opposing tissue heating of the endocardium during catheter ablation at any given fixed level of power delivery is convective cooling by the circulating blood pool. However, convective cooling also prevents excess heating at tissue surface, thereby preventing boiling of blood and charring of the tissue during radiofrequency ablation when temperatures exceed 100°C.[8] In turn, higher power can be delivered safely and, as a result, more volume heating and conductive heating occurs in deeper tissue layers. This heating translates directly into larger lesions. Because there is no circulating blood or fluid in the pericardial space, passive convective

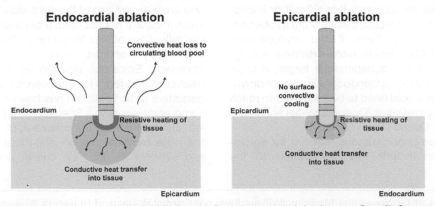

Fig. 1. Energy transfer during endocardial (*left panel*) and epicardial (*right panel*) radiofrequency ablation. During endocardial ablation, the convective heat loss to the circulating blood pool allows the operator to deliver high power, resulting in deep resistive and conductive heating. During epicardial ablation, absence of surface convective cooling results in rapid high surface temperatures and limits the amplitude of power that can be safely delivered, resulting in less resistive and conductive heating of the tissue, and a smaller lesion size.

cooling does not occur with epicardial ablation. The result is that high electrode-tissue interface temperatures are easily achieved, and power needs to be limited to avoid tissue charring. The lower power levels result in small lesions. Therefore, to achieve greater depths of tissue heating with epicardial radiofrequency ablation, cooled-tip catheters must be employed. Cooling can be achieved by either closed loop perfusion of the catheter tip or open loop irrigation. Both approaches allow the operator to deliver higher ablation power and create larger, more effective lesions. However, irrigated-tip catheters may pose an additional concern of fluid overload in the pericardial space that may compromise patient hemodynamics and result in pericardial tamponade. Specific differences between endocardial and epicardial ablation are outlined in **Table 1**.

ENERGY SOURCES FOR EPICARDIAL ABLATION

Radiofrequency Energy

Radiofrequency energy has been the primary energy source used in catheter ablation of cardiac arrhythmias. Radiofrequency energy is a form of alternating electrical current in which alternating current is transmitted through electrodes to cause hyperthermic ablation in myocardial tissue. The mechanism of heat generation is resistive heating; the current passes through tissue, which acts as a resistive medium, and as the voltage drops, heat is produced.[9] The resultant hyperthermic lesion is a result of the interplay between resistive volume heating, conductive heating, and convective cooling, as described earlier. The low electrical and thermal conductivity properties of fat make it a poor medium for resistive heating and subsequent heat conduction, which results in an inability of radiofrequency energy to penetrate the underlying myocardial tissue. Thus, epicardial fat acts as an insulator and limits the ability to ablate from some epicardial sites. High-amplitude power delivery using a cooled-tip catheter over regions of epicardial fat 2.6-mm thick created lesions similar in size to those generated by a standard catheter and low-amplitude power over regions without epicardial fat,[10] but smaller than high-powered cooled-tip lesions delivered directly to myocardium.

Radiofrequency energy can be delivered in unipolar or bipolar fashion for catheter ablation. Unipolar radiofrequency ablation focuses the current density at the catheter electrode-tissue interface; the energy is dispersed throughout the body and exits via a dispersive electrode applied to the patient's skin. This is the standard type of radiofrequency energy used for endocardial catheter ablation. Energy may be regulated by direct power control, or by temperature-feedback power control, in which power is automatically adjusted to maintain a preselected temperature measured within the electrode or at the electrode-tissue interface. If the ablation is power-limited, passive convective cooling from circulating blood with endocardial ablation, or active convective cooling with perfused tip catheters, decreases total energy delivery to the tissue and results in reduction of lesion size. However, if power can be increased to offset the energy dissipation by the circulating blood, then a greater depth of direct resistive heating is achieved and larger lesions are created. Irrigated or cooled-tip catheters increase lesion size by increasing the power that can be delivered. Because there is no circulating blood and no passive convective cooling in the pericardial space, the cooling effect on the surface of the

Table 1
Endocardial versus epicardial ablation

	Endocardial Ablation	Epicardial Ablation
Advantages	Minimally invasive Safe approach for most cardiac arrhythmias	Less effect of convective cooling from blood pool Possibility for failed endocardial ablations May allow direct visualization of epicardial structures
Disadvantages	Convective cooling from blood pool limits lesion size High risk of thermal injury to surrounding structures Inefficient lesion creation	Epicardial fat limits lesion size and mapping accuracy Risk of ablation over coronary arteries Access to epicardial structures may be limited Specific tools currently unavailable

tissue by irrigation serves to drive the focus of energy deeper into the tissue, providing deeper lesions. Standard radiofrequency energy delivery results in high-temperature, low-power lesions that are limited in size. Use of cooled-tip catheters significantly increases lesion size and ultimate efficacy of the ablative lesion.

Bipolar radiofrequency ablation is commonly used in surgical approaches to treat atrial arrhythmias. Bipolar radiofrequency ablation focuses energy between 2 closely spaced poles and can make discrete lesions rapidly. Direct contact with atrial tissue is required to maintain high current density and rapid resistive heating. Lall and colleagues[11] showed that bipolar energy application during the Cox-Maze procedure was equivalent to the traditional "cut and sew" technique, with similar outcomes at 12 months. The bipolar catheters currently available have impedance sensors to detect when transmural ablation has occurred. Because bipolar electrodes must be directly opposed to create adequate lesions, catheter flexibility and epicardial fat thickness may be limiting factors in epicardial lesion formation.[9] Bipolar clamps have been developed and used to isolate PVs during intraoperative ablation of atrial fibrillation. Clinical experience has shown that this design has limited maneuverability, and repeat ablation may be required to create continuous transmural lesions.[12]

A novel vacuum-stabilized saline-irrigated catheter has been developed to create epicardial lesions using unipolar radiofrequency energy. Tissue contact at the catheter tip is maintained by vacuum suction (−400 mm Hg). Normal saline is used to perfuse the electrode and tissue surface during vacuum stabilization and ablation. Radiofrequency energy is delivered to the tissue through an electrode coil measuring between 1 and 4 cm in length (**Fig. 2**). Conventional unipolar radiofrequency epicardial ablation fails to achieve significant lesion depth (or transmural lesions in atrial ablation) because surface heating limits power delivery. The perfused suction electrode achieves intimate electrode-tissue contact and bathes the ablation surface with saline to allow for high-power delivery to a large electrode. This delivery leads to lesions that are up to 8 mm deep, with lesion volumes significantly larger than those created by conventional irrigated catheters (**Fig. 3**).[13]

For clinical ablation, the perfused suction ablation device is introduced into the pericardial space by surgical port access without the need for a median sternotomy or cardiopulmonary bypass. Lesions are created with video-assisted guidance on a beating heart. Lesion continuity may be visualized by cardioscopy to avoid gaps in linear ablative lesions. This catheter has been employed clinically in the Ex-Maze procedure, an extracardiac biatrial ablation for atrial fibrillation treatment performed on the beating heart. The Ex-Maze epicardial lesion set approximates the surgical Cox-Maze III lesions with the supplementation of endocardial radiofrequency energy application in the PVs, coronary sinus, and cavotricuspid isthmus. The Ex-Maze procedure has been performed in a series of 54 patients with a predominance of persistent atrial fibrillation. Atrial fibrillation was noted in 48 patients at the time of the procedure. At a mean follow-up of 9 months, freedom from atrial fibrillation was noted in 88% of patients and sinus rhythm in 81% with

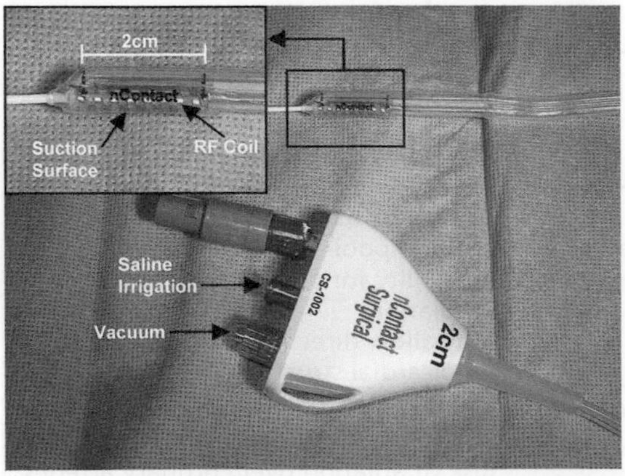

Fig. 2. A novel vacuum-stabilized saline-irrigated catheter designed for unipolar epicardial radiofrequency ablation. Inset: electrode coil with large surface area for tissue contact.

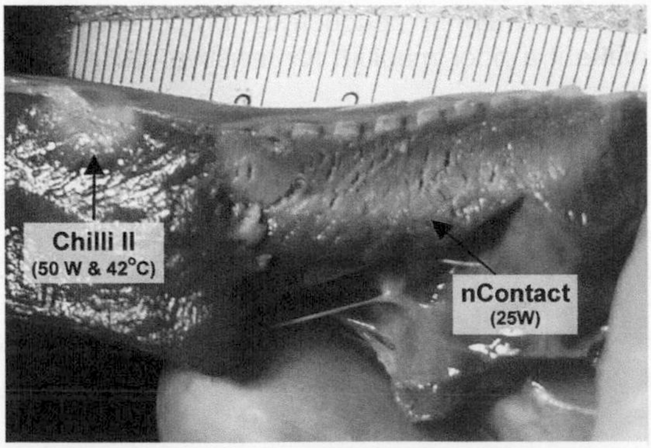

Fig. 3. Gross pathology sections of sheep myocardium after ablation in vitro. A lesion created with the vacuum-stabilized saline-irrigated catheter (nContact, Morrisville, NC, USA) is compared with a lesion created with a closed-irrigation 4-mm tip ablation catheter (Chilli II, Boston Scientific, Natick, MA, USA), and shows greater size and depth with low power delivery.

a single procedure.[14] Clinical experience with this catheter technology and hybrid endocardial-epicardial approach is growing, with promising initial outcomes. Experience with the clinical usefulness of the perfused suction ablation device for treatment of VT is growing, and this promising technology may evolve into a valuable treatment modality.

Microwave Energy

Electromagnetic waves radiated at a high frequency (915 or 2450 MHz) cause oscillation of water molecule dipoles within tissue, producing kinetic energy and heat generation. Microwave antenna ablation tools radially deliver the electromagnetic waves into the surrounding cardiac tissue. The antenna design (monopolar or helical coil) and its harmonic tuning with the generator determine the efficiency of microwave energy transfer to tissue, and ultimately the efficacy of the ablation system. No specific antenna design has been universally adopted. The microwave energy field generated around the ablation catheter antenna can create myocardial lesions up to 8 mm in depth,[8,15] and can theoretically create deeper lesions than radiofrequency energy because of greater volume heating and propagation through blood.[7] Initial studies documented feasibility of endocardial microwave ablation with the advantage of energy penetration into tissue without direct tissue contact; microwave ablation could achieve heating into deeper layers of the subepicardium and enabled ablation in regions of complex anatomy.[16] One disadvantage of microwave energy is that the energy can be delivered despite thrombus formation at the tissue surface; this may increase the thromboembolic risks. The safety of a temperature-controlled microwave system was evaluated and large lesions without significant catheter overheating or thrombus formation were found.[17] Another disadvantage of endocardial microwave energy application is that the energy may be absorbed by surrounding cardiac structures, causing damage to nontargeted structures. This effect can be overcome with use of shielded probes. However, damage to coronary arteries remains a concern, and left main coronary injury by incorrect catheter position has been reported.[18] Epicardial microwave ablation can be performed using an open surgical or minimally invasive thoracoscopic approach. A joint approach between electrophysiologists and surgeons for treatment of VT has been described during an open surgical procedure for coronary revascularization.[19] During open heart surgery, an electroanatomic mapping system was used and electrophysiologic testing was performed to identify and ablate VT using microwave energy. The thorascopic approach for the treatment of paroxysmal atrial fibrillation ablation requires port access and dissection of the pericardial reflections to allow access for the microwave ablation tool (**Fig. 4**). Epicardial microwave ablation has shown some early success, but rates of recurrence have approximated that of endocardial radiofrequency ablation at 1 year after a single procedure.[20] Although microwave energy can produce transmural lesions, these lesions are often incomplete over regions of thick epicardial fat.[15] Microwave energy has been used for ablation of VT on a limited basis, but similar concerns about coronary arterial injury and control of power delivery will also exist with this application if its use is expanded.

Laser Energy

Electromagnetic energy radiated in the frequency range of light induces harmonic vibrations in water molecules that create kinetic energy and produce heat.[9] Laser systems consist of a lasing medium of solid, liquid, or gas contained in a chamber of reflecting surfaces. Electricity is used to raise the energy state of the lasing medium, and photons are released as the energy falls to the baseline state. The difference between the 2 energy states determines the photon wavelength. Ablation using laser energy is wavelength dependent. Short

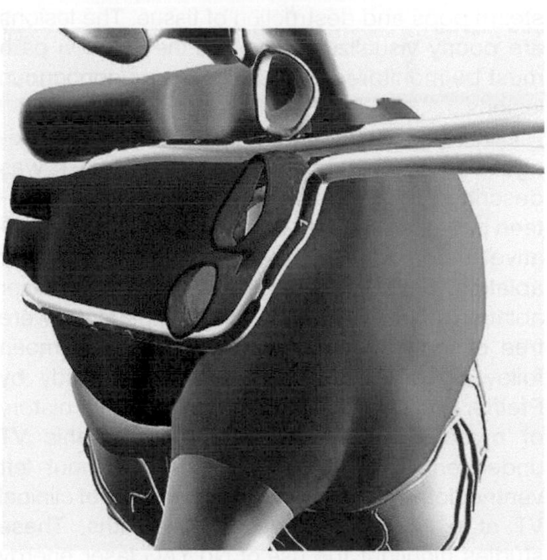

Fig. 4. The placement of a linear microwave ablation catheter designed for epicardial LA ablation. After dissection through the pericardial reflections superior and inferior to the right PVs, ablation devices can be carefully passed through the transverse sinus, around the left PVs, below the oblique sinus, and around the right PVs. Ablation along this line should result in electrical isolation of all PVs from the remainder of the atria.

wavelengths such as excimer (193 nm) have shallow skin depth and vaporize tissue with little or no deeper heating; energy is dissipated in the superficial layer of tissue. Longer wavelengths such as neodymium:yttrium-aluminum-garnet (Nd:YAG) (1064 nm) or solid state laser used in a laser balloon ablation system (980 nm) have greater depth of volume heating and allow for ablation of deeper substrates. Additional tissue injury occurs by conductive heating. Laser energy application can create transmural lesions from an epicardial approach, despite the presence of epicardial fat. In a study by Hong and colleagues[15] in vitro tissue models were used to compare the lesion characteristics of bipolar radiofrequency, microwave, and laser energy sources. Bipolar radiofrequency lesions were transmural in 83% of lesions without fat and in 0% of lesions with 2 mm of fat. Microwave lesions were transmural in tissue up to 5 mm in thickness without fat, and still capable of producing some transmural lesions in tissue with up to 2 mm of overlying fat. In comparison, laser energy was superior at producing transmural lesions in thick tissue (15 mm) with up to 4 mm of fat. In a canine model, epicardial laser ablation was performed by median sternotomy. Histology of the lesions showed large-volume transmural lesions without disruption of coronary vessels.[21] A disadvantage of laser ablation is its controllability. Laser ablation can create deep, uniform lesions, but excess heating can cause steam pops and destruction of tissue. The lesions are poorly visualized, therefore the ablation path must be monitored carefully to ensure contiguous lesions.

Clinical experience with Nd:YAG laser photocoagulation for intraoperative ablation of VT was described by Svenson and colleagues.[22] Seventeen patients with scar-based VT underwent operative mapping and endo- or epicardial laser ablation. Seven patients required epicardial laser ablation of the VT focus, and 13 patients were free of inducible or spontaneous VT at a mean follow-up of 11.8 months. In another study by Pfeiffer and colleagues,[23] 9 patients with a history of myocardial infarction and monomorphic VT underwent epicardial laser ablation without left ventriculotomy. Seven patients were free of clinical VT at a mean follow-up of 17 months. These studies highlight the use of Nd:YAG laser energy for deep tissue coagulation in epicardial applications. D'Avila and colleagues[24] showed that the optical properties of scar in Chagas disease differ from infarcted myocardium in that the fibrosis is less densely organized and can favorably scatter light, making it a suitable substrate for laser ablation. Nd:YAG laser ablation was seen to penetrate scarred Chagas myocardium, thus creating transmural endocardial lesions for treatment of an epicardial circuit.

Laser energy has been used in the treatment of atrial fibrillation for endocardial isolation of PVs. A balloon ablation catheter equipped with an endoscope allows direct visualization of the left atrium/PV junction. The catheter is delivered to the left atrium through a deflectable 15-Fr sheath; a fluid-filled balloon of maximum diameter 20 mm, 25 mm, or 30 mm is then inflated. An optical fiber within the balloon can then deliver an arc of ablative laser energy to the tissue visualized on the face of the balloon. In a multicenter clinical study, visually guided PV isolation with laser was technically feasible and clinically effective in patients with paroxysmal atrial fibrillation.[25] Laser energy has been extended to epicardial ablation of atrial fibrillation and has been described in animal models and small series of clinical experiences. Histologic examination of lesions from laser ablation in a canine model showed transmural lesions with preservation of atrial tissue at the lesion border and intact myocardium in the region of coronary vessels.[26]

Ultrasound Energy

Ultrasound produces mechanical heating through transmission of ultrasound waves through tissue. As the ultrasound wave disperses through tissue, harmonic oscillation of water generates thermal energy. With high-intensity focused ultrasound (HIFU), energy is highly concentrated and focused at a certain depth; HIFU can deliver enough energy to generate significant tissue heating and produce transmural lesions. Phased-array HIFU systems are composed of multiple ultrasound elements that are electronically focused (**Fig. 5**). Lesion depths up to 15 mm can be created. Ultrasound balloon delivery systems are being clinically evaluated for use in atrial endocardial ablation of PVs. An advantage of HIFU is that creation of transmural lesions is unimpeded by the presence of epicardial fat or the convective cooling of blood flow. A significant disadvantage of endocardial ablation with HIFU is that unfocused energy emanating from the transducer may still penetrate beyond the atrial or PV wall, causing unintentional damage to surrounding structures.

The multi-element phased-array system has been developed to deliver HIFU energy to ablate epicardial tissue. In the application of atrial fibrillation, this system produces transmural, circumferential LA lesions around the PVs. The transducers are positioned on the epicardium but are separated from direct tissue contact by

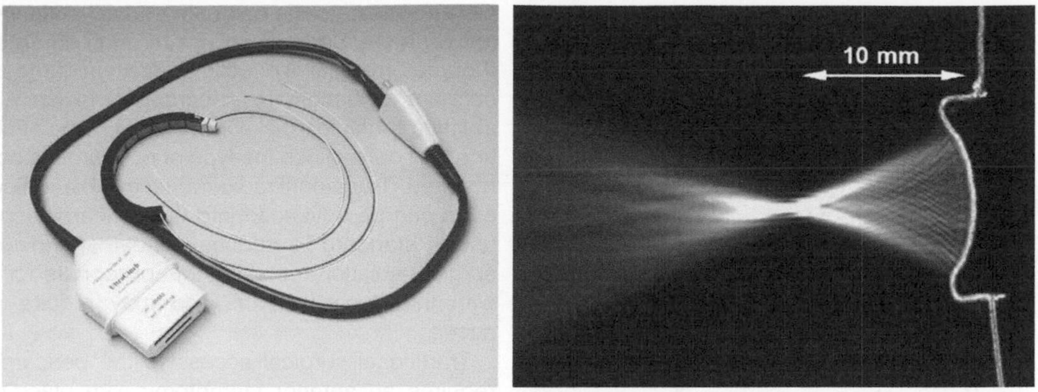

Fig. 5. A multiarray HIFU device for epicardial ablation of the posterior left atrium is shown in the left panel. The right panel shows the pattern of focused ultrasound energy originating from a concave transducer and visualized through a Schlieren effect (fluid-phase laser illumination to visualize the ultrasonic beam). The beam converges at the focal distance and dissipates beyond that point. The focal distance is fixed and determined only by the radius of the curvature of the transducer. (*From* Ninet J, Roques X, Seitelberger R, et al. Surgical ablation of atrial fibrillation with off-pump, epicardial, high-intensity focused ultrasound: results of a multicenter trial, J Thorac Cardiovasc Surg 2005;130:803–9; with permission.)

a perforated membrane. Saline is circulated between the membrane and the transducers during ablation to enhance acoustic coupling and surface cooling. The transducers are designed to deliver HIFU energy up to a distance of 10 mm. Beyond the focal point, energy dissipates within the blood pool without exposing surrounding structures to potential injury. In epicardial application, Mitnovetski and colleagues[27] showed that epicardial HIFU ablation was a safe and feasible alternative to the traditional Cox-Maze procedure for atrial fibrillation without risk of collateral damage. In addition, dissection of epicardial fat was not necessary as lesions created with HIFU were able to penetrate fat. Groh and colleagues[28] described epicardial HIFU ablation for atrial fibrillation on a beating heart in patients with ischemic heart disease undergoing concurrent coronary bypass surgery. There was a low incidence of postoperative atrial fibrillation, with freedom from arrhythmia of 84% at 6 months. HIFU has not been described as a modality used in epicardial ablation of VT, but theoretically, it should be well suited to this purpose.

Cryothermic Ablation

Cryoablation is an alternative energy source that was used commonly for surgical ablation. Cryoablation employs argon or helium delivered under high pressure to achieve temperatures of −55 to −90°C at the catheter tip. After the tissue is cooled for 2 minutes, the result is a discrete line of frozen tissue. During the freezing phase, intracellular and extracellular ice crystals form. Inflammation and fibrosis occur in the following hours or days. Transmural lesions are formed with preservation of the cellular architecture, and the integrity of adjacent tissue is not affected. Lesion size is affected by probe temperature and size and the duration and number of freeze cycles. Lower temperatures can generate larger lesions and repetitive cycles deepen lesions into the myocardium.

Cryoablation is approved by the US Food and Drug Administration to treat arrhythmias; it has several advantages and disadvantages. Cryoablation creates well-demarcated lesions and causes less structural damage to adjacent tissues, the catheter adheres to the tissue once ice forms, and transmural lesions can be created and monitored visually. Epicardial cryoenergy application has been shown in animal models to create similar lesions to an irrigated-tip radiofrequency energy catheter.[29,30] Lesions delivered over epicardial fat and coronary vessels showed a smaller depth and volume.[29] Epicardial cryoablation may not be practical because of the warming effect of endocardial blood flow. In addition, the cryoablation probes are rigid and their larger size may limit use in a minimally invasive approach. Cryoenergy is believed to have a lower risk of coronary artery injury than radiofrequency energy; however, there are reported cases of coronary stenosis.[31] Cryoenergy remains an alternative energy source for ablation during concomitant cardiac surgery.

PERICARDIAL ACCESS FOR NEW ABLATION TOOLS

The human heart has a visceral and parietal pericardial layer. The pericardial reflections form the

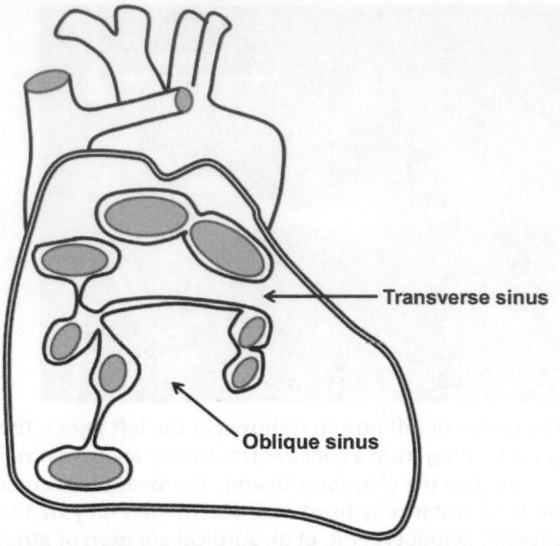

Fig. 6. Pericardial recesses and sinuses. The transverse sinus and oblique sinus are separated by pericardial reflections. The pulmonic vein recesses lie between the superior and inferior PVs. Pericardial reflections prevent free movement of ablation devices throughout the pericardial space, and dissection is required to complete an encircling PV lesion for atrial fibrillation ablation.

transverse and oblique sinuses (**Fig. 6**). The transverse sinus allows access to the epicardium between the great vessels. The oblique sinus allows access to the posterior LA wall and inferior left ventricle. Surgical access through an anterior thoracotomy allows direct visualization of the pericardium for access to epicardial surfaces. When ablating the epicardial surface, the choice of ablation tool determines the type of pericardial access required. Traditional radiofrequency ablation catheters can be advanced into the pericardial space using standard introducer sheaths; however, surgical ablation tools are not appropriate for use with introducer sheaths and may require port access.

Traditional surgical access to the pericardium requires an anterior sternotomy with placement of a left-sided chest tube and decompression of the lung for visualization and manipulation of cardiac structures. Subxyphoid video pericardioscopy is a minimally invasive approach for epicardial mapping that allows direct visualization of the left ventricular epicardium.[32,33] A 1.5-cm subxyphoid incision is made, and the tissue is dissected down to the pericardial level. A small (0.5 cm) pericardiotomy is performed under direct visualization. The subxyphoid video pericardioscopy device consists of a 7-mm extended length endoscope with 2 proximal entry service ports. The endoscope is inserted into the pericardial cavity and the anterior left ventricle is easily visualized for mapping and ablation.

Table 2
Energy sources for epicardial ablation

Energy Source	Frequency or Wavelength	Mechanism of Heating	Tissue Contact Needed	Advantages	Disadvantages
Radiofrequency	300–700 kHz	Resistive	Yes	Safe	Limited lesion size, unable to penetrate epicardial fat
Microwave	915–450 kHz	Dielectric	No	Penetrates scar and fat, creates large lesions	Complex catheter design
Laser	300–2000 nm	Photon absorption	No	Large lesions, penetrates fat	Difficulty controlling depth
Ultrasound	500 kHz to 20 MHz	Mechanical	No	Large lesions, penetrates fat, focal length of ablation is adjustable	Difficulty controlling depth
Cryothermal	−50 to −90°C	Freeze/thaw	Yes	Safe, stable tissue contact, reversibility of cryomapping	Rigid catheter design

A subxyphoid surgical approach to access the pericardial space in the electrophysiology laboratory was described by Soejima and colleagues.[34] They evaluated the feasibility of epicardial mapping and ablation in patients with failed percutaneous epicardial access or prior cardiac surgery. Under general anesthesia, a 7.5 cm (3-in) vertical incision was made in the midline epigastrium. The abdominal fascia was opened in the linea alba. The pericardium was exposed and opened horizontally, parallel to the diaphragmatic reflection. The pericardiotomy was extended to the patient's left to improve visualization of the ventricles. Adhesions were manually lysed to allow insertion of an 8-F sheath into the pericardial space. After ablation, the pericardial sheath was removed, the surgical incision was closed, and a Jackson-Pratt drain was left in the pericardial space overnight and removed the next morning, if there was no active drainage.

Percutaneous epicardial mapping and ablation was initially described by Sosa and colleagues[35] They successfully performed epicardial mapping and ablation in the pericardial space for the treatment of VTs.[1,35] Subsequently, epicardial catheter ablation has been employed in the treatment of atrial arrhythmias.[2] Percutaneous access to the pericardial space can be obtained through the subxyphoid approach, as described elsewhere is this issue.[35] With conventional dilators and vascular access sheaths, introducer sheaths for devices up to 18 Fr can be advanced over a wire into the pericardium. Care must be taken to use a stiff introducer wire, to upsize the dilators gradually, and to avoid forcing the introducer into the pericardium, because right ventricular or coronary arterial laceration is a possible complication of insertion of a large, stiff sheath.

SUMMARY

Advances in energy sources for ablation in the pericardial space will likely have great impact on management of cardiac arrhythmias (**Table 2**). Surgical tools provide direct visualization of epicardial structures; however, these techniques often require a more invasive approach, such as median sternotomy or thoracotomy. Electrophysiologists working in the pericardial space have to rely on fluoroscopic anatomy, intracardiac echocardiography, and electroanatomic mapping systems. At present, electrophysiologists have few dedicated tools for direct visualization or safe and effective energy delivery in the pericardial space. New delivery systems for time-tested energy sources will allow effective epicardial ablation for atrial fibrillation and ventricular arrhythmias with epicardial sites of origin. Hybrid procedures using an endocardial and epicardial ablation strategy may lead to improved clinical outcomes.

REFERENCES

1. Sosa E, Scanavacca M, D'Avila A, et al. Nonsurgical transthoracic epicardial catheter ablation to treat recurrent ventricular tachycardia occurring late after myocardial infarction. J Am Coll Cardiol 2000;35:1442–9.
2. Schweikert RA, Saliba WA, Tomassoni G, et al. Percutaneous pericardial instrumentation for endo-epicardial mapping of previously failed ablations. Circulation 2003;108:1329–35.
3. Pak HN, Hwang C, Lim HE, et al. Hybrid epicardial and endocardial ablation of persistent or permanent a trial fibrillation: a new approach for difficult cases. J Cardiovasc Electrophysiol 2007;18:917–23.
4. Saba MM, Akella J, Gammie J, et al. The influence of fat thickness on the human epicardial bipolar electrogram characteristics: measurements on patients undergoing open-heart surgery. Europace 2009; 11(7):949–53.
5. Fuller IA, Wood MA. Intramural coronary vasculature prevents trans-mural radio frequency lesion formation: implications for linear ablation. Circulation 2003;107:1797–803.
6. Haines DE, Watson DD. Tissue heating during radio frequency catheter ablation: a thermodynamic model and observations in isolated perfused and superfused canine right ventricular free wall. Pacing Clin Electrophysiol 1989;12:962–76.
7. Whayne JG, Nath S, Haines DE. Microwave catheter ablation of myocardium in vitro: assessment of the characteristics of tissue heating and injury. Circulation 1994;89:2390–5.
8. Haines DE, Verow AF. Observations on electrode-tissue interface temperature and effect on electrical impedance during radiofrequency ablation of ventricular myocardium. Circulation 1990;82:1034–8.
9. Williams MR, Garrido M, Oz MC, et al. Alternative energy sources for surgical a trial ablation. J Cardiovasc Surg 2004;19:201–6.
10. d'Avila A, Houghtaling C, Gutierrez P, et al. Catheter ablation of ventricular epicardial tissue: a comparison of standard and cooled-tip radio frequency energy. Circulation 2004;109:2363–9.
11. Lall SC, Melby SJ, Voeller RK. The effect of ablation technology on surgical outcomes after the Cox-maze procedure: a propensity analysis. J Thorac Cardiovasc Surg 2007;133(2):389–96.
12. Gillinov AM, McCarth PM. Atricure bipolar radio frequency clamp for intra-operative ablation of a trial fibrillation. Ann Thorac Surg 2002;74(6):2165–8.
13. Nori DN, Evonich RF, Ghia KK, et al. Acute lesion characteristics of a novel vacuum stabilized,

irrigated, epicardial radio frequency ablation probe [abstract]. Heart Rhythm 2007;4(5):S341.
14. Kiser AC, Wimmer-Greinecker G, Kapelak B. Achieving metrics during beating-heart ex-maze procedures improves outcomes. Heart Surg Forum 2008;11(4):E237–42.
15. Hong KN, Russo MJ, Liberman EA, et al. Effect of epicardial fat on ablation performance: a three-energy source comparison. J Cardiovasc Surg 2007;22(6):521–4.
16. Chan JY, Fung JW, Yu CM, et al. Preliminary results with percutaneous trans-catheter microwave ablation of typical a trial flutter. J Cardiovasc Electrophysiol 2007;18(3):286–9.
17. VanderBrink BA, Gilbride C, Aronovitz MJ, et al. Safety and efficacy of a steerable temperature monitoring microwave catheter system for ventricular myocardial ablation. J Cardiovasc Electrophysiol 2000;11(3):305–10.
18. Manasee E, Medici D, Ghiselli S, et al. Left main coronary arterial lesion after microwave epicardial ablation. Ann Thorac Surg 2003;76:276–7.
19. Braun MU, Knaut M, Rauwolf T, et al. Microwave ablation of an ischemic sustained ventricular tachycardia during aortocoronary bypass, mitral valve and tricuspid valve surgery guided by a three-dimensional non-fluoroscopic mapping system (CARTO). J Interv Card Electrophysiol 2005;13(3):243–7.
20. Salenger R, Lahey SJ, Saltman AE. The completely endoscopic treatment of a trial fibrillation: report on the first 14 patients with early results. Heart Surg Forum 2004;7(6):E555–8.
21. Weber HP, Heinze A, Enders S, et al. Laser catheter coagulation of normal and scarred ventricular myocardium in dogs. Lasers Surg Med 1998;22(2): 109–19.
22. Svenson RH, Gallagher JJ, Selle JG, et al. Neodymium:YAG laser photocoagulation: A successful new map-guided technique for the intra-operative ablation of ventricular tachycardia. Circulation 1987;76(6):1319–28.
23. Pfeiffer D, Moosdorf R, Svenson RH, et al. Epicardial neodymium: YAG laser photocoagulation of ventricular tachycardia without ventriculotomy in patients after myocardial infarction. Circulation 1996;94:3221–5.
24. d'Avila A, Splinter R, Svenson RH, et al. New perspectives on catheter-based ablation of ventricular tachycardia complicating Chagas' disease: experimental evidence of the efficacy of near infrared lasers for catheter ablation of Chagas' VT. J Interv Card Electrophysiol 2002;7(1):23–38.
25. Reddy VY, Neuzil P, Themistoclakis S, et al. Visually-guided balloon catheter ablation of atrial fibrillation: experimental feasibility and first-in-human multi-center clinical outcome. Circulation 2009;120:12–20.
26. Williams MR, Casher JM, Russo MJ, et al. Laser energy source in surgical atrial fibrillation ablation: preclinical experience. Ann Thorac Surg 2006;82: 2260–4.
27. Mitnovetski S, Almeida AA, Goldstein J, et al. Epicardial high-intensity focused ultrasound cardiac ablation for surgical treatment of atrial fibrillation. Heart Lung Circ 2009;18(1):28–31.
28. Groh MA, Binns OA, Burton HG 3rd, et al. Epicardial ultrasonic ablation of atrial fibrillation during concomitant cardiac surgery is a valid option in patients with ischemic heart disease. Circulation 2008;118(Suppl 14):S78–82.
29. Hashimoto K, Watanabe I, Okumura Y, et al. Comparison of endocardial and epicardial lesion size following large-tip and extra-large-tip trans-catheter cryoablation. J Circ 2009;73:1619–26.
30. d'Avila A, Gutierrez P, Scanavacca M, et al. Effects of radio frequency pulses delivered in the vicinity of the coronary arteries: implications for non-surgical trans-thoracic epicardial catheter ablation to treat ventricular tachycardia. Pacing Clin Electrophysiol 2002;25:1488–95.
31. Roberts-Thomson KC, Steven D, Seiler J, et al. Coronary artery injury due to catheter ablation in adults: presentation and outcomes. Circulation 2009;120: 1465–73.
32. Zenati MA, Bonanomi G, Chin AK, et al. Left heart pacing lead implantation using subxiphoid video-pericardioscopy. J Cardiovasc Electrophysiol 2003; 14:949–53.
33. Zenati MA, Shalaby A, Eisenman G, et al. Epicardial left ventricular mapping using subxyphoid video pericardioscopy. Ann Thorac Surg 2007;84:2106–7.
34. Soejima K, Couper G, Cooper JM, et al. Subxyphoid surgical approach for epicardial catheter-based mapping and ablation in patients with prior cardiac surgery or difficult pericardial access. Circulation 2004;110:1197–201.
35. Sosa E, Scanavacca M, D'Avila A, et al. A new technique to perform epicardial mapping in the electrophysiology laboratory. J Cardiovasc Electrophysiol 1996;7:531–6.

Epicardial Ablation of Ventricular Tachycardia in Chagas Heart Disease

Mauricio Scanavacca, MD, PhD*, Eduardo Sosa, MD, PhD

KEYWORDS

- Catheter ablation • Chagas heart disease
- Epicardial ablation • Ventricular tachycardia

American trypanozomiasis was first described 100 years ago by Carlos Chagas, a Brazilian physician, who did a comprehensive study of the disease. In a short period of 2 years he recognized the parasite, identified the vector, described the biologic cycle of the infection, and confirmed these findings by reproducing the disease in animals.[1,2] He subsequently described the clinical characteristics of each phase of human infection with trypanozomiasis.[2,3]

Chagas disease, caused by a flagellate protozoan parasite named *Trypanosoma cruzi* by Carlos Chagas, in honor to his mentor Osvaldo Cruz, is transmitted to humans in most cases through the feces of infected bloodsucking insects in endemic areas of Latin America. Other routes of infection are blood transfusion, congenital transmission, oral and accidental contamination, and by organ transplantation.[4] It is estimated that 75 to 90 million people are exposed to infection in Latin America; around 15 million are infected, causing 45,000 deaths per year, 90% by cardiac disease.[4,5] An important aspect for the disease diffusion in nonendemic countries is blood transfusion from contaminated immigrant blood donors.[6] In 2007, the Food and Drug Administration approved the Chagas disease ELISA test for all blood donor candidates in the United States to avoid diffusion of this disease.[7] In Latin America, governments have been working hard combating the vector and controlling blood transfusions. Vector transmission has been considered interrupted in Uruguay in 1997, in Chile in 1999, and in Brazil in 2006.[4] Despite the reduced *T cruzi* transmission in Latin America in recent years, however, it still is expected that many people will develop cardiac complications of the disease for a long period of time. After acute phase, 30% to 40% of contaminated people develop organ damage as late as 30 years.[8]

CLINICAL EVOLUTION AFTER INFECTION

The acute phase usually affects children or young adults in endemic areas. The mortality rate in this phase is around 5% because of acute myocarditis and meningoencephalitis. Benzonidazol, an antiparasitic drug, is effective treatment and usually cures those patients in this phase and prevents chronic manifestations of the disease.[8] If it is not treated, the acute phase resolves by itself within 4 to 8 weeks in approximately 90% of infected individuals. About 60% to 70% never develop symptoms. They can be recognized by serologic positive tests, but do not present any clinical or laboratorial manifestation of the disease.[9] Some affected individuals, however, develop cardiomyopathy, megaesophagus, megacolon, or a combination of these in 10 to 30 years after acute infection.[8–10]

The Cardiac Arrhythmia and Pacemaker Unit, The Heart Institute (INCOR) do Hospital das Clínicas da Faculdade de Medicina da Universidade de São Paulo, Av. Dr. Eneas de Carvalho Aguiar, 44, CEP: 05403-000, São Paulo, Brazil
* Corresponding author. Unidade Clínica de Arritmia e Marcapasso do Instituto do Coração da Faculdade de Medicina da Universidade de São Paulo, Av. Dr. Eneas de Carvalho Aguiar, 44, CEP: 05403-000, São Paulo, Brazil.
E-mail address: mauricio.scanavacca@incor.usp.br (M. Scanavacca).

Card Electrophysiol Clin 2 (2010) 55–67
doi:10.1016/j.ccep.2009.11.004
1877-9182/10/$ – see front matter

CHAGAS CARDIOMYOPATHY

Cardiac involvement is the most frequent and serious manifestation of chronic Chagas disease.[11] In acute phase, the myocardial fibers are invaded by the parasites, which replicate themselves in amastigote forms into pseudocysts, with small inflammatory response. The rupture of pseudocyst promotes intense lymphomononuclear inflammatory reaction. The chronic cardiac form is characterized by lymphomononuclear focal inflammatory process with progressive destruction of cardiac fibers and marked reactive and reparative fibrosis affecting multiple areas of the myocardium.[12] The pathogenesis of cardiac lesions appearing decades later after the initial infection is not completely understood. The failure of conventional histologic methods to find parasites in the myocardium led to the hypothesis that autoimmune responses are involved in the late clinical manifestations. Some studies have suggested involvement of cellular mechanisms, CD4 and CD8 T lymphocytes, along with macrophage activation and inflammatory cytokine mediators, which are also able to destroy nonparasitized myocardial cells increasing the myocardial damage.[13,14] Humoral immunity, expressed by a variety of antibodies against endothelium, vascular structures, and interstitium, has also been suggested to be implicated in the pathogenesis of Chagas myocarditis.[15,16] Using very sensitive immunohystochemical techniques, parasitic antigens have been found in the hearts of patients with Chagas disease.[17] In addition, an association between the presence of *T cruzi* and the intensity of the inflammatory process was observed, suggesting a direct participation of the parasite in the genesis of chronic myocarditis.[18] It is possible that even low-grade persistent parasitism behaves as a continuous antigenic stimulus and that both *T cruzi* inflammation and autoimmune response may play important roles in the pathogenesis of Chagas heart disease.

After infection, many patients remain asymptomatic throughout life; others develop multiple disturbances of rhythm, severe symptoms of heart failure, and thromboembolic phenomena. Focal myocardial fibrosis provides the anatomic substrate for ventricular arrhythmias and atrioventricular and intraventricular conduction disturbances; predisposes to cardiac dilatation; and leads to formation of ventricular aneurysms (**Fig. 1**).[19] An apical aneurysm is very common and a hallmark of Chagas heart disease. Thrombi are often present in the left ventricular aneurysm and in the atrial appendages that may explain the common occurrence of thromboembolic phenomena in the systemic and pulmonary circulation.[11] In general, sudden cardiac death is the main cause of death, occurring in 55% to 65% of patients, sometimes in the absence of previous cardiac symptoms. Death in consequence of congestive heart failure occurs in 25% to 30%, and for cerebral or pulmonary embolism in 10% to 15%.[8–12,19]

SUSTAINED VENTRICULAR TACHYCARDIA IN CHAGAS DISEASE

Ventricular arrhythmias are very common in patients with Chagas heart disease and the prevalence and complexity are related to the presence and extent of myocardial damage, particularly left ventricular dilatation.[20] Nonsustained ventricular tachycardia (VT) has been identified as an independent risk factor for death and included in a practical score for risk evaluation.[21] The prevalence of sustained VT in patients with Chagas disease is not well known, but it is considered the main cause of sudden death, inducing ventricular fibrillation.[22] It can occur in different functional phases of the disease, and even in patients without ventricular dysfunction. It can represent up to 50% of the patients with sustained VT attending tertiary centers.

TREATMENT OF SUSTAINED VT IN CHAGAS DISEASE

Amiodarone has been the most frequent drug prescribed in Latin America for patients with Chagas disease and ventricular arrhythmia. Implantable cardioverter defibrillators (ICDs) have been considered in patients with sustained VT and ventricular dysfunction. Radiofrequency (RF) ablation has been recommended for patients with recurrent VT, mainly for those receiving ICD shocks. Most Chagas disease patients probably receive a hybrid treatment combining all three strategies during their clinical evolution. The role of all these procedures in patients with Chagas disease, however, has still not been established by multicenter randomized studies. Clinical decisions have been made based on small cohort studies and data from multicenter studies involving nonchagasic patients. Some years ago the authors reported the evolution of 35 patients with Chagas disease and recurrent VTs, empirically treated with amiodarone, living in a metropolitan area and followed at a tertiary cardiovascular center.[23] It was observed that despite the high recurrence rate (50%) during follow-up, the annual mortality (5%) was low because many sustained VTs were well tolerated and sudden cardiac death

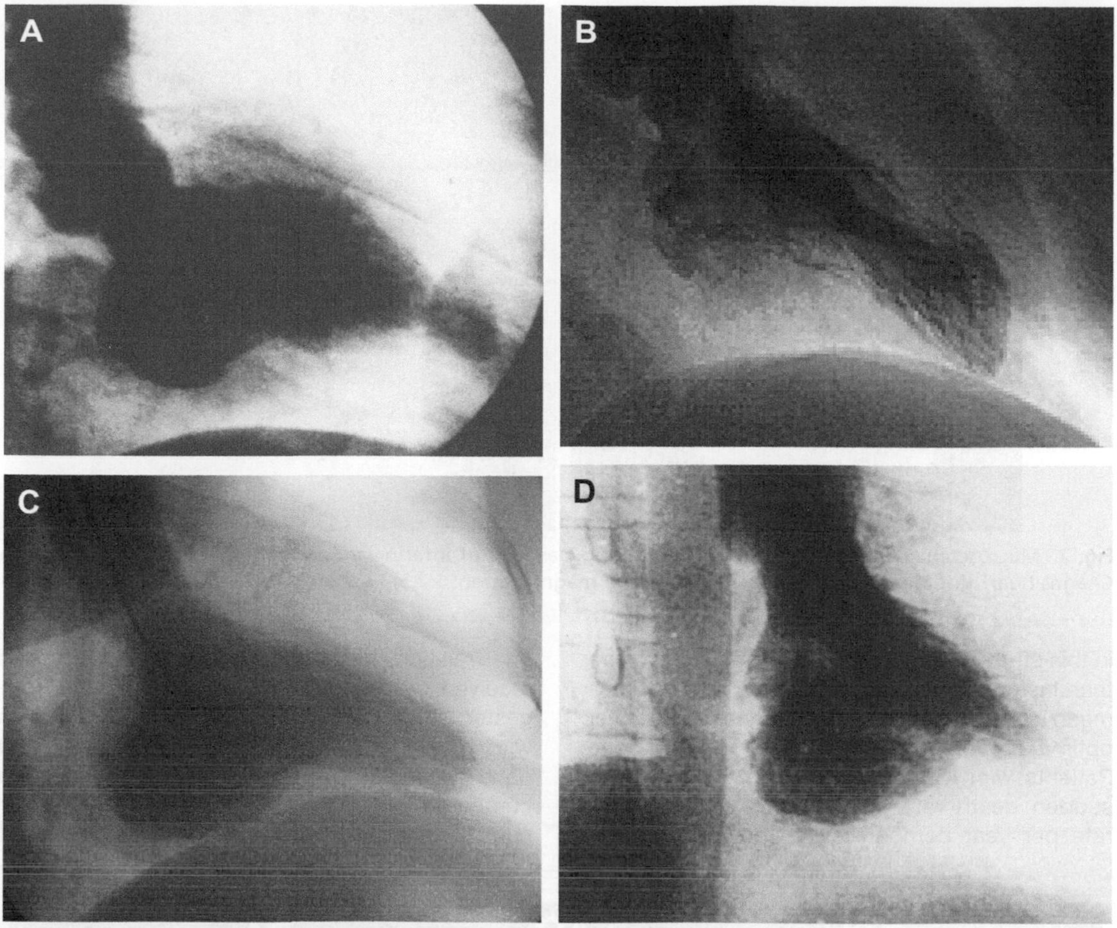

Fig. 1. Left ventricle angiographies of four different patients with Chagas heart disease and sustained ventricular tachycardia. (*A–C*) Combination of apical and inferior and lateral-basal aneurysms. (*D*) Isolated inferior aneurysm, which was the original site of sustained ventricular tachycardia in all cases.

occurred in few patients. It was also observed at that time that the most important variable related to VT recurrence and death was the degree of ventricular dysfunction. In patients with heart failure and functional class III or IV, 100% developed VT recurrence, 40% had sudden cardiac death, and there was 80% mortality in a mean follow-up of 27 months. In patients in functional class I or II, however, there was a 30% VT recurrence, with no mortality in the same period. Leite and colleagues[24] showed that electrophysiology (EP) testing can be useful to stratify patients with Chagas disease and sustained VT at higher risk for sudden death. Patients who had sustained VT inducible during the EP study and in whom class III antiarrhythmic drugs rendered VT not inducible or slower and well tolerated presented a lower probability of cardiac mortality and sudden death. Patients with positive EP test had a worse clinical evolution and significant higher probability of cardiac death, however, in most cases sudden. Other follow-up studies of patients with Chagas disease and sustained VT under antiarrhythmic drugs showed 10.7% to 11.9% annual mortality, with sudden death responsible for 61% to 78% of the cases.[25]

ICDs have been incorporated for the treatment of patients with Chagas disease in many areas in Latin America despite the economic problems. In a register study, Chagas disease was the second most common cause of ICD implantation from a specific company in seven countries of Latin America.[26] In this study, patients with Chagas disease received more ICD shocks within 6 months following the implantation than patients with coronary heart disease. The time course of VT recurrence was also different; most patients received a first shock in the first month after ICD implantation. This observation was confirmed by Cardinalli-Neto and colleagues,[27] who followed 90 patients with ICD implanted, with most patients also receiving amiodarone. An interesting aspect

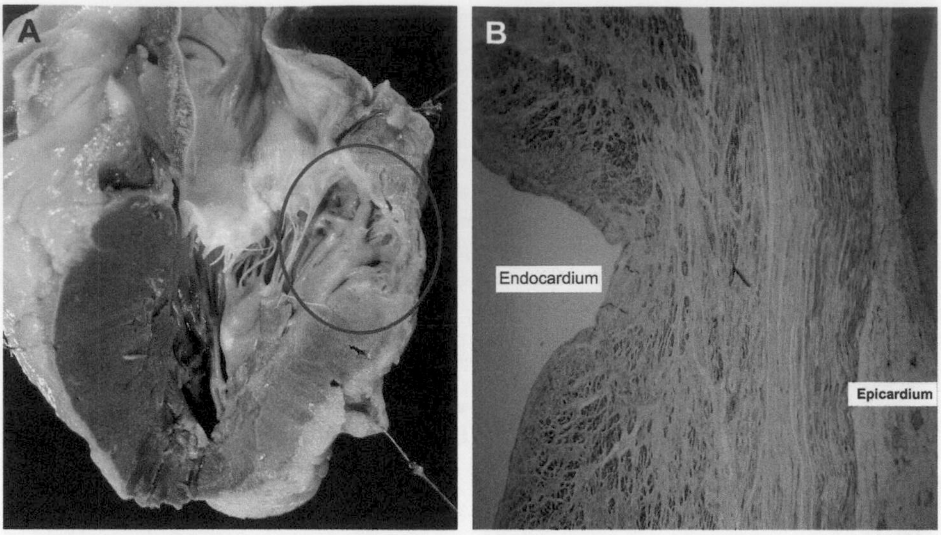

Fig. 2. Macroscopic (*A*) and microscopic (*B*) pathologic aspects of inferior and lateral basal segmental lesion in Chagas heart disease. (Masson trichrome, objective magnification: ×2.5).

in this study was a 16.6% annual mortality, higher than historical series in which patients had similar mean left ventricular ejection fraction and received optimal medical treatment with only amiodarone. Patients with ICD despite presenting a very low sudden death rate had a higher total mortality rate per year compared with the other groups. The relation between the number of shocks received by day 30 and survival has been suggested as indicating a worse prognosis. Patients with more than four shocks in a period of 30 days presented a higher mortality rate when compared with patients without or with a lower number of shocks. Because those patients died

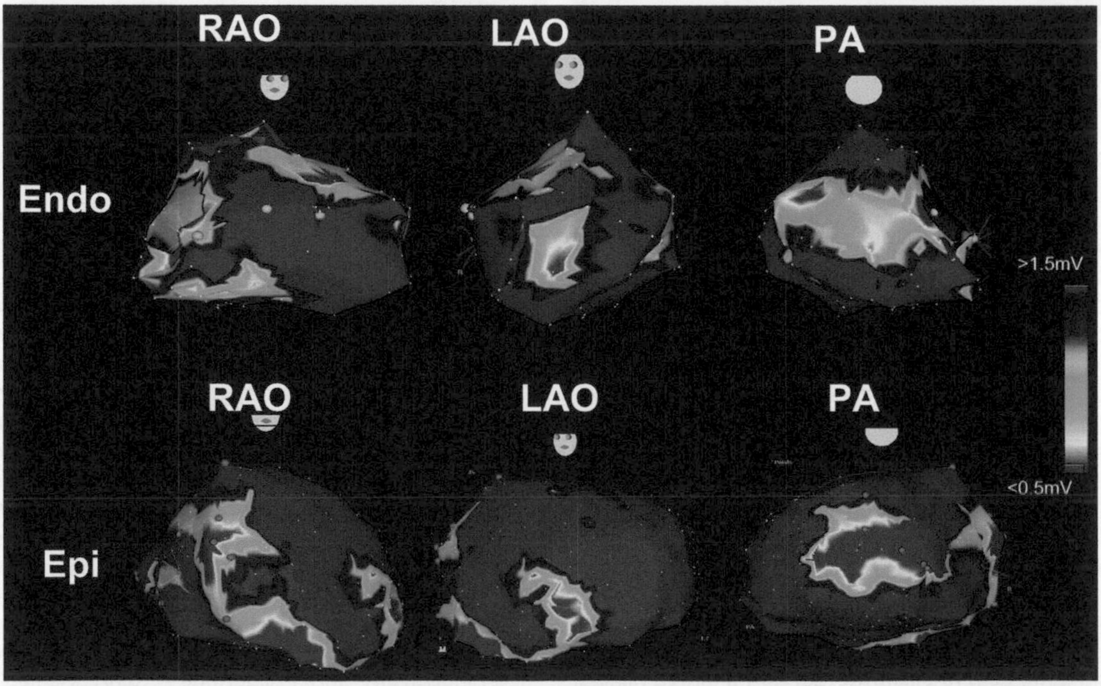

Fig. 3. Three different views of endocardial (Endo) and epicardial voltage mapping (Epi) in a patient with Chagas heart disease and recurrent sustained ventricular tachycardia. Note the epicardial mapping shows a denser scar compared with endocardial mapping. LAO, left anterior oblique; PA, posterior view; RAO, right anterior oblique.

predominately from heart failure, one can speculate that excessive shocks delivered by the ICD could depress left ventricular function and increase nonsudden mortality in this group of patients. Additionally, high doses of antiarrhythmic drugs can predispose to sinus bradycardia, increasing right ventricular pacing rate from the ICD, and promoting ventricular dyssynchronization. These data might suggest that a logical strategy to treat such patients is to reduce VT recurrence by changing the substrate for VT maintenance by catheter ablation to avoid ICD shocks.

CATHETER ABLATION OF CHAGAS VT

Chagas heart disease is the most frequent cause of VT ablation in the authors' center; in a series encompassing 698 patients with ischemic and nonischemic VTs, 274 (46%) were chagasic patients. In patients with Chagas disease, sustained VT is reproducible during programmed ventricular stimulation in almost all patients with recurrent VT, strongly suggesting a reentrant mechanism in such cases.[27,28] During electrophysiologic mapping, the left ventricle is the site of origin of sustained VT in more than 90% of the cases, and an inferolateral basal scar is the main substrate in around 70% of patients.[29,30] As demonstrated in Chagas disease and other structural heart diseases, most ventricular macroreentrant circuits are related to the arrangement of the surviving myocytes within dense ventricular scars. The critical fibers integrating the VT circuit can be localized in the subendocardial, subepicardial, or intramyocardial ventricular wall layers. In Chagas disease, some VT origin sites present thin wall with a discrete intramural scar between subendocardial and subepicardial fibers (**Fig. 2**). Hence, conventional RF pulses delivered from the endocardium can ablate subendocardial and subepicardial fibers potentially involved in reentrant circuit. In **Fig. 3**, a three-dimensional electroanatomic mapping shows the scar-related VT involving endocardial and epicardial surfaces of the posterior left ventricle. Note that the epicardial mapping shows a denser scar than the endocardial mapping. Continuous and fractionated electrograms were obtained during endocardial mapping (**Fig. 4**). RF pulses applied at that site interrupted the sustained VT. In some patients,

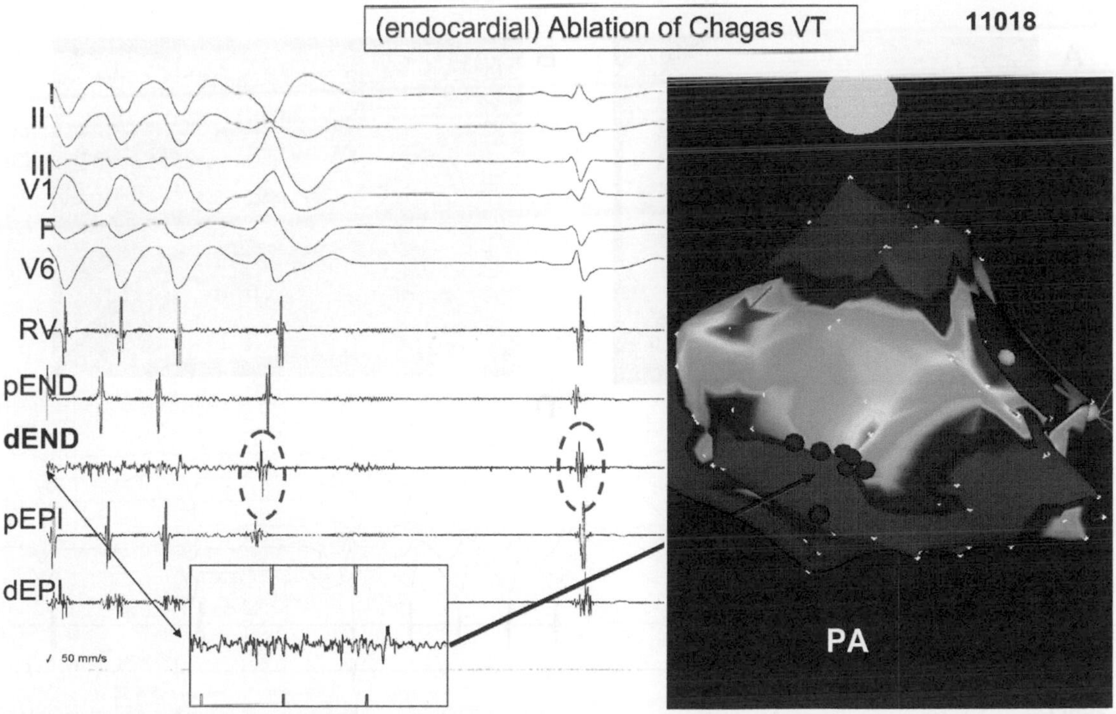

Fig. 4. Endocardial ablation of Chagas VT. Shown are reference ECG leads, I, II, III, V1, aVF, V6; RV electrogram, bipolar electrograms obtained from proximal and distal quadripolar catheter positioned on the endocardial surface of the left ventricle, pEND and dEND; and bipolar electrograms obtained from proximal and distal quadripolar catheter positioned on the epicardial surface of the left ventricle pEPI and dEPI. Note continuous and fractionated electrograms obtained during endocardial mapping at the site were RF delivery interrupted VT. Encircling electrograms show near normal electrograms at the ablation site after VT interruption.

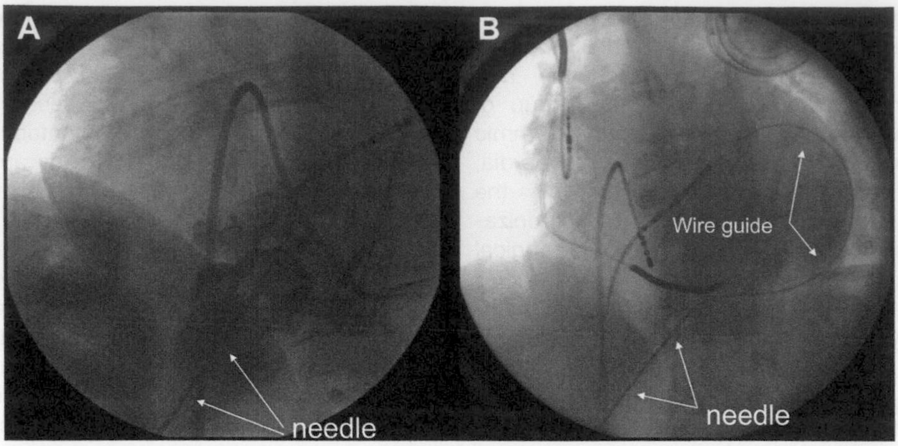

Fig. 5. Left anterior oblique views during subxiphoid pericardial puncture with Tuohy needle. (*A*) Needle tip position is monitored with contrast infusion. (*B*) Positioning of the guidewire into the pericardial space without contrast infusion.

however, the subendocardial tissue involved in the reentrant circuit is thick and relatively healthy and transmural lesions are very difficult to achieve with endocardial ablation. That was one of the authors' first observations to explain why VT ablation was unsuccessful in some patients. They decided to investigate the hypothesis that subepicardial circuits could be the origin of sustained VT in some Chagas patients using the transthoracic epicardial approach for epicardial mapping combined with endocardial mapping in most cases.[31–33]

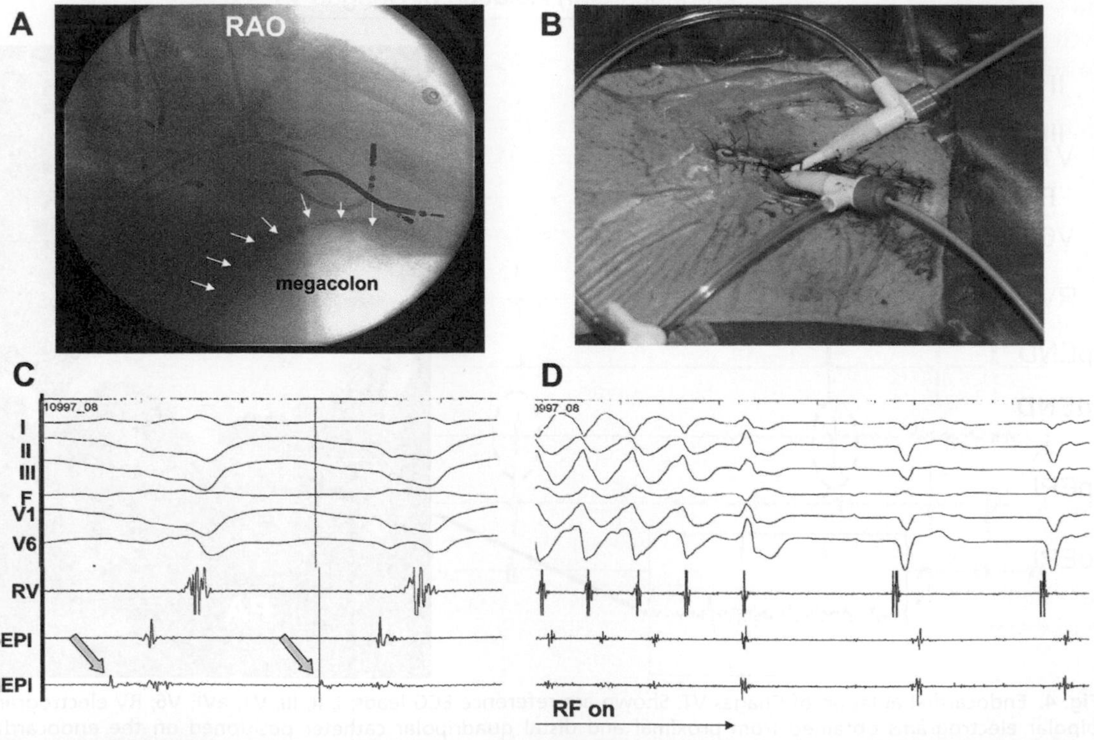

Fig. 6. Epicardial ventricular tachycardia mapping and ablation in a patient with Chagas disease with megacolon. (*A*) Right anterior oblique fluoroscopic projection showing the relationship of the megacolon, diaphragm and the heart. (*B*) Subxyphoid surgical approach. (*C*) I, II, III, F, V1, V6 reference ECG leads. Arrows show mid-diastolic electrograms. (*D*) Interruption of VT during RF pulse delivering.

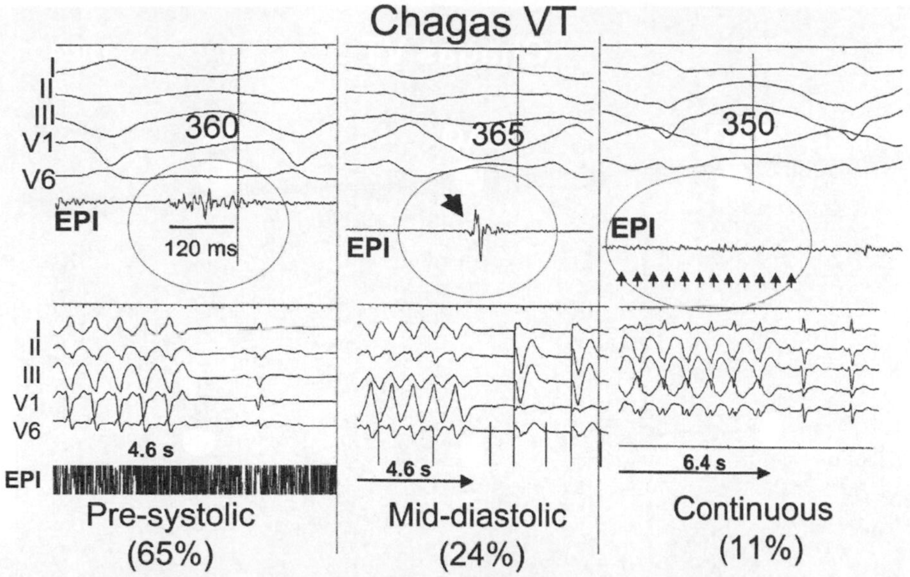

Fig. 7. Electrogram patterns obtained during sustained VT in Chagas disease in which RF pulse delivery interrupted VT.

EPICARDIAL ABLATION OF CHAGAS VT

The transthoracic epicardial approach has been used by the authors in the last 14 years to assess and ablate epicardial circuits in patients with Chagas VT.[31–33] This technique has changed a little with the experience acquired; however, the tools to access the pericardial space have not changed. The Tuohy needle is the main tool to reach the pericardial space. It has a curved and blunt tip. These characteristics facilitate needle introduction between the pericardial membranes with low risk of ventricular perforation. In using this technique a 10% risk of pericardial bleeding is expected, which is mostly small and transitory and does not prevent procedure conclusion. The risk of persistent bleeding requiring surgical repair is around 1% to 2%. Monitoring of the needle tip position was traditionally confirmed by infusing some iodine contrast during left and right anterior oblique fluoroscopic views; however, in some cases too much contrast infusion makes needle tip visualization difficult (**Fig. 5**A). The authors have avoided contrast infusion and intrapericardial needle tip position has been confirmed by advancing the regular guidewire when the needle tip is believed to have crossed the parietal pericardial (**Fig. 5**B). A left lateral border guidewire positioning confirms intrapericardial needle position avoiding pericardial contrast infusion. Epicarditis is frequently observed in pathologic specimens in Chagas heart disease; despite this, pericardial adhesions precluding pericardial space access are uncommon. In most of the patients this approach allows wide area epicardial mapping and ablation. Pericardial adhesions are also uncommon after prior ablation procedures. In 70 consecutive patients reviewed, nine (13%) underwent a redo procedure for simultaneous epicardial and endocardial ablation, seven patients had one previous procedure, and two had three and four procedures before, respectively. No limitations were observed by pericardial adhesions in those patients.

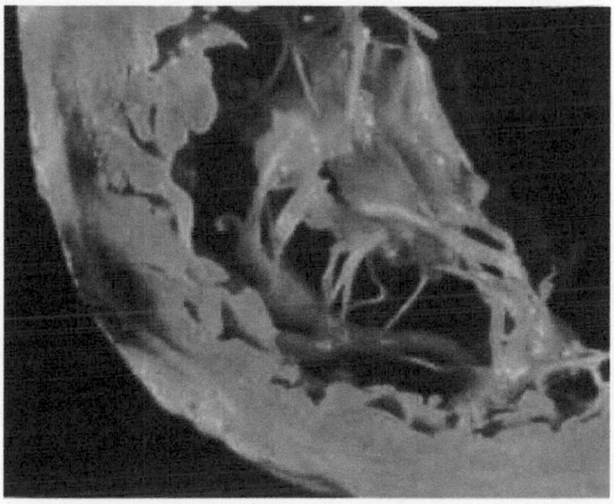

Fig. 8. Pathologic aspect of a successful epicardial ventricular ablation site in a patient with Chagas disease documented after cardiac transplantation. Note the linear subepicardial scar relationship with the ablation site and a normally thick left ventricle wall.

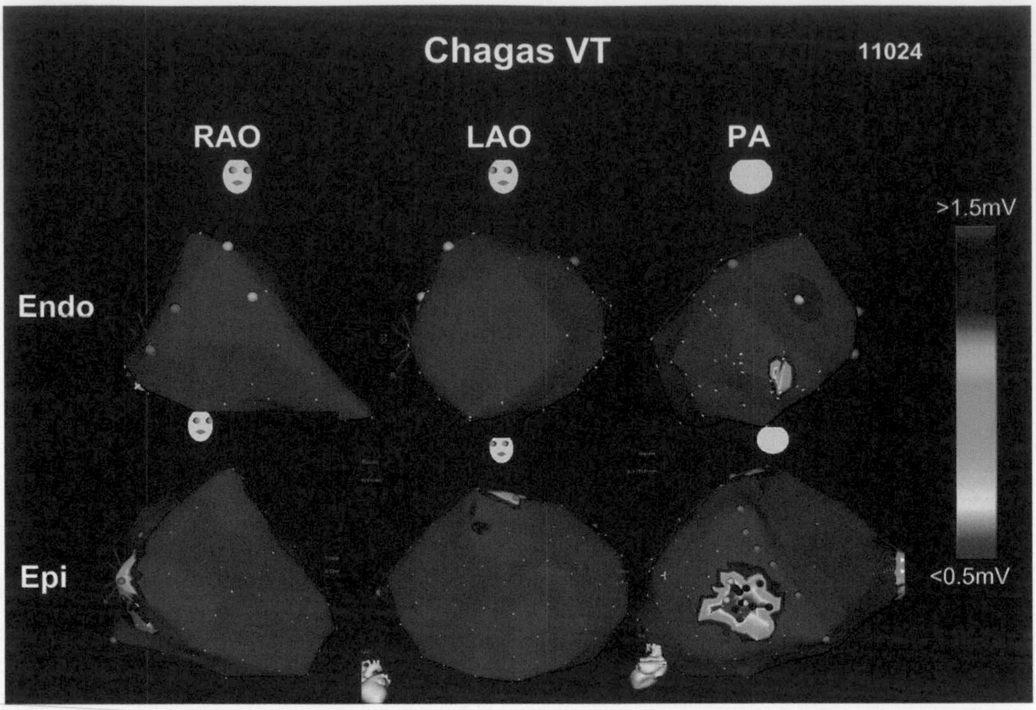

Fig. 9. Endocardial (Endo) and Epicardial (Epi) voltage mapping in a patient with Chagas heart disease with very well preserved systolic function with recurrent sustained ventricular tachycardia (VT). Note that scar related to VT is predominantly subepicardial.

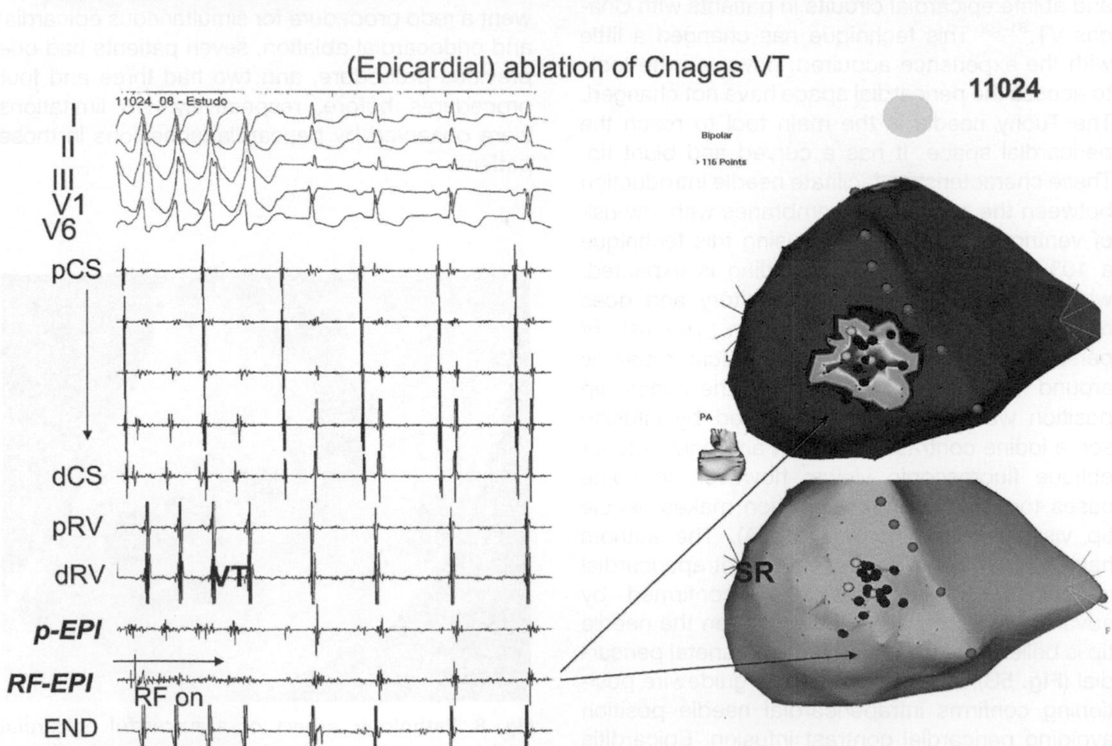

Fig. 10. Epicardial radiofrequency ablation (RF-EPI) of sustained ventricular tachycardia in the same patient shown in **Fig. 9.** Epicardial mapping at the epicardial scar area showed continuous and fractionated electrograms. RF delivered at that site interrupted sustained VT. Note that local electrograms presented relatively high amplitude after VT interruption, suggesting relatively health tissue near the macro reentrant circuit.

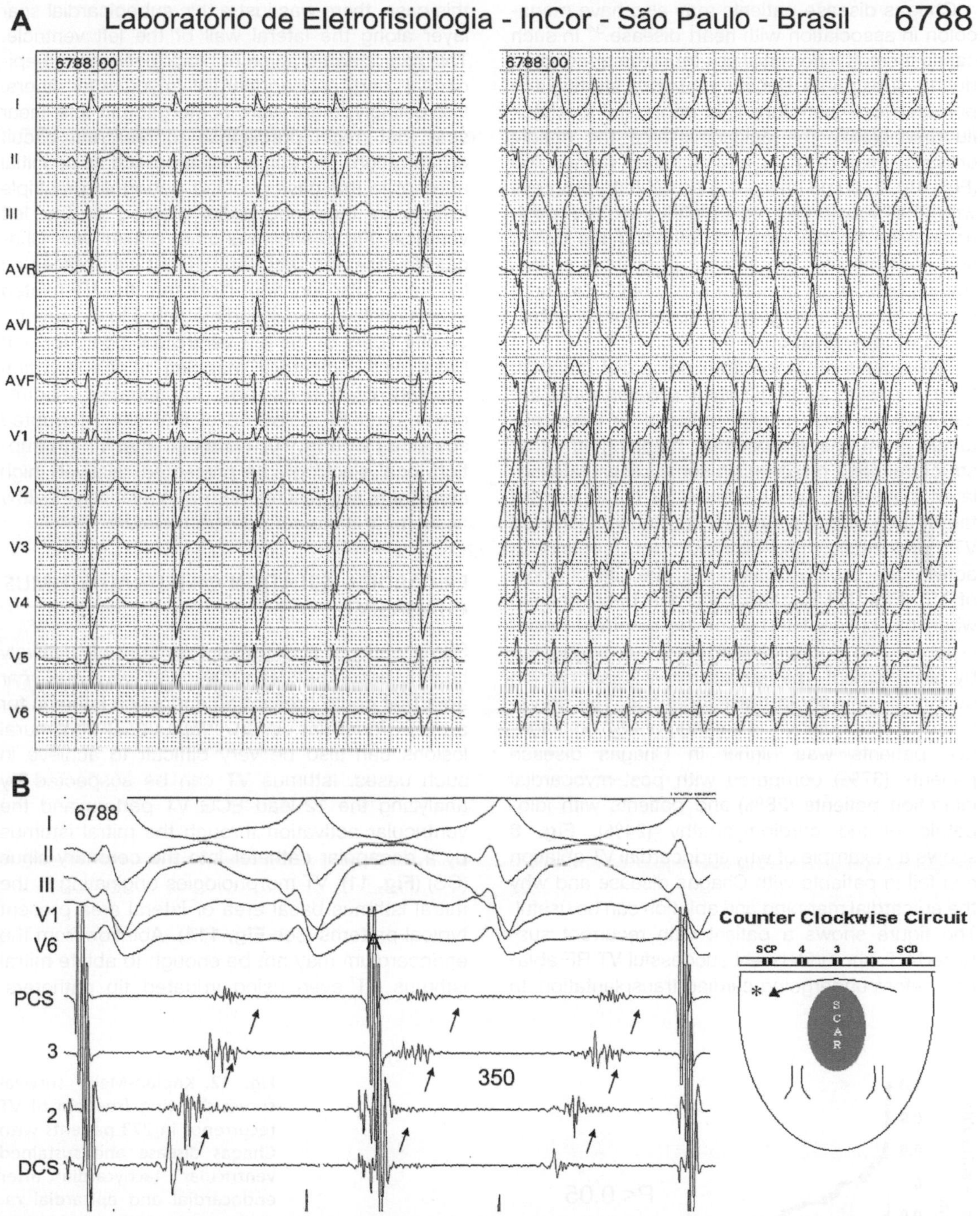

Fig. 11. Sustained ventricular tachycardia related to mitral isthmus in Chagas disease. Superior panel shows 12-lead ECGs in sinus rhythm (*A*) and sustained ventricular tachycardia (*B*) in a patient with Chagas cardiomyopathy. VT ECG pattern suggests left inferior and septal basal wall origin. The inferior panel shows mid-diastolic electrograms obtained by a decapolar catheter positioned into the coronary sinus. Ventricular activation sequence through the mitral isthmus comes from the lateral wall to the septal (exit site) wall strongly suggesting the mitral isthmus as an essential part of the reentry circuit. In this condition, a linear lesion connecting the mitral annulus to the ventricular scar is essential to interrupt VT.

Chagas disease patients may also have megacolon in association with heart disease.[34] In such cases there is a potential risk for colon perforation during subxiphoid puncture. Before starting the percutaneous puncture it is important to check fluoroscopically the epigastric area the needle crosses, searching for an insufflated megacolon (**Fig. 6**A). In some cases it is possible to progress with the subxiphoid pericardial puncture positioning the needle very flat, avoiding the colon, and searching for the anterior pericardial space. Rarely, pericardial puncture is too high risk and it is safer to ask a surgeon to open a small subxiphoid window (**Fig. 6**B).

The signals obtained from epicardial mapping from a possible VT origin site in patients with Chagas disease show similar patterns as those obtained from the endocardial mapping in other structural heart diseases. In some cases, late isolated potentials can be found in the epicardial target area during sinus rhythm; during sustained VT, presystolic, mid-diastolic, and continuous activity are usually observed at the site of origin of VT (**Fig. 7**). Epicardial VT has been defined when the critical isthmus of the reentrant circuit is located in subepicardial tissue as suggested by entrainment maneuvers or VT interruption during RF delivery in these locations. The prevalence of epicardial VT in a series of 257 consecutive patients was higher in Chagas disease patients (37%) compared with post–myocardial infarction patients (28%) and patients with idiopathic dilated cardiomyopathy (24%). **Fig. 8** shows an example of why endocardial VT ablation can fail in patients with Chagas disease and why the epicardial mapping and ablation can be useful. The figure shows a patient with recurrent sustained VT who underwent successful VT RF ablation before undergoing cardiac transplantation. In this case, there was just a thin subepicardial scar layer along the lateral wall of the left ventricle. This scar created a line of block between subepicardial and subendocardial myocardial fibers. Interestingly, there were some gaps in this linear scar that might predispose to reentrant circuit organization. The epicardial approach as an initial attempt in this case avoided performing multiple lesions in the endocardial surface of the left ventricle. **Fig. 9** shows another patient with Chagas disease and recurrent VT but with preserved left ventricular function. Note that the VT-related scar is relatively small and restricted to the subepicardial fibers of the left ventricular posterior and basal wall. Epicardial mapping at that location showed continuous and fractionated electrograms, and RF delivered at that site interrupted sustained VT (**Fig. 10**). Note that after VT interruption local electrograms presented relatively high amplitude, suggesting there was relatively healthy tissue near the macroreentrant circuit.

EPICARDIAL ABLATION OF MITRAL ISTHMUS CHAGAS VT

Some patients also present an area of relatively healthy tissue between the mitral valve and scar area that could present a conduction isthmus for a macroreentrant circuit.[35] Epicardial transmural lesions can also be very difficult to achieve in such cases. Isthmus VT can be suspected by analyzing the 12-lead ECG VT pattern and the ventricular activation through the mitral isthmus by a decapolar catheter into the coronary sinus (CS) (**Fig. 11**). VT morphologies originating in the mitral isthmus basal area or lateral area present typical patterns (see **Fig. 11**A). Ablation from the endocardium may not be enough to ablate mitral isthmus VT even using irrigated tip catheters.

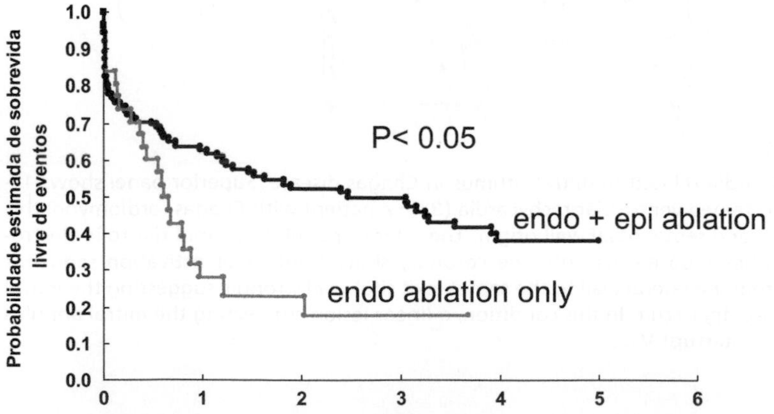

Fig. 12. Kaplan-Meier survival curves showing freedom of VT recurrence in 273 patients with Chagas disease and sustained ventricular tachycardia after endocardial and epicardial radiofrequency catheter ablation.

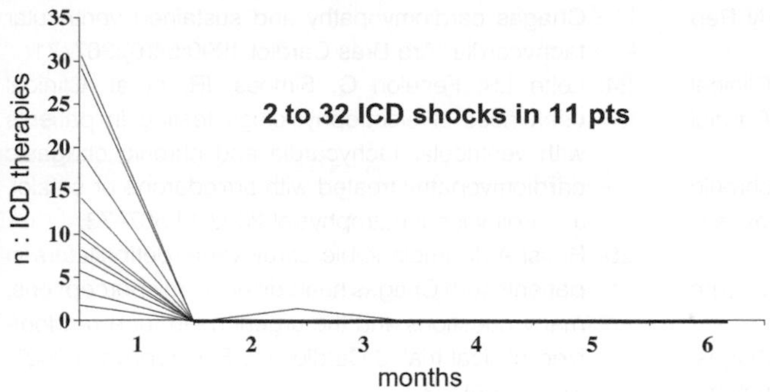

Fig. 13. Therapies from implantable cardioverter defibrillator before and after combining endocardial and epicardial radiofrequency ablation in 11 patients with Chagas disease and recurrent VT. Patients with two or more shocks in the month before the catheter ablation showed significant decrease in the number of therapies.

Although epicardial ablation is useful, epicardial fat and coronary artery location could be a limitation to delivering RF energy. RF delivered from the CS could make adjunctive lesions to help complete the line of block.

Fig. 12 shows long-term outcome of the authors' largest series encompassing 273 chagasic patients with combined epicardial and endocardial RF ablation at their institution. These patients underwent RF ablation with regular 4-mm tip electrodes, target mapping based on local electrograms obtained during sustained VT, and delivering few RF lesions without electroanatomic mapping assistance. Even with a better understanding of the mechanisms evolved in Chagas VT, the clinical results still seems to be worse than expected and may be dependent of limited ablation or disease evolution. Epicardial RF ablation based on electroanatomic mapping and irrigated tip catheter ablation might be more effective to control VT recurrences.[36–38] Performing extensive and deep lesions for substrate modification from the epicardial approach might increase the risk for damaging coronary arteries and extracardiac structures.[39–41] A randomized prospective study to evaluate the role of different strategies during catheter ablation in patients with Chagas disease is still needed. There is a specific group of patients in whom catheter ablation even using regular tools shows an important benefit: patients with ICD receiving multiple shocks, despite adjunctive therapy with antiarrhythmic drugs. In such cases, clinical results are clear in the short-term evaluation (**Fig. 13**). Despite successful VT treatment, Chagas heart disease is a progressive disease. It is not uncommon to see patients who had a successful VT ablation with good left ventricular function present after 5 to 10 years following ablation with left ventricular dysfunction and recurrence of a new sustained VT.

SUMMARY

Chagas heart disease is a chronic diffuse inflammatory cardiomyopathy with focal aspects. A wide spectrum of cardiac involvement can be found over time and these pathologic aspects determine different clinical presentations of the disease. The peculiar progress of the anatomic substrate may predispose the patient to a progressive cardiomyopathy, complex arrhythmias, and thromboembolic phenomena. Chagas VT is a reentrant and scar-related tachycardia and epicardial circuits are frequently found that substrate predominantly related to the inferior and lateral basal walls. Catheter ablation is successful in the short term, but late arrhythmia recurrence is common, suggesting an incomplete or reversible target elimination or further disease progression. Catheter ablation is a useful treatment for selected patients with recurrent Chagas VT. Combining endocardial and epicardial mapping and ablation could improve the results of conventional endocardial VT ablation.

REFERENCES

1. Chagas C. Nova tripanozomiaze humana. Estudos sobre a morfolojia e o ciclo evolutivo do Schizotrypanum cruzi n.gen. n.sp., ajente etiolojico de nova entidade morbida do homem. Mem Inst Oswaldo Cruz 1909;1:159–218 [in Portuguese].
2. Chagas C. Nova entidade morbida do homem. Rezumo geral de estudos etiolojicos e clínicos. Mem Inst Oswaldo Cruz 1911;3:219–75 [in Portuguese].
3. Chagas C, Villela E. Forma cardíaca da tripanosomíase Americana. Mem Inst Oswaldo Cruz 1922; 14:5–61 [in Portuguese].
4. Coura JR, Dias JCP. Epidemiology, control and surveillance of Chagas disease: 100 years after its discovery. Mem Inst Oswaldo Cruz 2009;104(I):31–40.
5. World Health Organization. Control of Chagas disease. Second report of the WHO Expert Committee. Technical report Series. 2002;905:192
6. Schmunis GA. Epidemiology of Chagas disease in non-endemic countries: the role of international migration. Mem Inst Oswaldo Cruz 2007;102(I): 75–85.
7. Centers for Disease Control and Prevention (CDC). Blood donor screening for Chagas disease—United

States, 2006–2007. MMWR Morb Mortal Wkly Rep 2007;56(7):141–3.
8. Punukollu G, Gowda RM, Khan IA, et al. Clinical aspects of the Chagas' heart disease. Int J Cardiol 2007;115(3):279–83.
9. Dias JCP. The indeterminate form of human chronic Chagas' disease: a clinical epidemiological review. Rev Soc Bras Med Trop 1989;22:147–56.
10. Barret MP, Burchmore RJ, Stich A, et al. The trypanosomiases. Lancet 2003;362:1469–80.
11. Laranja FS, Dias E, Nobrega G, et al. Chagas' disease: a clinical, epidemiologic and pathologic study. Circulation 1956;14:1035–60.
12. Köberle F. Chagas' heart disease and Chagas' syndromes: the pathology of American trypanosomiasis. Adv Parasitol 1968;6:63–116.
13. Andrade ZA. Immunopathology of Chagas disease. Mem Inst Oswaldo Cruz 1999;94:71–80.
14. Higuchi ML, Reis MM, Aiello VD, et al. Human chronic chagasic myocarditis is T. cruzi antigen and CD8 + T cell dependent. Am J Trop Med Hyg 1997;56:485–9.
15. Brener Z, Ramirez LE, Krettli AU, et al. EVI antibodies in patients with Chagas' disease: relationship with anti-Trypanosoma cruzi immunoglobulins and effects of specific treatment. Mem Inst Oswaldo Cruz 1983;78(4):437–42.
16. Cossio PM, Diez C, Szarfman A. Chagasic cardiopathy: demonstration of a serum gamma globulin factor which reacts with endicardium and ascular structures. Circulation 1974;49:13–21.
17. Higuchi ML, Brito T, Reis MM, et al. Correlation between T. cruzi parasitism and myocardia inflammation in human chronic chagasic myocarditis: light microscopy and immunohistochemical findings. Cardiovasc Pathol 1993;2:101–2.
18. Palomino AS, Aiello VD, Higuchi ML, et al. Systematic mapping of hearts from chronic chagasic patients: the association between the occurrence of histopathological lesions and Trypanosoma cruzi antigens. Ann Trop Med Parasitol 2000;94:571–9.
19. Marin-Neto JA, Cunha-Neto E, Maciel BC, et al. Pathogenesis of chronic Chagas heart disease. Circulation 2007;115:1109–23.
20. Carrasco HA, Guerrero L, Parada H, et al. Ventricular arrhythmias and left ventricular myocardial function in chronic chagasic patients. Int J Cardiol 1990; 28(1):35–41.
21. Rassi A Jr, Rassi A, Little WC, et al. Development and validation of a risk score for predicting death in Chagas' heart disease. N Engl J Med 2006;355: 799–808.
22. Rassi A Jr, Rassi SG, Rassi A. Sudden death in Chagas'disease. Arq Bras Cardiol 2001;76:75–96.
23. Scanavacca MI, Sosa EA, Lee JH, et al. Empiric therapy with amiodarone in patients with chronic Chagas cardiomyopathy and sustained ventricular tachycardia. Arq Bras Cardiol 1990;54(6):367–71.
24. Leite LR, Fenelon G, Simões JR, et al. Clinical usefulness of electrophysiology testing in patients with ventricular tachycardia and chronic chagasic cardiomyopathy treated with amiodarone or sotalol. J Cardiovasc Electrophysiol 2003;14:567–73.
25. Rassi A Jr. Implantable cardioverter-defibrillators in patients with Chagas heart disease: misperceptions, many questions and the urgent need for a randomized clinical trial. J Cardiovasc Electrophysiol 2007; 18(12):1241–3.
26. Rabinovich R, Muratore C, Iglesias R, et al. Time to first shock in implantable cardioverter defibrillator (ICD) patients with Chagas cardiomyopathy. Pacing Clin Electrophysiol 1999;22:202–5.
27. Cardinalli-Neto A, Bestetti RB, Cordeiro JA, et al. Predictors of all-cause mortality for patients with chronic Chagas' heart disease receiving implantable cardioverter defibrillator therapy. J Cardiovasc Electrophysiol 2007;18(12):1236–40.
28. de Paola AA, Horowitz LN, Miyamoto MH, et al. Angiographic and electrophysiologic substrates of ventricular tachycardia in chronic chagasic myocarditis. Am J Cardiol 1990;65(5):360–3.
29. Sarabanda AV, Sosa E, Simões MV, et al. Ventricular tachycardia in Chagas' disease: a comparison of clinical, angiographic, electrophysiologic and myocardial perfusion disturbances between patients presenting with either sustained or nonsustained forms. Int J Cardiol 2005;102(1):9–19.
30. d'Avila A, Splinter R, Svenson RH, et al. New perspectives on catheter-based ablation of ventricular tachycardia complicating Chagas' disease: experimental evidence of the efficacy of near infrared lasers for catheter ablation of Chagas' VT. J Interv Card Electrophysiol 2002;7(1):23–38.
31. Sosa E, Scanavacca M, d'Avila A, et al. A new technique to perform epicardial mapping in the electrophysiology laboratory. J Cardiovasc Electrophysiol 1996;7(6):531–6.
32. Sosa E, Scanavacca M, D'Avila A, et al. Radiofrequency catheter ablation of ventricular tachycardia guided by nonsurgical epicardial mapping in chronic chagasic heart disease. Pacing Clin Electrophysiol 1999;22:128–30.
33. Sosa E, Scanavacca M. Epicardial mapping and ablation techniques to control ventricular tachycardia. J Cardiovasc Electrophysiol 2005;16(4): 449–52.
34. de Rezende JM, Moreira H. Chagasic megaesophagus and megacolon: historical review and present concepts. Arq Gastroenterol 1988;25:32–43.
35. Scanavacca M, Sosa E, d'Avila A, et al. Radiofrequency ablation of sustained ventricular tachycardia related to the mitral isthmus in Chagas' disease. Pacing Clin Electrophysiol 2002;25(3):368–71.

36. d'Avila A, Houghtaling C, Gutierrez P, et al. Catheter ablation of ventricular epicardial tissue: a comparison of standard and cooled-tip radiofrequency energy. Circulation 2004;109(19):2363–9.
37. Aryana A, d'Avila A, Heist EK, et al. Remote magnetic navigation to guide endocardial and epicardial catheter mapping of scar-related ventricular tachycardia. Circulation 2007;115(10): 1191–200.
38. Garcia FC, Bazan V, Zado ES, et al. Epicardial substrate and outcome with epicardial ablation of ventricular tachycardia in arrhythmogenic right ventricular cardiomyopathy/dysplasia. Circulation 2009;120(5):366–75.
39. D'Avila A, Gutierrez P, Scanavacca M, et al. Effects of radiofrequency pulses delivered in the vicinity of the coronary arteries: implications for nonsurgical transthoracic epicardial catheter ablation to treat ventricular tachycardia. Pacing Clin Electrophysiol 2002;25(10):1488–95.
40. Sánchez-Quintana D, Ho SY, Climent V, et al. Anatomic evaluation of the left phrenic nerve relevant to epicardial and endocardial catheter ablation: implications for phrenic nerve injury. Heart Rhythm 2009;6(6):764–8.
41. Buch E, Vaseghi M, Cesario DA, et al. A novel method for preventing phrenic nerve injury during catheter ablation. Heart Rhythm 2007;4(1):95–8.

Epicardial Ablation of Ischemic Ventricular Tachycardia

Usha Tedrow, MD, MSc*, William G. Stevenson, MD

KEYWORDS

- Epicardium • Ventricular tachycardia
- Ischemic cardiomyopathy • Ablation

Ventricular tachycardia (VT) is a major cause of morbidity and mortality in patients with ischemic heart disease.[1,2] Reentry related to ventricular scars is the most common cause of sustained monomorphic VT associated with ischemic cardiomyopathy. Implantable cardioverter-defibrillators can be lifesaving, but they expose the patient to shocks, which can be painful and are also associated with exacerbations of underlying heart failure.[3] Catheter ablation for VT is an important therapy for patients with drug-refractory ventricular arrhythmias[4,5] and can be immediately lifesaving when VT is incessant.[6] Although most VTs in patients with coronary artery disease and prior infarction originate from reentry circuits in the subendocardium, endocardial mapping fails to identify a clinically important reentry circuit in approximately 20% of patients. Furthermore, during follow-up, approximately one-half of patients experience at least one VT recurrence. Epicardial and intramural reentry circuit locations are well recognized from surgical mapping and ablation and are an important cause of failure of endocardial ablation.[7]

The method of percutaneous access to the pericardial space for mapping and ablation developed by Sosa and colleagues[8] now allows epicardial reentry circuits to be treated with catheter ablation. Pericardial adhesions after cardiac surgery often prevent percutaneous access, although limited access is possible in some patients.[9,10] A direct surgical approach to the pericardial space via a subxiphoid pericardial window or thoracotomy can achieve access in most patients. It is important to recognize and take precautions to minimize potential risks inherent in epicardial access and ablation. There is risk of injury to an epicardial coronary artery if catheter position is in close proximity and the coronary vessel diameter is small. Overlying epicardial fat can potentially be protective. Proximity to the coronary arteries is assessed most commonly by angiography. Phrenic nerve injury, subdiaphragmatic vascular injury, and intraabdominal and pericardial bleeding are also potential risks.

INDICATIONS FOR EPICARDIAL MAPPING AND ABLATION

A recent review of VT ablation cases from 3 tertiary centers found that epicardial mapping and ablation was performed in 17% of 913 VI ablation procedures. A prior endocardial ablation had failed in 86% of patients. VT was due to ischemic heart disease in 38% of patients undergoing epicardial procedures.[11]

Epicardial origin of VT should be suspected when endocardial mapping fails to identify the reentry circuits or substrate-guided endocardial ablation fails. Most of the patients in reported series of epicardial mapping and ablation have failed endocardial ablation.[12] Thus, reported patients are a selected population. In general there is a perception that epicardial reentry circuits are more frequent with inferior wall (**Fig. 1**), as opposed to anterior wall infarctions, although epicardial circuits can occur with anterior wall infarctions.[13,14]

The Cardiovascular Division, Department of Medicine, Brigham and Women's Hospital, Harvard Medical School, 75 Francis Street, Boston, MA 02115, USA
* Corresponding author.
E-mail address: utedrow@partners.org (U. Tedrow).

Card Electrophysiol Clin 2 (2010) 69–79
doi:10.1016/j.ccep.2009.11.005
1877-9182/10/$ – see front matter

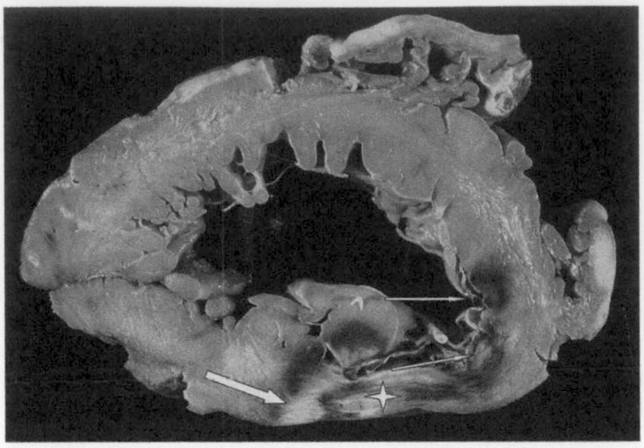

Fig. 1. Endocardial and epicardial ablation shown is a gross pathology specimen of a patient with an inferior wall scar (marked with the *star*), whose VT could not be terminated with endocardial ablation (*thin arrows*). Note the myocardial thickness relative to the size of the endocardial ablation lesions. Epicardial ablation did control the patient's arrhythmia. The epicardial lesions are indicated by the thicker arrow.

Several electrocardiographic features of VT that suggest an epicardial origin have been described. These criteria generally reflect the reasonable physiologic consideration that endocardial circuits have more rapid access to the Purkinje system along the endocardium than epicardial circuits, resulting in more rapid initial spread of myocardial activation.[12] Epicardial origin is suggested by (1) the presence of a pseudodelta wave or by time to earliest rapid deflection in the precordial leads of 34 milliseconds or more and (2) prolonged intrinsicoid deflection, for example, time to peak R wave in V_2 of more than 85 milliseconds and time to earliest QRS nadir of more than 121 milliseconds in the precordial leads.[15] Infarct scar-related VTs usually have a right bundle branch block configuration in V_1, but left bundle branch block configuration VTs also occur.[6]

Given the 3-dimensional nature of VT circuits, these ECG criteria probably indicate the exit for a VT reentry circuit. It is possible for a circuit to have an epicardial exit but with other portions of the circuit being intramural or endocardial (where they can be interrupted with endocardial ablation). In some cases, broad endocardial exits may be identified, but the reentry circuit isthmus may be intramural or epicardial. Thus, patients who have failed an endocardial attempt are reasonable candidates for an epicardial approach independent of the VT QRS morphology.[5] Epicardial mapping can be considered as the first approach in patients with left ventricular (LV) thrombus if their anticoagulation can be safely interrupted for the procedure.[15] If no prior ablation has been performed, limited transvenous mapping of induced VT via the coronary sinus and accessible LV branches can suggest an epicardial VT circuit.[9]

EPICARDIAL ACCESS

Percutaneous epicardial access adopts the approach developed by Sosa and colleagues,[8] using a Tuohy needle designed for epidural access (Codman & Shurtleff Inc, Raynham, MA, USA) and a soft-tipped guidewire with firm body, such as a Bentson wire (Cook Medical Inc, Bloomington, IN, USA). Access can be achieved in more than 90% of patients who have not had prior cardiac surgery.[9,16] Skin entry is generally 2 to 3 cm below the xiphoid process.[5] There are 2 approaches. Directing the needle superiorly at a fairly shallow angle, aiming for the right ventricular (RV) apex in the right anterior oblique (RAO) projection generally enters the pericardial space anteriorly over the right ventricle. This approach facilitates access to the anterior aspect of the ventricles and may be may be more likely to avoid the rare reported inadvertent puncture of subdiaphragmatic vessels than a posterior puncture. Directing the needle more posteriorly and toward the left shoulder, one enters the pericardium over the inferior aspect of the ventricles, such that the sheath typically tracks along the posterior aspect of the LV as observed in the left anterior oblique (LAO) projection. The authors use biplane RAO and LAO fluoroscopy (**Fig. 2**) to facilitate anatomic localization. As the needle approaches the pericardium, injection of a small amount (<1 mL) of contrast can help assess the relation of the needle to the parietal pericardium. Once tenting of the pericardium is seen, a slight advance achieves entry into the space and is palpable. Aspiration without blood indicates that the needle has not entered the RV. Injected contrast should layer in the pericardial space. The guidewire is then advanced generously into the pericardial space. It is essential to observe the wire in the LAO projection, ensuring that it hugs the cardiac silhouette, crossing more than one chamber circumferential to the right and left heart.[8] Observation in the RAO or anteroposterior projection alone can be misleading, because a wire that enters the RV and passes into the right atrium or pulmonary artery can be misinterpreted as intrapericardial. It is critical to ensure that the wire is in the pericardial space and has not entered the RV. Inadvertent RV puncture is not uncommon, but it is usually benign if only the needle or wire has entered the chamber in a patient who is not anticoagulated.

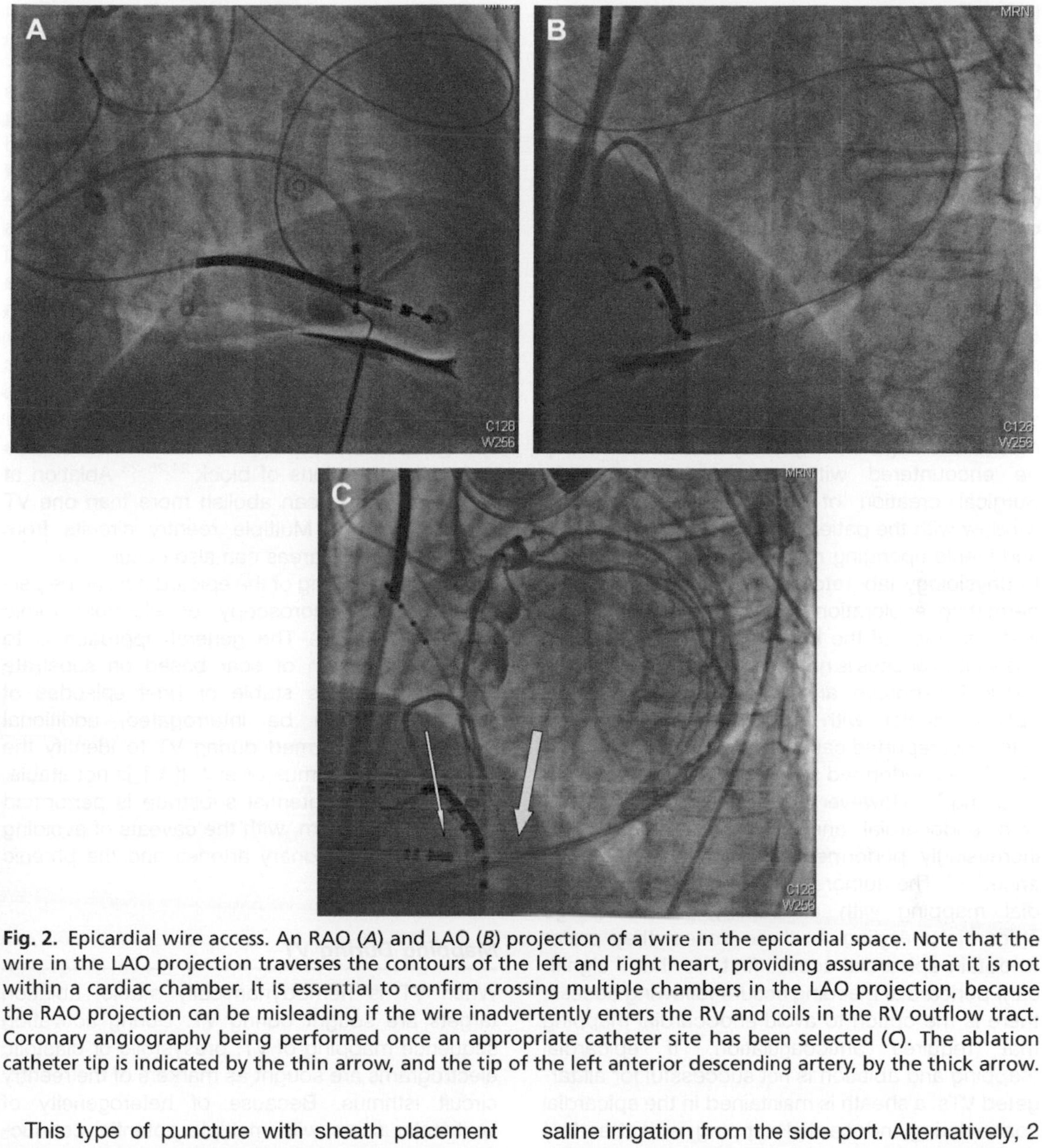

Fig. 2. Epicardial wire access. An RAO (*A*) and LAO (*B*) projection of a wire in the epicardial space. Note that the wire in the LAO projection traverses the contours of the left and right heart, providing assurance that it is not within a cardiac chamber. It is essential to confirm crossing multiple chambers in the LAO projection, because the RAO projection can be misleading if the wire inadvertently enters the RV and coils in the RV outflow tract. Coronary angiography being performed once an appropriate catheter site has been selected (*C*). The ablation catheter tip is indicated by the thin arrow, and the tip of the left anterior descending artery, by the thick arrow.

This type of puncture with sheath placement and mapping can be performed under conscious sedation. Many centers use general anesthesia, allowing control of respiratory movement, which may make access easier but introduces the potential problems of positive pressure ventilation for patients who often have severe structural heart disease or underlying pulmonary disease.[5]

Sheath selection depends on the size of the patient and VT location. For inferior wall VT circuits, a 15-cm, 8F sheath may be sufficient. For more extensive mapping, the authors generally use a deflectable sheath (Agilis sheath; St Jude Medical, St Paul, MN, USA). Using a sheath with a lumen larger than the ablation catheter (eg, 8F with a 7.5F catheter) allows aspiration of blood or saline irrigation from the side port. Alternatively, 2 guidewires can be inserted into a single sheath and exchanged for a mapping sheath and a separate pericardial catheter for drainage of pericardial fluid during the procedure if an ablation catheter with external irrigation is used. Once an introducer sheath and catheter are in place, the catheter moves freely, constrained only by the reflections of the pericardial membrane located around the pulmonary veins and the great vessels.

Inadvertent puncture of a vessel or cardiac chamber is a concern. Approximately 10% to 20% of patients experience pericardial bleeding, particularly if inadvertent RV or LV puncture has occurred. Bleeding is managed by frequent aspiration from the pericardial access sheath. This type of bleeding does not usually preclude mapping and catheter ablation. It is not uncommon to aspirate 10 to 40 mL of bloody drainage from the pericardial sheath early in the procedure, but with no evidence of continued bleeding, the authors routinely use systemic anticoagulation with heparin if subsequent LV endocardial mapping or coronary angiography is desired.

In patients who have previously had cardiac surgery, a percutaneous approach is not always feasible because of pericardial adhesions. Percutaneous epicardial access was attempted in 30 patients with VT related to coronary artery disease and it failed in 6, all of whom had prior cardiac surgery.[10] In addition, bypass grafts to the posterior descending coronary artery could conceivably be encountered with a posterior approach. Surgical creation of a subxiphoid pericardial window with the patient under general anesthesia and sterile operating room conditions in the electrophysiology laboratory is an alternative option, permitting exploration of at least the diaphragmatic surface of the heart.[17] For those in whom this limited access is not an option, more extensive surgical exposure and surgical ablation is an option in centers with experience.[9,18]

In most reported cases, epicardial mapping and ablation is performed separately from endocardial mapping.[19] However, combination procedures with endocardial and epicardial mapping are increasingly performed at centers with experience.[14,20] The authors are prepared for endocardial mapping with all patients who undergo epicardial mapping. In these cases, they prefer to obtain epicardial access first, so that if significant pericardial bleeding occurs following access, there is the option to avoid endocardial mapping that requires anticoagulation. If epicardial mapping and ablation is not successful for all targeted VTs, a sheath is maintained in the epicardial space during endocardial mapping, with attendant anticoagulation to allow for careful monitoring and removal of any fluid that might accumulate. When epicardial mapping follows endocardial mapping, LV catheters are removed and heparin anticoagulation is reversed with protamine for epicardial access.

MAPPING BASED ON THE VT MECHANISM AND SUBSTRATE

Mapping approaches based on the mechanisms of VT are similar for endocardial and epicardial VTs. Reentry related to a chronic infarct scar is the most common mechanism of monomorphic VT associated with ischemic cardiomyopathy.[21] Infarct scars are composed of variable regions of dense fibrosis that create conduction block with interposed surviving myocyte bundles and interstitial fibrosis. Diminished cellular coupling produces circuitous paths and zones of slow conduction that promote reentry.[22] These circuits can be modeled as having an isthmus or channel composed of a small mass of tissue that does not contribute to the surface ECG. The QRS complex begins when the excitation wave front emerges from an exit along the border of the scar and spreads across the ventricles. Scars related to VT often border a valve annulus that forms a border segment for part of the circuit.[23–25] Multiple VTs with different QRS morphologies can be due to multiple exits from the same region of scar or changes in activation remote from the circuit due to functional regions of block.[24,26–28] Ablation at one region often can abolish more than one VT morphology.[28–31] Multiple reentry circuits from widely separated areas can also occur.

Catheter mapping of the epicardium can be performed using fluoroscopy or electroanatomic mapping systems. The general approach is to identify the region of scar based on substrate mapping. If VT is stable or brief episodes of induced VT can be interrogated, additional mapping is performed during VT to identify the reentry circuit isthmus or exit. If VT is not stable, ablation of the potential substrate is performed during sinus rhythm, with the caveats of avoiding the epicardial coronary arteries and the phrenic nerves.

Mapping During VT

When VT is hemodynamically stable, ablation targets are sought during VT. During activation sequence mapping of VT, presystolic or diastolic electrograms are sought as markers of the reentry circuit isthmus. Because of heterogeneity of ventricular scars with multiple potential conduction paths and channels, electrogram timing alone is not a reliable guide for targeting a specific reentry circuit isthmus.[32] Confirmation that a site is involved in the reentry circuit can be obtained by entrainment mapping.[24,32–34] At pacing sites in the reentry circuit, stimuli that are captured during VT can reset the circuit. The conduction time required for the stimulated wave front to complete one revolution through the circuit is equal to the tachycardia cycle length, and thus, the postpacing interval (PPI) following the pacing train approximates the tachycardia cycle length. At pacing sites removed from the circuit, the PPI increases as a function of the conduction time between the site and the reentry circuit. If the site is a reentry circuit isthmus, entrainment occurs without changing the QRS morphology (entrainment with concealed fusion), because the stimulated wave fronts follow the path of the reentry circuit and propagate through its exit. In this case, the S-QRS interval indicates the conduction time from the pacing site to the reentry circuit exit and matches the electrogram to QRS interval during VT.

Other features that indicate that a site is in the reentry circuit include reproducible VT termination by catheter-induced mechanical pressure; termination by ablation during VT; and termination by a pacing stimulus that does not produce a response that propagates away from the pacing site; such that there is no QRS complex following the pacing stimulus.[33,35,36] It is not necessary to define the entire circuit if an isthmus can be identified for ablation.

Inability to identify the reentry circuit isthmus on the endocardium by entrainment mapping suggests that the isthmus is epicardial or intramural. Often a focal point of earliest endocardial activation is identified in these cases, where entrainment indicates a potential exit or outer loop site but ablation fails to interrupt VT, suggesting that there is an epicardial or intramural circuit with a broad endocardial exit.

Substrate Mapping

Substrate mapping is the identification of the scar and likely portions of the reentry circuit that constitute the substrate for reentry circuits during stable sinus or paced rhythm (**Fig. 3**).[12] Areas of infarction or scar have low-amplitude electrograms similar to findings during endocardial mapping (see **Fig. 3**).[19,25,37] However, at some sites, epicardial fat creates low-amplitude regions.[38] Epicardial fat is also a potential barrier to pacing and ablation.[39] Normal endocardial bipolar electrograms filtered at 20 to 400 Hz have an amplitude greater than 1.55 mV.[27] These values have been extrapolated to epicardial mapping. Recently, Marchlinski and colleagues[40] also evaluated epicardial bipolar electrograms (4 mm tip and 2 mm ring electrode with 1 mm interelectrode distance, filtered at 30 to 400 Hz) in patients with structurally normal hearts. The mean amplitude was 3.2 mV, and 95% of signals had amplitudes exceeding 0.61 mV. Excluding regions along the atrioventricular groove and large coronary vessels, the mean amplitude was 3.6 mV, and 95% of electrograms had amplitudes exceeding 0.94 mV. They suggest a threshold of less than 1.0 mV to designate scar during epicardial mapping. In most infarct scars, confluent regions of low voltage much lower than this value are identified. The border area can contain electrograms that are greater than 1.0 mV but with fractionated or split potentials. The presence of fractionated or split potentials and late potentials may be more specific to scar regions as opposed to fat. The authors' approach to epicardial substrate mapping is essentially the same as for endocardial substrate mapping. An epicardial voltage map is created (see **Fig. 3**A), and areas with fractionated and split electrograms are tagged during the process.

Pace mapping is used to confirm the presence of viable tissue. With unipolar pacing, the pacing threshold is generally less than 10mA at a pulse width of 2 milliseconds in normal tissue. Therefore, the authors can usually perform standard pace mapping and entrainment mapping. Areas of high threshold can be due to fat, scar, or poor contact. Inability to capture during bipolar epicardial pacing can limit the use of pace mapping and entrainment mapping.[12,38,40] Sites where pacing replicates the QRS morphology of VT indicate proximity to an exit. Areas of slow conduction are indicated with S-QRS delays greater than 40 milliseconds, and those where the QRS also matches a VT are potential isthmus regions that are desirable targets for ablation.

EPICARDIAL ABLATION

Radiofrequency (RF) energy remains the primary ablative energy source. The absence of circulating blood flow often allows electrode temperature to increase substantially during low-power applications, potentially limiting lesion formation. Heating to the point of thrombus formation and charring is of less concern, because there is no potential for arterial embolization from the epicardial space; therefore, a higher temperature (>60°C) can be tolerated, but lesion size often seemed inadequate with standard 4- or 5-mm solid electrodes. Active cooling of the RF ablation electrode increases lesion size in animal models, consistent with the impression that cooling creates more effective lesions in the epicardium in humans.[13] Therefore, the authors use an internally irrigated cooled-tip catheter (Chilli; Boston Scientific, Natick, MA, USA) or externally irrigated catheters (Thermocool; Biosense Webster Inc, Diamond Bar, CA, USA) for epicardial ablation. The authors typically ablate at 30 to 50 watts for 60 to 120 seconds. With external irrigation, they reduce the flow during mapping to 1mL/min and increase it during ablation to 10 to 17 mL/min. These lower flow rates, as compared with those used during endocardial mapping and ablation, are acceptable because thrombus formation does not pose a risk of embolization

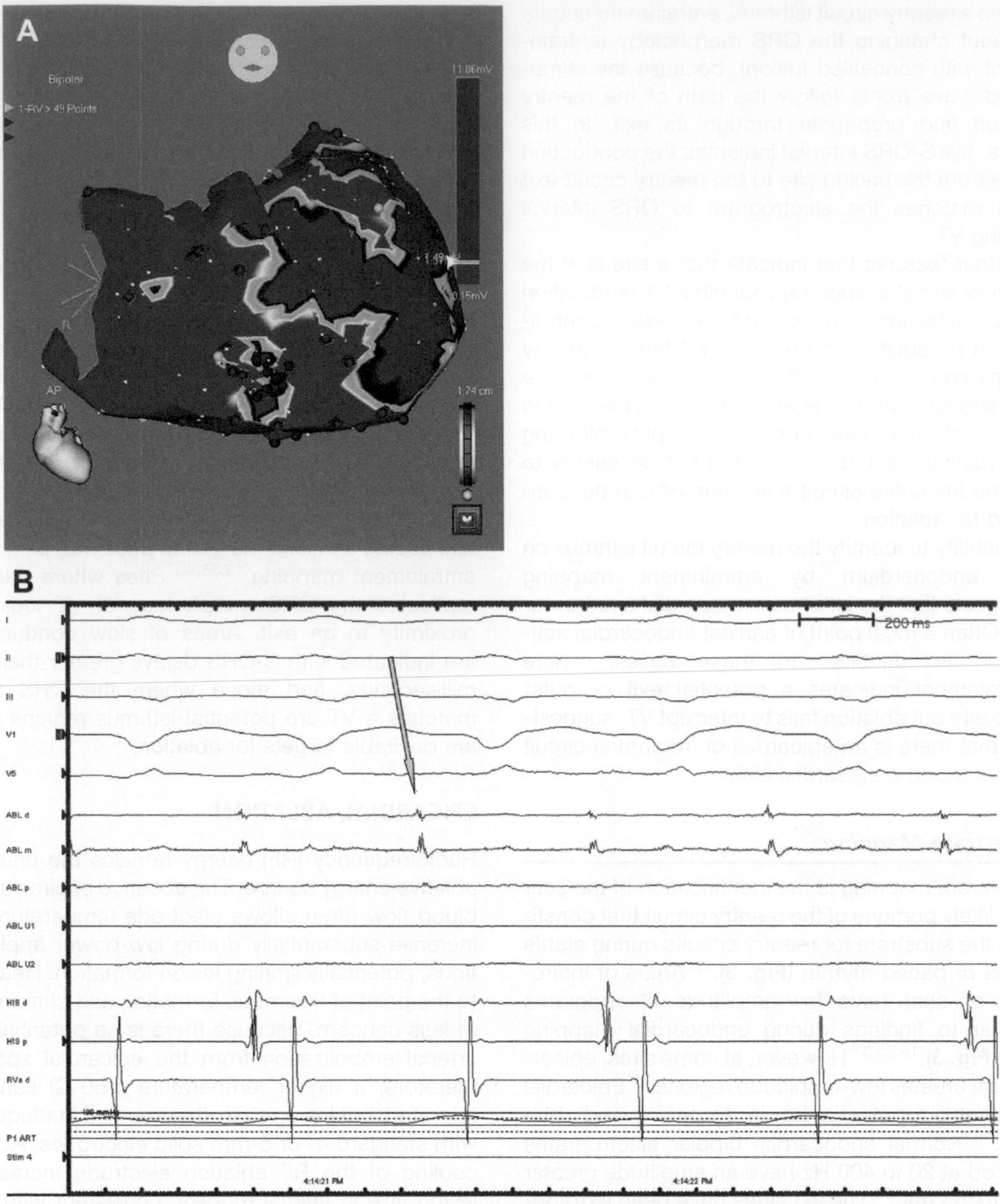

Fig. 3. An electroanatomic map of the epicardium (*A*). This patient had VT storm and a prior anteroapical infarction, but endocardial mapping showed only a small area of scar. Percutaneous epicardial mapping and ablation was performed after extensive endocardial mapping. Low-voltage areas are indicated in red, and purple areas indicate normal voltage. The border zone is at the edge of the red area, and electrically unexcitable areas are indicated with gray dots. In this case, distinguishing epicardial fat (likely to be seen in a typical peri-coronary distribution, for example, at the mustard dot and overlying the RV) from myocardial scar was exceedingly challenging. (*B*) The induced VT with low amplitude mid-diastolic fractionated signals on the distal ablation catheter. (*C*) Entrainment of the tachycardia at a cycle length of 460 milliseconds, with a postpacing interval of 510 milliseconds and tachycardia cycle length of 490 milliseconds. Ablation at this site terminated the tachycardia (*D*).

and it is desirable to limit infusion of fluid into the pericardial space. It is important to periodically drain the pericardial space after every few RF applications or every 15 to 20 minutes to avoid accumulation of pericardial fluid from the irrigant. Ablation with irrigated RF typically renders the pacing threshold at the target area greater than 10 mA.

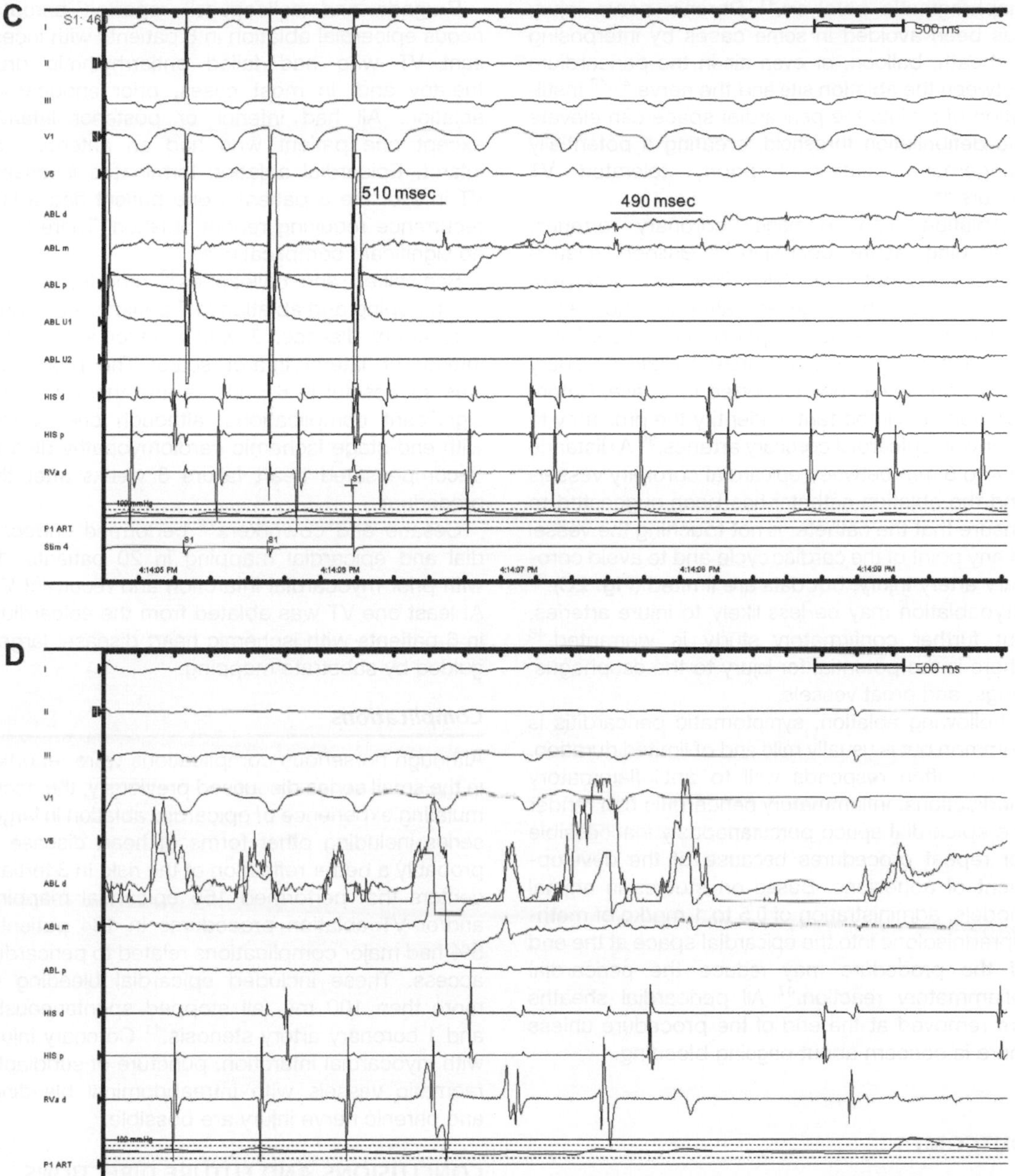

Fig. 3. *(continued)*

Freezing with a cryoablation catheter also is feasible, but there is limited data regarding efficacy. Absence of circulating blood should favor creation of cryolesions while it impairs creation of RF ablation lesions, but more study is needed to assess safety and efficacy. Surgical cryoablation with handheld operating room probes achieves much lower temperatures (<−150°C) and generates larger lesions than small electrophysiology catheters. Cryoablation is the authors' modality of choice in the operating room.

Several precautions are important to avoid injury to adjacent structures. Over the lateral LV, pacing should be used to identify phrenic nerve capture, indicating where ablation might cause diaphragmatic paralysis.[41] Phrenic nerve injury has been avoided in some cases by interposing a sheath, balloon, or even air in the pericardium between the ablation site and the nerve.[42,43] Instillation of air into the pericardial space can elevate the defibrillation threshold, creating a potentially dangerous situation if poorly tolerated VT occurs.[44]

Ablation can damage coronary arteries, producing acute occlusion.[45] Balloon dilation alone does not reestablish flow and emergent stenting may be required, although no reflow phenomena have been reported in 1 case. Injury to the coronary wall may lead to late coronary occlusion, as has been reported in 1 case. Before ablation, it is important to identify the proximity to overlying epicardial coronary arteries.[39] A distance of 4 to 5 mm between epicardial coronary vessels and the ablation catheter has been suggested to ensure that the catheter is not touching the vessel at any point of the cardiac cycle and to avoid coronary artery injury, but data are limited (**Fig. 2**C).[39] Cryoablation may be less likely to injure arteries, but further confirmatory study is warranted.[46] There is the potential for injury to the esophagus, lungs, and great vessels.

Following ablation, symptomatic pericarditis is common but is usually mild and of limited duration, and it often responds well to antiinflammatory medications. Inflammatory pericarditis can render the epicardial space percutaneously inaccessible for repeat procedures because of the development of adhesions. Based on studies in animal models, administration of 0.5 to 1 mg/kg of methylprednisolone into the epicardial space at the end of the procedure may reduce the pericardial inflammatory reaction.[47] All pericardial sheaths are removed at the end of the procedure unless there is concern about ongoing bleeding.

OUTCOMES

Published outcome data is limited to small case series of selected patients. Sosa and colleagues[12] performed epicardial mapping in 14 consecutive patients with recurrent sustained monomorphic VT due to prior inferior wall myocardial infarction. Of 30 induced VTs mapping was performed in 18; 7 were interrupted with epicardial ablation (39% of all mappable VTs) and 3 were interrupted by endocardial ablation. Both epicardial and endocardial ablation failed for 8 VTs, suggesting an intramural origin. None of the 7 VTs that were ablated from the epicardium recurred during a mean follow-up of 14 months. There were no significant complications.

Brugada and colleagues[6] reported percutaneous epicardial ablation in 8 patients with incessant VT who had failed antiarrhythmic drug therapy and, in most cases, prior endocardial ablation. All had inferior or posterior infarcts except one patient who had an anterior wall infarct. Epicardial ablation terminated incessant VT in 7 of the 8 patients; one patient had a late recurrence requiring repeat ablation. There were no significant complications.

Schweikert and colleagues[48] reported epicardial mapping and ablation in 7 patients with coronary artery disease, 3 with anterior and 4 with inferior or lateral infarct scars. The procedure was successful in 6 patients and there were no significant complications, although one patient with end-stage ischemic cardiomyopathy died of decompensated heart failure 6 weeks after the procedure.

Cesario and coworkers[19] performed endocardial and epicardial mapping in 20 patients, 12 with prior myocardial infarction and recurrent VT. At least one VT was ablated from the epicardium in 6 patients with ischemic heart disease, largely guided by substrate mapping.

Complications

Although no serious complications were reported in the small series discussed previously, the accumulating experience of epicardial ablation in larger series including other forms of heart disease is probably a better reflection of the risk. In 3 tertiary centers that performed 156 epicardial mapping and/or VT ablation procedures in 134 patients, 5% had major complications related to pericardial access. These included epicardial bleeding of more than 100 mL (all stopped spontaneously) and 1 coronary artery stenosis.[11] Coronary injury with myocardial infarction, puncture of subdiaphragmatic vessels with intraabdominal bleeding, and phrenic nerve injury are possible.[5]

CONCLUSIONS AND FUTURE DIRECTIONS

Percutaneous epicardial catheter techniques expand the options for investigating and treating arrhythmias in patients with ischemic heart disease. Epicardial catheter mapping and ablation are increasingly common in tertiary centers, providing an option that can be life-saving when endocardial ablation is not adequate to control the arrhythmia. The prevalence of epicardial reentry circuits in patients with coronary artery disease and monomorphic VT is not yet clear, but it is probably between 5% and 15% depending on infarct location and greater in patients who have already failed an endocardial ablation attempt. Although safety and outcomes appear acceptable, it should be recognized that available information is from experience in tertiary centers.

Several advances are needed. Better methods for assessing coronary artery location and risk of injury would be welcome. Epicardial mapping in combination with endocardial mapping does not render all scar-related VTs accessible for catheter ablation. Tachycardia circuits can originate intramurally or from deep within the ventricular septum and may require transcoronary ethanol ablation or future irrigated needle catheters. Ablation can be limited by epicardial fat and proximity to coronary arteries and other structures, even when the arrhythmia originates from the epicardium. Methods of better characterizing epicardial fat distribution in patients undergoing epicardial VT ablation need to be developed.

Correlation of epicardial with endocardial data could lead to new insights into transmural myocardial properties influencing repolarization and arrhythmogenesis, facilitating better understanding and treatment of arrhythmias from body surface recordings. Minimally invasive surgical techniques also need to evolve to facilitate electrophysiologic investigation of the epicardium.

REFERENCES

1. Moss AJ, Greenberg H, Case RB, et al. Long-term clinical course of patients after termination of ventricular tachyarrhythmia by an implanted defibrillator. Circulation 2004;110(25):3760–5.
2. Schron EB, Exner DV, Yao Q, et al. Quality of life in the antiarrhythmics versus implantable defibrillators trial: impact of therapy and influence of adverse symptoms and defibrillator shocks. Circulation 2002;105(5):589–94.
3. Poole JE, Johnson GW, Hellkamp AS, et al. Prognostic importance of defibrillator shocks in patients with heart failure. N Engl J Med 2008;359(10): 1009–17.
4. Reddy VY, Reynolds MR, Neuzil P, et al. Prophylactic catheter ablation for the prevention of defibrillator therapy. N Engl J Med 2007;357(26):2657–65.
5. Aliot EM, Stevenson WG, Almendral-Garrote JM, et al. EHRA/HRS Expert Consensus on Catheter Ablation of Ventricular Arrhythmias: developed in a partnership with the European Heart Rhythm Association (EHRA), a Registered Branch of the European Society of Cardiology (ESC), and the Heart Rhythm Society (HRS); in collaboration with the American College of Cardiology (ACC) and the American Heart Association (AHA). Heart Rhythm 2009;6(6):886–933.
6. Brugada J, Berruezo A, Cuesta A, et al. Nonsurgical transthoracic epicardial radiofrequency ablation: an alternative in incessant ventricular tachycardia. J Am Coll Cardiol 2003;41(11):2036–43.
7. Svenson RH, Littmann L, Colavita PG, et al. Laser photoablation of ventricular tachycardia: correlation of diastolic activation times and photoablation effects on cycle length and termination–observations supporting a macroreentrant mechanism. J Am Coll Cardiol 1992;19(3):607–13.
8. Sosa E, Scanavacca M, d'Avila A, et al. A new technique to perform epicardial mapping in the electrophysiology laboratory. J Cardiovasc Electrophysiol 1996;7(6):531–6.
9. Tedrow U, Stevenson WG. Strategies for epicardial mapping and ablation of ventricular tachycardia. J Cardiovasc Electrophysiol 2009;20(6):710–3.
10. Roberts-Thomson KC, Seiler J, Steven D, et al. Percutaneous access of the epicardial space for mapping ventricular and supraventricular arrhythmias in patients with and without prior cardiac surgery. J Cardiovasc Electrophysiol 2009. [Epub ahead of print].
11. Sacher F, Roberts-Thomson K, Maury P, et al. Epicardial VT ablation: a multicenter safety study. in press.
12. Sosa E, Scanavacca M, d'Avila A, et al. Nonsurgical transthoracic epicardial catheter ablation to treat recurrent ventricular tachycardia occurring late after myocardial infarction. J Am Coll Cardiol 2000;35(6): 1442–9.
13. d'Avila A, Houghtaling C, Gutierrez P, et al. Catheter ablation of ventricular epicardial tissue: a comparison of standard and cooled-tip radiofrequency energy. Circulation 2004;109(19):2363–9.
14. Sosa E, Scanavacca M, D'Avila A, et al. Nonsurgical transthoracic epicardial approach in patients with ventricular tachycardia and previous cardiac surgery. J Interv Card Electrophysiol 2004;10(3): 281–8.
15. Berruezo A, Mont L, Nava S, et al. Electrocardiographic recognition of the epicardial origin of ventricular tachycardias. Circulation 2004;109(15): 1842–7.
16. d'Avila A. Epicardial catheter ablation of ventricular tachycardia. Heart Rhythm 2008;5(Suppl 6): S73–5.
17. Soejima K, Couper G, Cooper JM, et al. Subxiphoid surgical approach for epicardial catheter-based mapping and ablation in patients with prior cardiac surgery or difficult pericardial access. Circulation 2004;110(10):1197–201.
18. Page PL, Cardinal R, Shenasa M, et al. Surgical treatment of ventricular tachycardia. Regional cryoablation guided by computerized epicardial and endocardial mapping. Circulation 1989;80(3 Pt 1): I124–34.
19. Cesario DA, Vaseghi M, Boyle NG, et al. Value of high-density endocardial and epicardial mapping for

catheter ablation of hemodynamically unstable ventricular tachycardia. Heart Rhythm 2006;3(1):1–10.
20. Verma A, Marrouche NF, Schweikert RA, et al. Relationship between successful ablation sites and the scar border zone defined by substrate mapping for ventricular tachycardia post-myocardial infarction. J Cardiovasc Electrophysiol 2005; 16(5):465–71.
21. Stevenson WG. Functional approach to site-by-site catheter mapping of ventricular reentry circuits in chronic infarctions. J Electrocardiol 1994; 27(Suppl):130–8.
22. de Bakker JM, van Capelle FJ, Janse MJ, et al. Slow conduction in the infarcted human heart. 'Zigzag' course of activation. Circulation 1993; 88(3):915–26.
23. Marchlinski FE, Zado E, Dixit S, et al. Electroanatomic substrate and outcome of catheter ablative therapy for ventricular tachycardia in setting of right ventricular cardiomyopathy. Circulation 2004; 110(16):2293–8.
24. Soejima K, Suzuki M, Maisel WH, et al. Catheter ablation in patients with multiple and unstable ventricular tachycardias after myocardial infarction: short ablation lines guided by reentry circuit isthmuses and sinus rhythm mapping. Circulation 2001;104(6):664–9.
25. Soejima K, Stevenson WG, Sapp JL, et al. Endocardial and epicardial radiofrequency ablation of ventricular tachycardia associated with dilated cardiomyopathy: the importance of low-voltage scars. J Am Coll Cardiol 2004;43(10):1834–42.
26. de Chillou C, Lacroix D, Klug D, et al. Isthmus characteristics of reentrant ventricular tachycardia after myocardial infarction. Circulation 2002; 105(6):726–31.
27. Marchlinski FE, Callans DJ, Gottlieb CD, et al. Linear ablation lesions for control of unmappable ventricular tachycardia in patients with ischemic and nonischemic cardiomyopathy. Circulation 2000;101(11): 1288–96.
28. Klemm HU, Ventura R, Steven D, et al. Catheter ablation of multiple ventricular tachycardias after myocardial infarction guided by combined contact and noncontact mapping. Circulation 2007; 115(21):2697–704.
29. Soejima K, Stevenson WG, Maisel WH, et al. Electrically unexcitable scar mapping based on pacing threshold for identification of the reentry circuit isthmus: feasibility for guiding ventricular tachycardia ablation. Circulation 2002;106(13): 1678–83.
30. Della Bella P, Riva S, Fassini G, et al. Incidence and significance of pleomorphism in patients with postmyocardial infarction ventricular tachycardia. Acute and long-term outcome of radiofrequency catheter ablation. Eur Heart J 2004;25(13):1127–38.
31. Bogun F, Li YG, Groenefeld G, et al. Prevalence of a shared isthmus in postinfarction patients with pleiomorphic, hemodynamically tolerated ventricular tachycardias. J Cardiovasc Electrophysiol 2002; 13(3):237–41.
32. Delacretaz E, Stevenson WG. Catheter ablation of ventricular tachycardia in patients with coronary heart disease: part I: mapping. Pacing Clin Electrophysiol 2001;24(8 Pt 1):1261–77.
33. Bogun F, Kim HM, Han J, et al. Comparison of mapping criteria for hemodynamically tolerated, postinfarction ventricular tachycardia. Heart Rhythm 2006;3(1):20–6.
34. El-Shalakany A, Hadjis T, Papageorgiou P, et al. Entrainment/mapping criteria for the prediction of termination of ventricular tachycardia by single radiofrequency lesion in patients with coronary artery disease. Circulation 1999;99(17):2283–9.
35. Bogun F, Good E, Han J, et al. Mechanical interruption of postinfarction ventricular tachycardia as a guide for catheter ablation. Heart Rhythm 2005; 2(7):687–91.
36. Soejima K, Delacretaz E, Suzuki M, et al. Saline-cooled versus standard radiofrequency catheter ablation for infarct-related ventricular tachycardias. Circulation 2001;103(14):1858–62.
37. Reddy VY, Wrobleski D, Houghtaling C, et al. Combined epicardial and endocardial electroanatomic mapping in a porcine model of healed myocardial infarction. Circulation 2003;107(25): 3236–42.
38. Dixit S, Narula N, Callans DJ, et al. Electroanatomic mapping of human heart: epicardial fat can mimic scar. J Cardiovasc Electrophysiol 2003; 14(10):1128.
39. D'Avila A, Gutierrez P, Scanavacca M, et al. Effects of radiofrequency pulses delivered in the vicinity of the coronary arteries: implications for nonsurgical transthoracic epicardial catheter ablation to treat ventricular tachycardia. Pacing Clin Electrophysiol 2002;25(10):1488–95.
40. Cano O, Hutchinson M, Lin D, et al. Electroanatomic substrate and ablation outcome for suspected epicardial ventricular tachycardia in left ventricular nonischemic cardiomyopathy. J Am Coll Cardiol 2009;54(9):799–808.
41. Fan R, Cano O, Ho SY, et al. Characterization of the phrenic nerve course within the epicardial substrate of patients with nonischemic cardiomyopathy and ventricular tachycardia. Heart Rhythm 2009;6(1): 59–64.
42. Matsuo S, Jais P, Knecht S, et al. Images in cardiovascular medicine. Novel technique to prevent left

phrenic nerve injury during epicardial catheter ablation. Circulation 2008;117(22):e471.
43. Buch E, Vaseghi M, Cesario DA, et al. A novel method for preventing phrenic nerve injury during catheter ablation. Heart Rhythm 2007;4(1):95–8.
44. Yamada T, McElderry HT, Platonov M, et al. Aspirated air in the pericardial space during epicardial catheterization may elevate the defibrillation threshold. Int J Cardiol 2009;135(1):e34–5.
45. Roberts-Thomson K, Steven D, Seiler J, et al. Coronary artery injury due to catheter ablation in adults: presentations and outcomes. Circulation 2009; 120(15):1465–73.
46. Lustgarten DL, Bell S, Hardin N, et al. Safety and efficacy of epicardial cryoablation in a canine model. Heart Rhythm 2005;2(1):82–90.
47. d'Avila A, Neuzil P, Thiagalingam A, et al. Experimental efficacy of pericardial instillation of anti-inflammatory agents during percutaneous epicardial catheter ablation to prevent postprocedure pericarditis. J Cardiovasc Electrophysiol 2007;18(11):1178–83.
48. Schweikert RA, Saliba WI, Tomassoni G, et al. Percutaneous pericardial instrumentation for endo-epicardial mapping of previously failed ablations. Circulation 2003;108(11):1329–35.

Epicardial Ablation of Idiopathic Ventricular Tachycardia

Alexander I. Green, MD*, David J. Wilber, MD

KEYWORDS

- Arrhythmia • Ventricular tachycardia
- Ablation • Epicardium

Idiopathic ventricular tachycardia (VT) describes ventricular arrhythmias in the absence of structural heart disease. Most idiopathic VT originates from the right ventricular (RV) outflow tract (OT) in close proximity to the pulmonic valve. However, idiopathic VT may arise from other right ventricular sites, including the pulmonary artery[1,2] and tricuspid annulus,[3] and left ventricular sites, predominately the left ventricular (LV) outflow tract (OT). VT from the aortic sinus cusps (ASC)[4] and the epicardium (EPI) remote from the ASCs has been increasingly reported. In the authors' experience, approximately 10% of patients referred for ablation of ventricular arrhythmias have an epicardial focus. As with typical RVOT VT, radiofrequency ablation (RFA) of EPI-VT is a safe and effective means of treating these arrhythmias.

ELECTROPHYSIOLOGICAL CHARACTERISTICS

Idiopathic VT arising from the RVOT and LVOT shares a common mechanism consistent with cyclic adenosine monophosphate (cAMP)-mediated triggered activity,[5] despite varied clinical presentations of sustained VT, bursts of nonsustained monomorphic VT, or frequent premature ventricular contractions (PVCs).[6] Characteristic findings of triggered arrhythmias include inability to entrain VT, catecholamine enhancement, and termination with adenosine. In the authors' initial experience, they noted catecholaminergic facilitation of sustained VT in 11 of 12 patients and termination of tachycardia with adenosine in 8 of 9 patients. Stellbrink and colleagues[7] also reported a case of EPI-VT terminated with adenosine. These findings support triggered activity as the mechanism of EPI-VT. Unique to EPI-VT, however, is the apparent perivascular origin of tachycardia, which has been widely reported.[8–11] Although atrial fibrillation is often associated with the musculature of the thoracic veins and the ligament of Marshall, the anterior interventricular vein (AIV) and distal great cardiac vein (GCV) from which EPI-VT frequently arises do not have a muscular coat. The proximal coronary sinus, a few millimeters proximal to the GCV, and the proximal middle cardiac vein (MCV) have a muscular coat and are reported, albeit infrequent, sites of origin for EPI-VT.[12] The media of the coronary veins do contain myocytes derived from primitive right atrial cells, but their role in the genesis of VT has not been well elucidated.[13] Further research is needed to clarify the mechanistic relationship between EPI-VT and the coronary veins.

ELECTROCARDIOGRAPHIC ANALYSIS

Analysis of the surface electrocardiogram (ECG) remains the first method of VT localization and is invaluable in planning an ablation strategy. EPI-VT most often originates from the anterior summit of the heart at the AIV, distal GCV, or AIV-GCV junction. As such, a left bundle branch

Department of Cardiology, Cardiovascular Institute, Loyola University Medical Center, 2160 South First Avenue, Maywood, IL 60153, USA
* Corresponding author.
E-mail address: aigreen1075@yahoo.com (A.I. Green).

Card Electrophysiol Clin 2 (2010) 81–91
doi:10.1016/j.ccep.2009.11.006
1877-9182/10/$ – see front matter

block (LBBB) inferior axis QRS morphology grossly similar to RVOT VT is frequently observed. EPI-VT originating from the MCV or proximal coronary sinus may have a right bundle branch block (RBBB) or LBBB and superior axis morphology, and it must be distinguished from inferior mitral annular or posterior papillary muscle VT.

Algorithms for localization of VT within the outflow tracts have relied on several criteria, none of which reliably identifies EPI-VT. The precordial transition is defined by the precordial lead in which the R/S ratio is greater than or equal to 1. Tanner and colleagues[14] described 3 different ablation approaches for patients in whom the precordial transition was observed in V_3 including ablation from the epicardium, RVOT, and LVOT. A late transition greater than or equal to V_4 is observed exclusively in RVOT VT.[15,16] An S wave in leads V_5 and V_6 is reported to distinguish endocardial LVOT VT from foci above the aortic valve.[17] However, more proximal coronary venous foci, including MCV EPI-VT, may inscribe a V_6 S wave.[7,11] A prominent S wave in lead I may be observed in anteroseptal RVOT VT, ASC-VT, and EPI-VT.[14,18–20] Ouyang and colleagues[21] proposed the R/S amplitude index greater than or equal to 0.3 and the R-wave duration index greater than or equal to 0.5 in leads V_1 or V_2 to identify ASC-VT, but these criteria are typically met for most left ventricular VTs, including EPI-VT.[15] In the authors' experience, however, some EPI-VT foci in the distal AIV and AIV-GCV junction may not satisfy either precordial R wave criteria and may be virtually indistinguishable from RVOT VT. A Q-wave ratio of leads aVL to aVR greater than 1.4 and an S-wave amplitude in V_1 greater than or equal to 1.2mV may distinguish EPI-VT from ASC-VT when the precordial R-wave indices are met. These criteria are derived in part from pace-mapping studies performed from the AIV-GCV junction, and extrapolation to all EPI-VT may not be justified.[19] The authors have seen one patient with EPI-VT in whom the V_1 S wave was greater than 1.2mV, but the precordial R-wave indices were not fulfilled. In their patients, no statistically significant difference was observed in the Q-wave ratio of aVL to aVR between EPI-VT and ASC-VT, although a larger value was observed for ASC-VT, contradicting previously reported data (1.13 ± 0.34 vs 1.48 ± 1.70, $P = .3$).[19]

In their laboratory, the authors apply the metric of the maximum deflection index (MDI) to identify EPI-VT.[22] It is calculated as follows. The QRS duration is measured as the interval between the earliest rapid deflection of the ventricular complex in any of the simultaneous leads to the latest offset in any lead. Time to maximum deflection is measured from the onset of the QRS complex to the maximum deflection in each of the precordial leads; the timing of the maximum deflection is at the largest amplitude deflection above or below the isoelectric line. The time to maximum deflection is divided by the QRS duration to obtain the MDI for each precordial lead (**Fig. 1**). The earliest precordial maximum deflection (shortest precordial MDI) is used to classify the tracing. In the authors' initial experience, an MDI of 0.55 or greater was identified as the optimal cutoff point for the detection of EPI-VT remote from the ASCs.[22] When applied to their current data set of 240 cases of idiopathic VT, the earliest precordial MDI remains a reasonable discriminator of EPI-VT (sensitivity 79.1%, specificity 93.3%). Ventricular arrhythmias arising from the pulmonary artery (PA) or ASCs represent the greatest number of false-positives, although occasionally, a prolonged MDI may be observed in VT of right ventricular endocardial origin (**Fig. 2**).

Additional ECG criteria have been proposed for identification of EPI-VT in the setting of ischemic or nonischemic cardiomyopathy[23,24] but appear to be less useful in patients with idiopathic VT.

Future directions for the noninvasive localization of EPI-VT may include electrocardiographic imaging (ECGi). ECGi uses 250 electrodes to record body-surface potentials in conjunction with a heart-torso computed tomography registration to construct epicardial activation and repolarization and to permit construction of virtual epicardial electrograms. An exclusively negative QS complex without an initial R wave in virtual electrograms at the site of origin may signify an epicardial focus. However, experience with ECGi imaging for idiopathic VT is limited,[25,26] and further experience will be required to validate this concept.

CATHETER ABLATION

Patients with a prolonged MDI on the surface ECG and those in whom prior comprehensive endocardial mapping and ablation were unsuccessful are the most likely to have an epicardial origin of VT. In these patients, the authors find it useful to place a 3.5F, 16-pole microwire with 2-6-2–mm spacing (Pathfinder; Cardima Inc, Fremont, CA, USA) through the coronary sinus and position it to span the distal GCV, AIV-GCV junction, and distal AIV at the start of the study (**Fig. 3**B). This region represents the most common origin of idiopathic epicardial VT with an inferior axis. For patients with a high probability of an epicardial origin whose limb-lead axis is superior, the microwire is best positioned in the middle cardiac vein. An electrogram to QRS onset in the microwire of

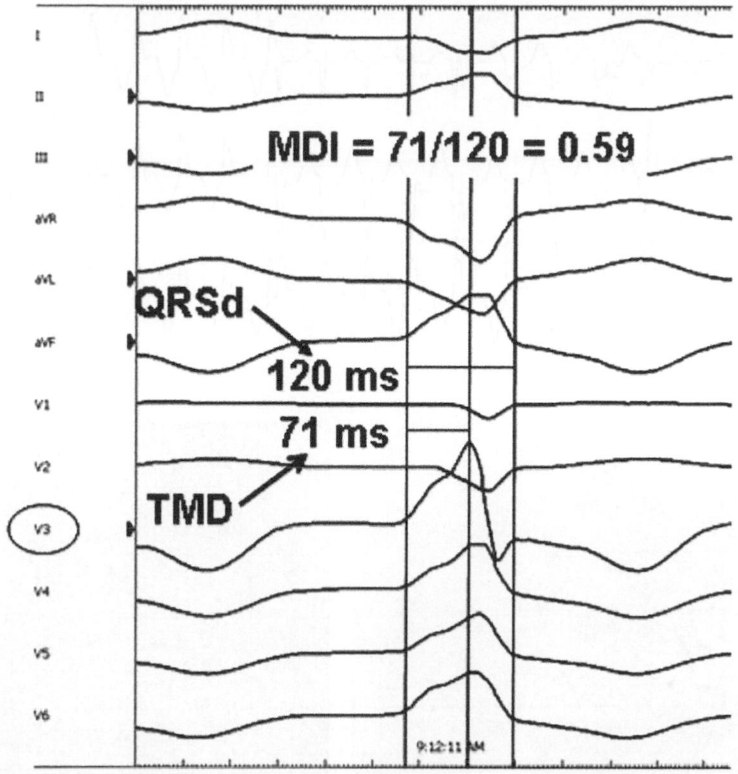

Fig. 1. Calculation of the MDI. The earliest time to maximum deflection (TMD) in any of the precordial leads (in this example, lead V3) is measured and divided by total QRS duration (QRSd). (Reprinted with permission).

approximately 35 to 40 milliseconds pre-QRS suggests an epicardial focus and permits a more focused and efficient approach to mapping. However, to confirm the epicardium as the earliest activation site before ablation, the coronary venous activation must still be carefully compared with activation in the ASC, RV, PA, and LV endocardium for inferior axis VTs and with the RV and LV endocardium for superior axis VTs. When the suspicion of an epicardial origin is high and the

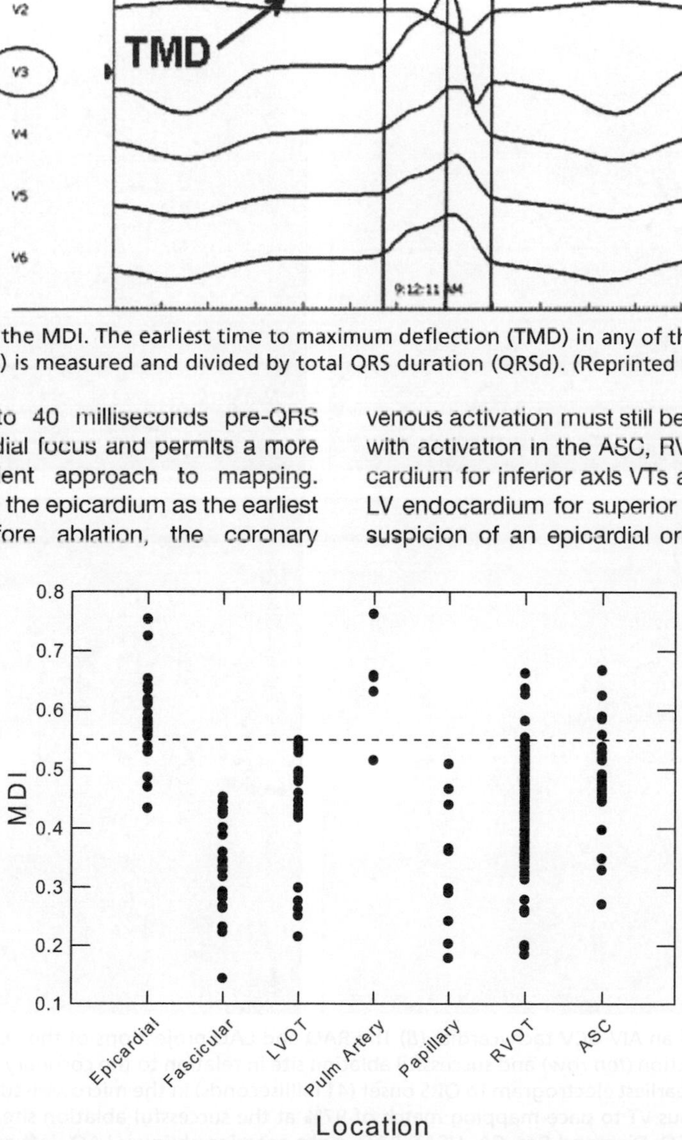

Fig. 2. The distribution of values for MDI for the different anatomic locations. The dashed line demarcates an MDI of 0.55.

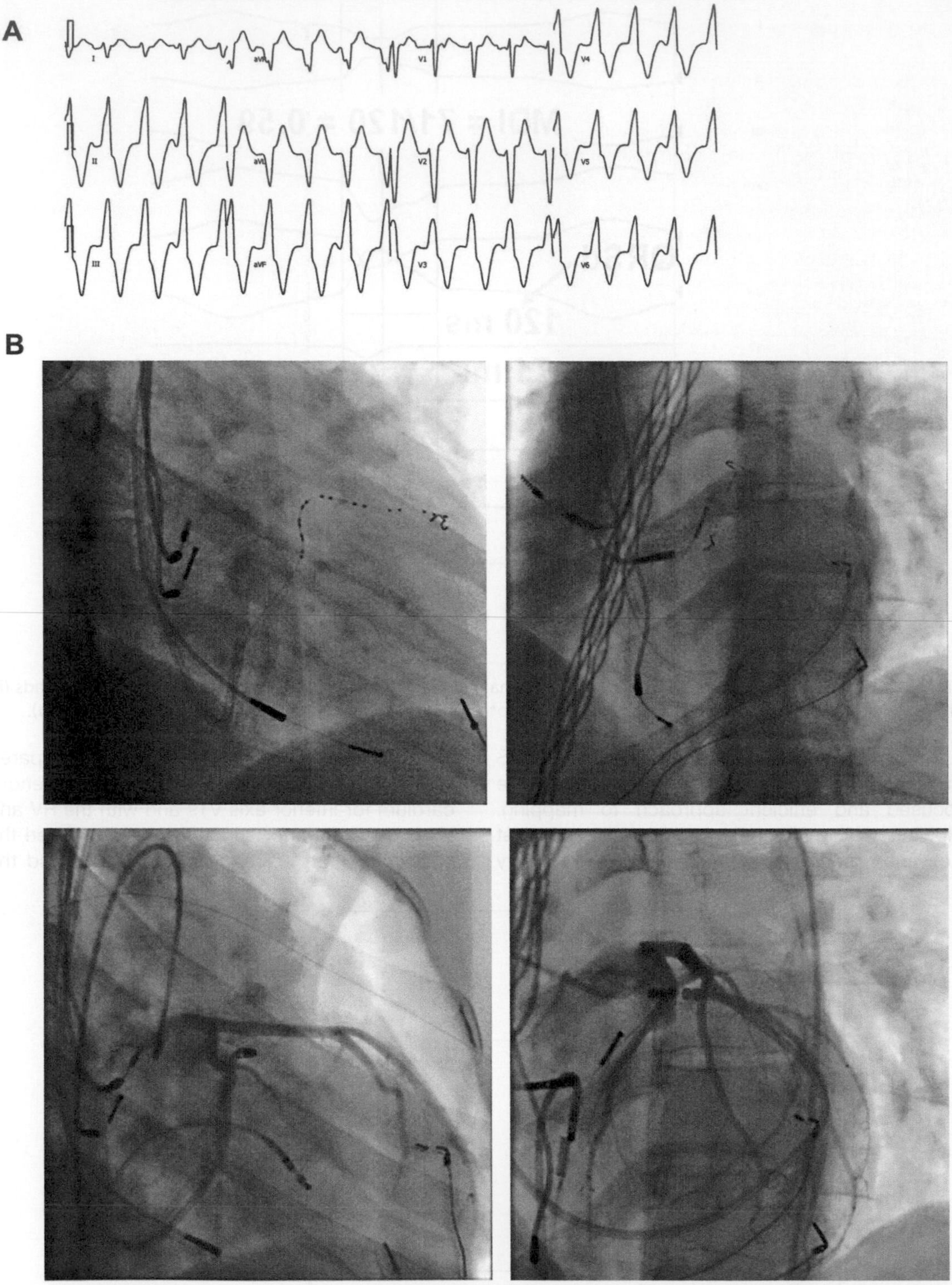

Fig. 3. (*A*) The ECG of an AIV-GCV tachycardia. (*B*) The RAO and LAO projections of the 16-pole microwire spanning the AIV-GCV junction (*top row*) and successful ablation site in relation to the coronary arteries (*bottom row*). (*C*) The timing of the earliest electrogram to QRS onset (41 milliseconds) in the microwire suggesting an epicardial origin. (*D*) Spontaneous VT to pace-mapping match of 97% at the successful ablation site with the use of automated software (PASSO, Diamond Bar, CA, USA). RAO, right anterior oblique; LAO, left anterior oblique.

C

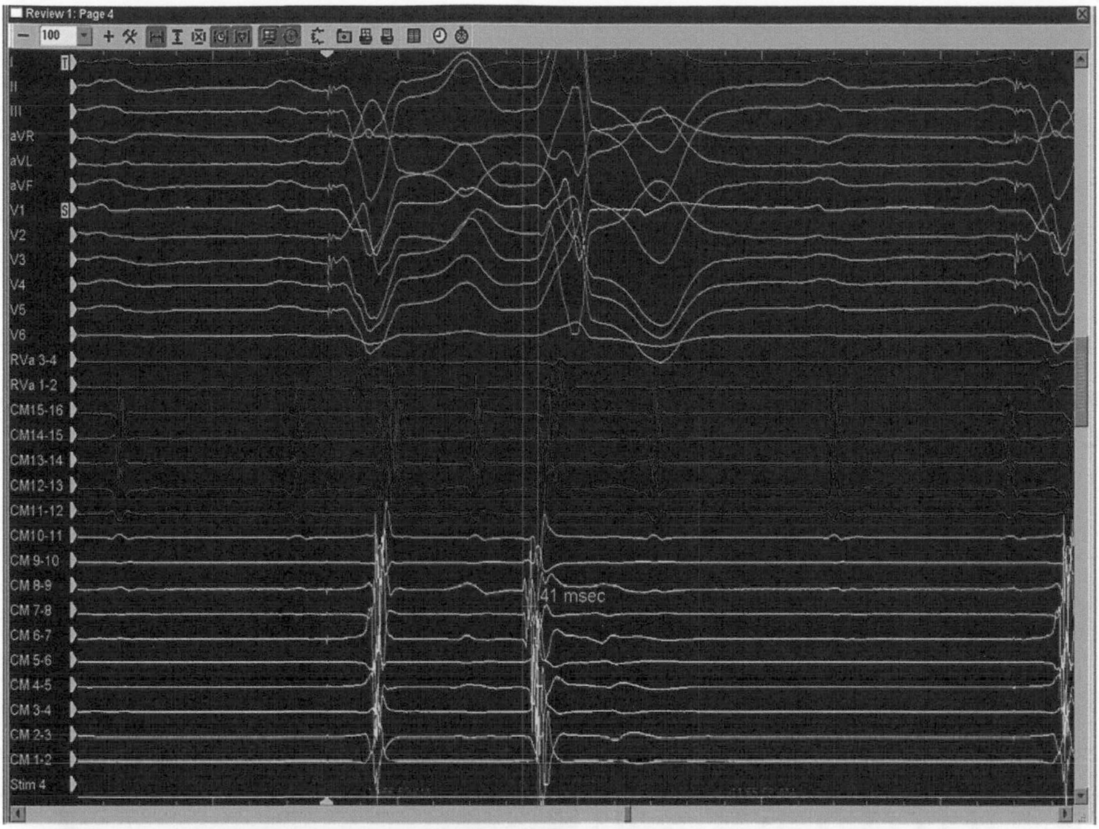

D

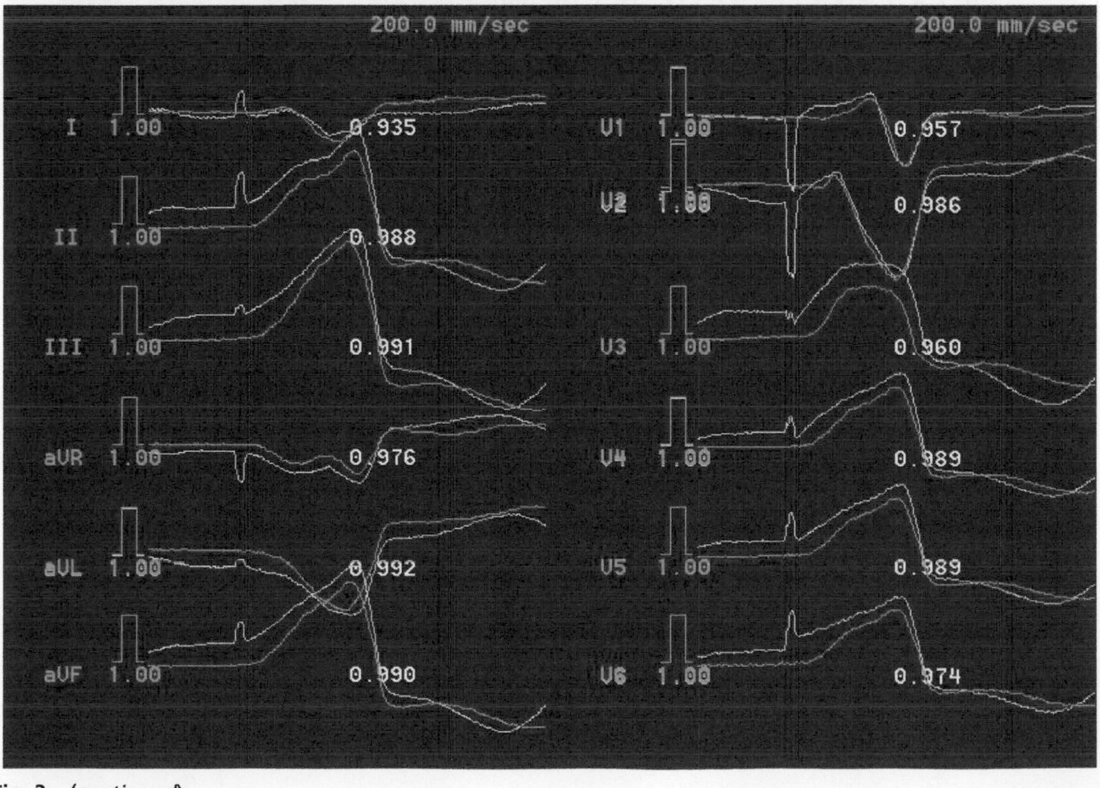

Fig. 3. *(continued)*

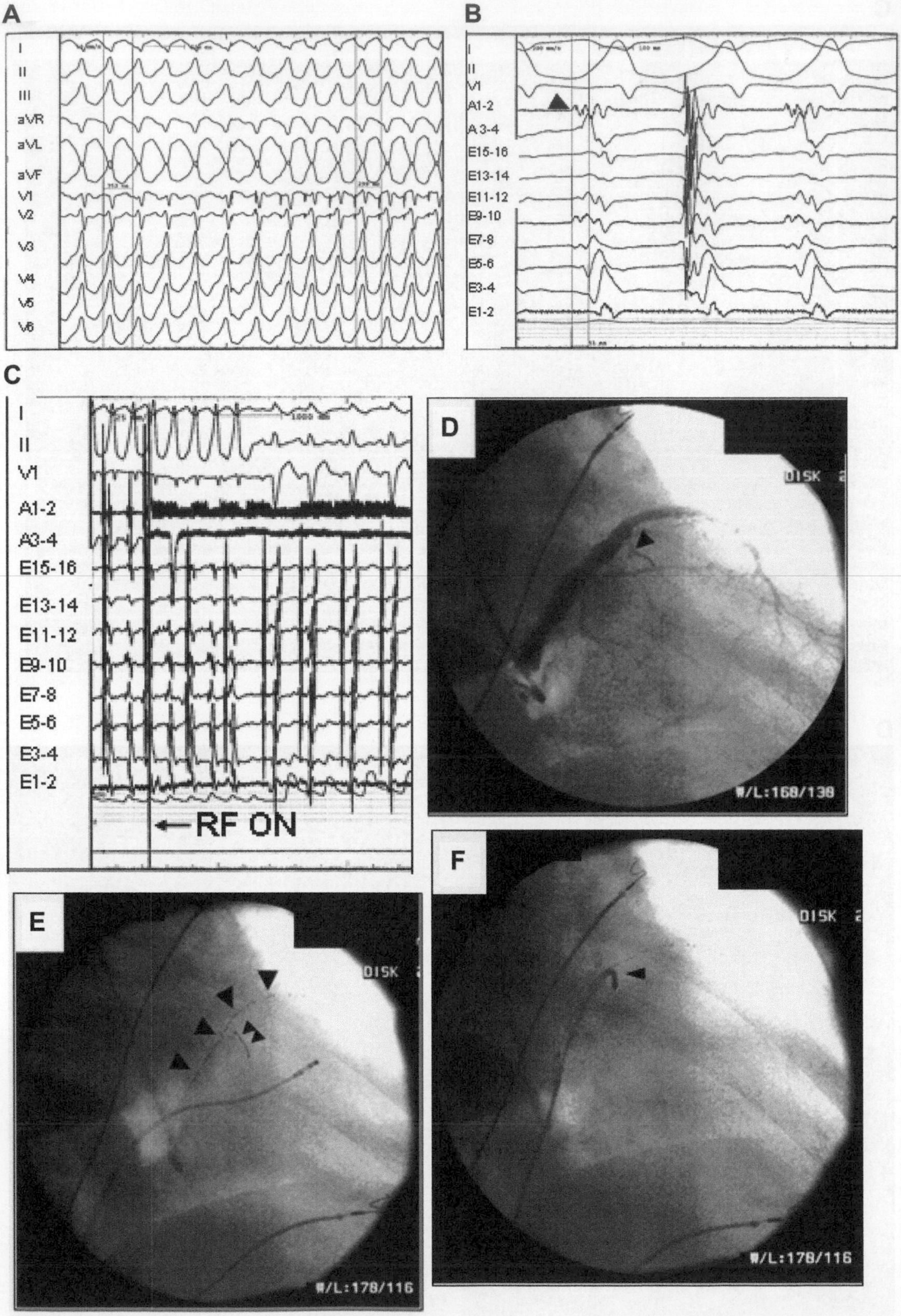

Fig. 2 (continued).

authors anticipate a subxyphoid approach, this is generally performed before the administration of heparin and mapping of the left ventricle and aortic root. Once epicardial access is obtained, the patient may be given heparin to achieve an activated clotting time of 250 milliseconds or greater.

An epicardial origin is confirmed via a combination of multichamber electroanatomic mapping and pace mapping, the latter being particularly valuable when there is little spontaneous ventricular ectopy. However, caution should be exercised in proceeding with epicardial ablation based on pace mapping alone in the absence of confirmatory activation mapping. Pace mapping has, at best, modest spatial resolution, and pacing over a fairly large area (up to 2–3 cm^2) may produce excellent pace-map matches.[27,28] These studies address pace mapping as a means of localizing RVOT-VT and may not apply directly to EPI-VT. The authors have occasionally observed excellent pace-map matches from the epicardium or ASC in sites successfully ablated from the endocardium, and vice versa, pace mapping from the epicardium and ASCs frequently requires pacing at high outputs that may influence the QRS morphology. Finally, the absence of noninducibility or abolition of spontaneous arrhythmias as a procedural endpoint is suboptimal. It is therefore the authors' practice to make vigorous attempts to reproduce the clinical arrhythmia (stimulation from multiple sites and use of intravenous isoproterenol, epinephrine, or phenylephrine) for activation mapping, and to use pace mapping predominantly as a corroborative measure. Phenylephrine is particularly useful for long-coupled PVCs and bradycardia-dependent arrhythmias.

Catheter ablation of EPI-VT may be attempted via 2 different approaches. The first approach is to map the coronary sinus and its tributaries. Given the perivenous origin of most idiopathic EPI-VT, ablation from within the veins may be successful, although maximum delivery of power with 4-mm electrodes may not exceed 15 to 20 W. The use of irrigated tip catheters to improve power delivery in the coronary sinus may be reasonable before a subxiphoid approach. It has been recommended by some investigators that a maximum of 20 W be used in the coronary veins to limit the risk of coronary injury or hemopericardium.[9] The tortuosity, angulation, and small caliber of the coronary veins often limits successful navigation to the site of origin. The distal GCV and AIV-GCV junction run parallel with the proximal circumflex coronary artery and the distal AIV, with the left anterior descending artery. For this reason, angiography should be performed before and following ablation. **Figs. 3** and **4** demonstrate examples of transvenous ablation of EPI-VT from the AIV-GCV junction and more proximal GCV.

When venous mapping and ablation are unable to eliminate VT, direct pericardial access is accomplished by a subxiphoid approach as described by Sosa and colleagues.[29] Patients with EPI-VT and structurally normal hearts in whom prior sternotomy has been performed may require a combined approach of surgical subxiphoid epicardial exposure. Even then, dense adhesion may limit access to the anterior, superior epicardial surface.[30] Ablation in the pericardial space carries important limitations in the delivery of adequate power as compared with the endocardial surface. Specifically, the lack of convective cooling of the ablation electrode by the blood and the relatively thick layer of adipose tissue that often overlays the perivenous VT foci may hamper ablation attempts. In animal models, d'Avila and colleagues[31] demonstrated that standard RFA produced significant lesions (3.7 ± 1.2 mm thick) on epicardial tissue without an interposing adipose layer, but they were unable to produce myocardial lesions when applied to normal tissue with epicardial fat (3.1 ± 1.2 mm thick). However, the use of cooled-tip RFA in a closed chest animal model resulted in appreciable myocardial lesions (4.07 ± 2 mm depth) when applied to tissue with overlying fat (2.6 ± 1.2 mm thick). The volume of epicardial fat has been correlated to visceral adiposity, increased body mass index, female gender, and increased age. Cardiovascular magnetic resonance imaging and multi-detector computed tomography to

Fig. 4. (*A, B*) Surface ECG and intracardiac electrograms from a patient with VT from the distal great cardiac vein. (*A*) The left half of the panel demonstrates the 12-lead ECG during tachycardia. Note the slight irregularity of cycle length. Pacing from the ablation site (*right half of panel*) results in an exact match of QRS morphology in all 12 leads. (*B*) Recordings from the distal bipole of the ablation catheter (*arrowhead*) and bipolar pairs of the venous epicardial mapping catheter in the GCV. Activation at this site is 53 milliseconds before QRS onset. (*C*) Termination of VT in 2 seconds after onset of radiofrequency energy application of 5 W and a temperature of 60°C. (*D*) Occlusive venogram demonstrating the coronary sinus and proximal GCV. There is a small marginal vein with a takeoff from the proximal GCV (*small arrowhead*). (*E*) RAO radiographs of coronary venous mapping. Multipolar microcatheters in the GCV (*large arrowheads*) and marginal branch (*small arrowheads*) are demonstrated. (*F*) 6F 4-mm electrode catheter positioned in the proximal portion of the marginal branch at the site of successful VT ablation (*small arrowhead*).

quantify the distribution and thickness of epicardial adipose tissue may prove beneficial in planning epicardial procedures.[32,33]

Thermal injury to adjacent coronary vessels with the potential for acute thrombosis or future stenosis is important to consider during ablation. In addition to applied power, the main factors predicting coronary injury are the distance from the ablation catheter to the arterial wall and the size of the arterial vessel. It has been empirically recommended that ablation within 5 to 10 mm of a coronary vessel be avoided. Animal studies have demonstrated that standard RFA within approximately 0.3 mm of the arterial wall has the potential to cause intravascular thrombosis or significant intimal hyperplasia, whereas RFA delivered from distances greater than 0.3 mm may cause replacement of the arterial media with extracellular matrix.[34] The long-term consequences of the latter are unknown, and extrapolation to patients should be made with caution. Additionally, these studies were not performed with irrigated tip catheters where greater lesion size may be achieved. It is the authors' practice to perform coronary angiography before ablation to assess the proximity of the coronary arteries. Ablation is then performed with initially low power and titration of power, with careful attention paid to hemodynamic stability and the ST segments for any evidence of acute elevation or depression suggestive of myocardial injury. A repeat angiogram is performed within 30 minutes following ablation. The overall risk of coronary injury is estimated at less than 1%. Intracoronary irrigation with chilled saline has been proposed as a mechanism for reducing the risk of heat-related coronary injury, although this maneuver has not been widely adopted in clinical practice.[35]

Ablation within the epicardial space can also cause phrenic nerve injury, and high output pacing to identify phrenic capture is advisable to avoid this complication. A recent cadaveric study demonstrated that the phrenic nerve may run in an anterior course parallel to the anterior interventricular within 4 mm of the left main coronary artery.[36,37] This highlights the proximity of the AIV-GCV junction to the pericardiophrenic neurovascular bundle. Several strategies, including the infusion of saline or air into the pericardial space or the use of large-diameter balloons to "lift" the nerve from the epicardial surface, have been proposed to avoid phrenic nerve injury. The introduction of a combination of air and saline to create an iatrogenic "hydropneumopericardium" has also been proposed.[36]

In the authors' experience, an epicardial approach is useful in 3 different clinical scenarios (**Table 1**). The first was in 21 patients (mean age 39 years, range 11–74 years) with 22 tachycardias that were perivenous in origin typical of those previously reported. In this population, the earliest epicardial local activation times (42 ± 5 milliseconds) significantly preceded endocardial activation times (22 ± 5 milliseconds). In patients in whom VT was localized to the AIV or AIV-GCV junction, local activation times in the ASCs were significantly later than those recorded from the epicardium (13 ± 18 milliseconds). Ablation was successful in the elimination of 17 of 22 ventricular arrhythmias via a coronary venous approach in 8 cases, percutaneous epicardial approach in 7, and open surgical approach in 2. In 5 patients, the elimination of VT was ultimately unsuccessful. One patient refused a percutaneous epicardial approach following failed ablation via a coronary venous approach. In one patient, the left main coronary artery and AIV-GCV junction were too closely approximated to allow safe RFA. Phrenic nerve capture limited ablation in one patient. The authors were unable to access the pericardial space in one patient; however, the PVC burden on subsequent ambulatory monitoring was less than 1% off all antiarrhythmic medications despite ectopy at the end of the procedure. The last patient had persistent ectopy following transpericardial ablation despite the use of an irrigated tip catheter and cryoablation.

Table 1
Location of ablation sites for idiopathic epicardial VT (N=30)

I. Epicardial sites adjacent to the coronary vasculature	
a. Proximal AIV	6
b. AIV-GCV junction	9
c. GCV	4
d. MCV	3
II. Intramural sites	
a. Anterobasal left ventricle	5
b. Base of the papillary muscle	2
III. Other	
Tricuspid annular	1

The second scenario in which epicardial ablation has a role is in patients with an apparent intramural ectopic focus. These sites were usually not intimately associated with the coronary vasculature. The authors performed ablation of 7 VT morphologies in 7 patients (mean age 29 years, range 14–53 years). The distribution of VT was the anterior base of the left ventricle in 5 patients and the base of the papillary muscle in 2 patients

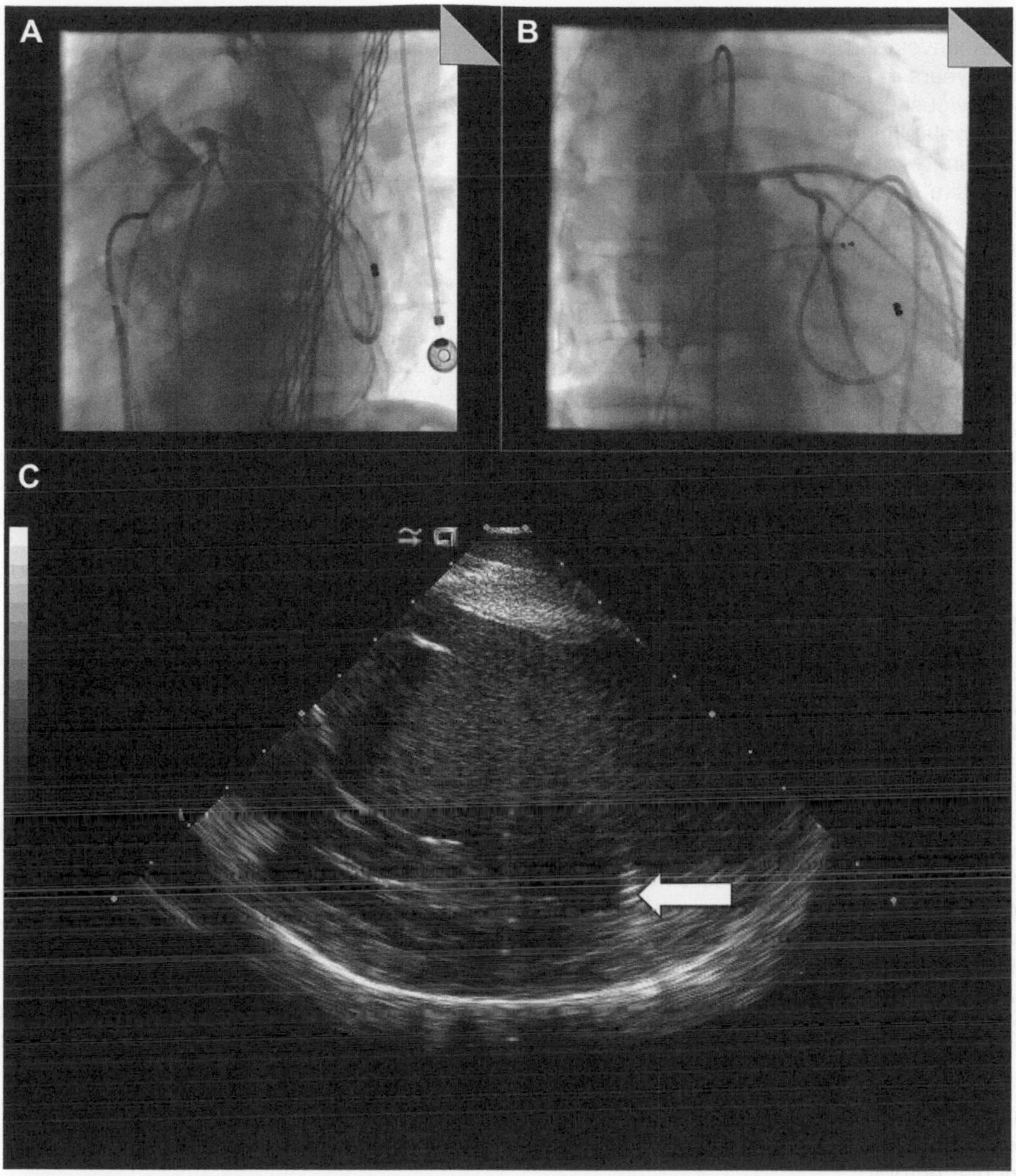

Fig. 5. Radiographs (*A*) and (*B*) demonstrate the epicardial catheter position in relation to the coronary arteries before ablation in a patient with intramural VT localized to the base of the anterolateral papillary muscle. (*C*) The intracardiac echocardiogram demonstrated the ablation catheter tip (*large, white arrow*) at the base of the papillary muscle.

(**Fig. 5**). The earliest local activation times from the epicardial and endocardium were nearly equal and within 10 milliseconds of each other (38 $\pm$ 4 milliseconds EPI vs 35 $\pm$ 7 milliseconds endocardium). In each case, ablation at the site with the earliest time (either epicardial or endocardial) was not successful. The authors' ablation approach was to "sandwich" the putative VT focus via a combined endocardial and epicardial approach. Ablation was successful in 3 of 5 patients ablated at anterobasal LV sites and both patients with papillary muscle VT. The latter 2 patients were part of 10 patients with idiopathic papillary muscle VT undergoing ablation at the authors' institution. Prior reports on idiopathic papillary muscle VT have not described this approach.[36]

In a final patient, VT originated from the superior lateral aspect of the right ventricle, adjacent to the tricuspid annulus. This VT was reentrant as determined by entrainment and originated from a small region of epicardial low voltage. The patient had undergone an extensive and repeated workup for arrhythmogenic right ventricular cardiomyopathy and has developed no other task force criteria during 5 years of follow-up.

As previously mentioned, the authors routinely perform preablation angiography to demonstrate the proximity of the coronary arteries to the planned site of ablation and perform high-output pacing to document the presence of absence of phrenic nerve capture. During ablation, they limit their power settings to 20 to 30 W in the coronary veins, but up to 50 W may be required on the epicardial surface at sites remote from epicardial vasculature. During coronary venous ablation, standard RFA catheters are often unable to effectively deliver power, necessitating the use of an irrigated tip catheter. When ablating from the epicardium via a subxyphoid approach, the authors typically use irrigated tip catheter ablation from the outset.

SUMMARY

Epicardial VT is an increasingly recognized arrhythmia in clinical practice. ECG algorithms to identify epicardial VT should be used with the understanding that they are an initial guide to localization and do not exclude an epicardial origin of VT, particularly when endocardial approaches are unsuccessful. Ablation using a transvenous approach or direct epicardial access may produce favorable results, although care must be taken to avoid coronary artery or phrenic nerve injury. A subset of patients require a combined endocardial and epicardial approach to eliminate VT. Although these ablation strategies are generally well tolerated, they should be limited to patients with highly symptomatic arrhythmias or those in whom myocardial depression is thought to be related to prolonged tachycardia or repetitive ventricular ectopy.

REFERENCES

1. Sekiguchi Y, Aonuma K, Takahashi A, et al. Electrocardiographic and electrophysiologic characteristics of ventricular tachycardia originating within the pulmonary artery. J Am Coll Cardiol 2005;45(6): 887–95.
2. Tada H, Tadokoro K, Miyaji K, et al. Idiopathic ventricular arrhythmias arising from the pulmonary artery: prevalence, characteristics, and topography of the arrhythmia origin. Heart Rhythm 2008;5(3): 419–26.
3. Tada H, Tadokoro K, Ito S, et al. Idiopathic ventricular arrhythmias originating from the tricuspid annulus: prevalence, electrocardiographic characteristics, and results of radiofrequency catheter ablation. Heart Rhythm 2007;4(1):7–16.
4. Kanagaratnam L, Tomassoni G, Schweikert R, et al. Ventricular tachycardias arising from the aortic sinus of valsalva: an under-recognized variant of left outflow tract ventricular tachycardia. J Am Coll Cardiol 2001;37(5):1408–14.
5. Iwai S, Cantillon DJ, Kim RJ, et al. Right and left ventricular outflow tract tachycardias: evidence for a common electrophysiologic mechanism. J Cardiovasc Electrophysiol 2006;17(10):1052–8.
6. Kim RJ, Iwai S, Markowitz SM, et al. Clinical and electrophysiological spectrum of idiopathic ventricular outflow tract arrhythmias. J Am Coll Cardiol 2007;49(20):2035–43.
7. Stellbrink C, Diem B, Schauerte P, et al. Transcoronary venous radiofrequency catheter ablation of ventricular tachycardia. J Cardiovasc Electrophysiol 1997;8(8):916–21.
8. Meininger GR, Berger RD. Idiopathic ventricular tachycardia originating in the great cardiac vein. Heart Rhythm 2006;3(4):464–6.
9. Obel OA, d'Avila A, Neuzil P, et al. Ablation of left ventricular epicardial outflow tract tachycardia from the distal great cardiac vein. J Am Coll Cardiol 2006;48(9):1813–7.
10. Wright M, Hocini M, Ho SY, et al. Epicardial ablation of left ventricular outflow tract tachycardia via the coronary sinus. Heart Rhythm 2009;6(2): 290–1.
11. Doppalapudi H, Yamada T, Ramaswamy K, et al. Idiopathic focal epicardial ventricular tachycardia originating from the crux of the heart. Heart Rhythm 2009;6(1):44–50.
12. von Ludinghausen M. The venous drainage of the human myocardium. Adv Anat Embryol Cell Biol 2003;168:1–104.
13. Vrancken Peeters MP, Gittenberger-de Groot AC, Mentink MM, et al. Differences in development of coronary arteries and veins. Cardiovasc Res 1997; 36(1):101–10.
14. Tanner H, Hindricks G, Schirdewahn P, et al. Outflow tract tachycardia with R/S transition in lead V3: Six different anatomic approaches for successful ablation. J Am Coll Cardiol 2005; 45(3):418–23.
15. Ito S, Tada H, Naito S, et al. Development and validation of an ECG algorithm for identifying the optimal ablation site for idiopathic ventricular outflow tract tachycardia. J Cardiovasc Electrophysiol 2003; 14(12):1280–6.
16. Tanner H, Wolber T, Schwick N, et al. Electrocardiographic pattern as a guide for management and radiofrequency ablation of idiopathic ventricular tachycardia. Cardiology 2005;103(1):30–6.
17. Hachiya H, Aonuma K, Yamauchi Y, et al. How to diagnose, locate, and ablate coronary cusp

ventricular tachycardia. J Cardiovasc Electrophysiol 2002;13(6):551–6.
18. Wilber DJ, Baerman J, Olshansky B, et al. Adenosine-sensitive ventricular tachycardia. clinical characteristics and response to catheter ablation. Circulation 1993;87(1):126–34.
19. Tada H, Nogami A, Naito S, et al. Left ventricular epicardial outflow tract tachycardia: A new distinct subgroup of outflow tract tachycardia. Jpn Circ J 2001;65(8):723–30.
20. Kaseno K, Tada H, Tanaka S, et al. Successful catheter ablation of left ventricular epicardial tachycardia originating from the great cardiac vein: a case report and review of the literature. Circ J 2007;71(12):1983–8.
21. Ouyang F, Fotuhi P, Ho SY, et al. Repetitive monomorphic ventricular tachycardia originating from the aortic sinus cusp: electrocardiographic characterization for guiding catheter ablation. J Am Coll Cardiol 2002;39(3):500–8.
22. Daniels DV, Lu YY, Morton JB, et al. Idiopathic epicardial left ventricular tachycardia originating remote from the sinus of valsalva: electrophysiological characteristics, catheter ablation, and identification from the 12-lead electrocardiogram. Circulation 2006;113(13):1659–66.
23. Bazan V, Gerstenfeld EP, Garcia FC, et al. Site-specific twelve-lead ECG features to identify an epicardial origin for left ventricular tachycardia in the absence of myocardial infarction. Heart Rhythm 2007;4(11):1403–10.
24. Berruezo A, Mont L, Nava S, et al. Electrocardiographic recognition of the epicardial origin of ventricular tachycardias. Circulation 2004;109(15):1842–7.
25. Intini A, Goldstein RN, Jia P, et al. Electrocardiographic imaging (ECGI), a novel diagnostic modality used for mapping of focal left ventricular tachycardia in a young athlete. Heart Rhythm 2005;2(11):1250–2.
26. Green A, Brysiewicz N, Finn C, et al. Preliminary experience with noninvasive electrocardiographic imaging in patients with idiopathic ventricular tachycardia [abstract]. Circulation 2008;118:S985.
27. Azegami K, Wilber DJ, Arruda M, et al. Spatial resolution of pacemapping and activation mapping in patients with idiopathic right ventricular outflow tract tachycardia. J Cardiovasc Electrophysiol 2005; 16(8):823–9.
28. Bogun F, Taj M, Ting M, et al. Spatial resolution of pace mapping of idiopathic ventricular tachycardia/ectopy originating in the right ventricular outflow tract. Heart Rhythm 2008;5(3):339–44.
29. Sosa E, Scanavacca M, d'Avila A, et al. A new technique to perform epicardial mapping in the electrophysiology laboratory. J Cardiovasc Electrophysiol 1996;7(6):531–6.
30. Soejima K, Couper G, Cooper JM, et al. Subxiphoid surgical approach for epicardial catheter-based mapping and ablation in patients with prior cardiac surgery or difficult pericardial access. Circulation 2004;110(10):1197–201.
31. d'Avila A, Houghtaling C, Gutierrez P, et al. Catheter ablation of ventricular epicardial tissue: A comparison of standard and cooled-tip radiofrequency energy. Circulation 2004;109(19):2363–9.
32. Abbara S, Desai JC, Cury RC, et al. Mapping epicardial fat with multi-detector computed tomography to facilitate percutaneous transepicardial arrhythmia ablation. Eur J Radiol 2006;57(3):417–22.
33. Sarin S, Wenger C, Marwaha A, et al. Clinical significance of epicardial fat measured using cardiac multislice computed tomography. Am J Cardiol 2008;102(6):767–71.
34. D'Avila A, Gutierrez P, Scanavacca M, et al. Effects of radiofrequency pulses delivered in the vicinity of the coronary arteries: Implications for nonsurgical transthoracic epicardial catheter ablation to treat ventricular tachycardia. Pacing Clin Electrophysiol 2002;25(10):1488–95.
35. Thyer IA, Kovoor P, Barry MA, et al. Protection of the coronary arteries during epicardial radiofrequency ablation with intracoronary chilled saline irrigation: assessment in an in vitro model. J Cardiovasc Electrophysiol 2006;17(5):544–9.
36. Di Biase L, Burkhardt JD, Pelargonio G, et al. Prevention of phrenic nerve injury during epicardial ablation: comparison of methods for separating the phrenic nerve from the epicardial surface. Heart Rhythm 2009;6(7):957–61.
37. Good E, Desjardins B, Oral H, et al. Ventricular arrhythmias originating from a papillary muscle in patients without prior infarction: a comparison with fascicular arrhythmias. Heart Rhythm 2008;5: 1530–7.

Epicardial Ablation of VT in Patients with Nonischemic LV Cardiomyopathy

Mathew D. Hutchinson, MD*, Francis E. Marchlinski, MD

KEYWORDS

- Ventricular tachycardia • Radiofrequency ablation
- Left ventricular cardiomyopathy • Epicardial ablation

Despite considerable investigation and clinical experience, the ablation of ventricular tachycardia (VT) in patients with nonischemic left ventricular (LV) cardiomyopathy (CM) remains a significant challenge. These patients were historically treated in the context of experience with postinfarction VT, with an approach centered on endocardial mapping and ablation. Several observations have greatly enhanced our understanding of the LVCM VT substrate distribution and disease mechanism, and the advent of percutaneous epicardial mapping and ablation strategies have greatly improved procedural outcomes. Nevertheless several stumbling blocks still confound the treatment of this increasingly prevalent patient population.

This article reviews the ablative approach to VT in LVCM, focusing on epicardial mapping and ablation. Specific topics addressed include:

- Epidemiology and prevalence of VT
- Common substrate distribution
- VT electrocardiographic (ECG) morphology and mechanism
- Mapping and ablative techniques
- Common pitfalls.

EPIDEMIOLOGY

Despite remarkable progress in the treatment of coronary heart disease and modifiable cardiac risk factors, the incidence of sudden cardiac death (SCD) continues to increase.[1] This may be partly due to the increased prevalence of noncoronary heart disease. The dominant clinical risk factor for SCD in patients with LVCM is depressed LV ejection fraction (EF).[2] Despite the prognostic importance of LVEF, more than two-thirds of sudden deaths occur in the absence of known cardiac disease.[3] Thus, the use of adjunctive risk assessment tools in selected patients with only modestly impaired LV function may help identify patients at risk of SCD without traditional indications for device therapy. Some of these tests include microvolt T-wave alternans, signal-averaged ECG, QRS duration, and myocardial imaging.[4–7] For example, the ongoing Defibrillators to Reduce Risk by Magnetic Resonance Imaging Evaluation (DETERMINE) trial is assessing the value of myocardial scar burden as measured by magnetic resonance imaging (MRI) for predicting SCD risk.[8]

Patients with LVCM and depressed LVEF have a high prevalence of frequent premature ventricular contractions (PVCs) and nonsustained VT.[9–11] In the absence of sustained arrhythmias, the routine use of electrophysiologic study (EPS) as a risk stratification technique in patients with LVCM is not recommended. However, patients presenting with sustained VT have a high rate of inducibility during EPS.[12,13]

Disclosures: Mathew D. Hutchinson MD and Francis E. Marchlinski have participated in clinical research protocols for ventricular tachycardia ablation sponsored by Biosense Webster that are unrelated to the content of this article. Mathew D. Hutchinson receives modest lecture honoraria from Siemens Acuson.

Cardiovascular Division, Department of Medicine, University of Pennsylvania, 9 Founders Pavilion, The Hospital of the University of Pennsylvania, 3400 Spruce Street, Philadelphia, PA 19104, USA
* Corresponding author.
E-mail address: Mathew.Hutchinson@uphs.upenn.edu (M.D. Hutchinson).

Card Electrophysiol Clin 2 (2010) 93–103
doi:10.1016/j.ccep.2009.11.007

Most patients referred for VT ablation present with frequent implantable cardioverter defibrillator (ICD) shocks. In addition to the obvious psychological effect on the patient, the presence of recurrent ICD therapies is associated with significantly increased mortality and worsening heart failure symptoms.[14,15] Patients receiving an ICD for secondary prevention of sudden death have a high rate of recurrent arrhythmias, up to 68% at 12 months.[16] In contrast, the large primary prevention trials that enrolled patients with nonischemic LVCM (ie, Sudden Cardiac Death in Heart Failure trial [SCD-HeFT], DEFINITE, and Comparison of Medical Therapy, Pacing, and Defibrillation in Heart Failure [COMPANION]) revealed the annualized incidence of appropriate ICD therapies at 5% to 7.4%.[2,17,18] Patients with LVCM presenting with syncope have a substantially higher rate of sustained VT/ventricular fibrillation; 2 retrospective studies estimated the annualized incidence of appropriate ICD therapies in this group at 23%.[19,20] The Optimal Pharmacological Therapy in Implantable Cardioverter Defibrillator Patients (OPTIC) study showed a significant reduction in ICD shocks with amiodarone (28% absolute reduction at 12 months); however, the drug was discontinued in nearly one-fifth of patients because of excessive side effects.[21]

Although the relative efficacy of ablation compared with drug therapy has not been tested, most patients referred for VT ablation have failed multiple antiarrhythmic drug trials. Several studies have demonstrated a dramatic reduction in ICD therapies after ablation in patients with structural heart disease presenting with either tolerated or hemodynamically unstable VT.[22–25]

SUBSTRATE CHARACTERISTICS IN PATIENTS WITH VT AND NONISCHEMIC LVCM

Characteristics of Endocardial Electrogram

The hallmark feature of abnormal myocardium in patients with structural heart disease is bipolar voltage attenuation. The authors' group previously explained that with detailed mapping, the mean bipolar LV electrogram amplitude in normal ventricles is 4.8 ± 3.1 mV, with 95% of normal LV recordings having a bipolar voltage greater than 1.55 mV.[26] Patients with structural heart disease presenting with VT commonly have fractionated electrograms (EGMs) representing nonuniform activation within scar and late potentials representing delayed activation within the relatively insulated scar tissue. The original description of endocardial mapping in patients with structural heart disease by Cassidy and colleagues[27] found strikingly different bipolar EGM characteristics in LVCM versus postinfarction patients. In ischemic and nonischemic patients, abnormal bipolar EGMs were found within the scar boundary; however abnormal EGMs (defined as amplitude less than 3.0 mV, fractionated or late potentials) were seen significantly more frequently in postinfarction patients when compared with nonischemic patients with LVCM (43 ± 21 vs 15 ± 18%, *P*<.001). Patients with nonischemic LVCM in this series who presented with sustained VT had significantly more abnormal endocardial EGM sites compared with those without VT (37 ± 27 vs 13 ± 7%, *P*<.01).

Electroanatomic Mapping

The consistency in substrate distribution for the spectrum of diseases comprising the common clinical phenotype of nonischemic LV cardiomyopathy is remarkable. The initial experience of the authors' group with LV endocardial electroanatomic mapping in 19 Patients with LVCM found a uniform pattern of abnormal tissue characteristics (defined as bipolar amplitude <1.8 mV) extending from the mitral annulus in all 19 patients; apical involvement was uncommon in this cohort (1 of 19, 5.2%) (**Fig. 1**).[22] The substrate distribution differs fundamentally from patients with prior infarction, whose low-voltage abnormality subtends a coronary arterial distribution. The mean surface area of the abnormal substrate region was 41 ± 28 cm^2; this represented less than 25% of the total endocardial surface area in 14 of 19 patients. The presence of dense endocardial scar (defined as bipolar amplitude <0.5 mV) was also unusual in these patients, comprising only 27 ± 20% of the total low-voltage region.

Epicardial Substrate

Early reports of poor outcomes with endocardial VT ablation in patients with nonischemic cardiomyopathy have spurred investigation into the importance of epicardial substrate abnormalities in patients with nonischemic LVCM.[22,23,28,29] The development of percutaneous epicardial access and mapping techniques by Sosa and colleagues[30] has allowed these procedures to be performed in the electrophysiology (EP) laboratory instead of the operating room. Previous reports of VT ablation in LVCM used epicardial mapping and ablation in a minority of cases, usually in patients with limited endocardial voltage abnormalities or in those whose VT was not suppressed with endocardial ablation.[22,23] Soejima and colleagues[23] were the first to describe improved outcome in 7 patients who underwent combined endocardial and epicardial mapping and ablation.

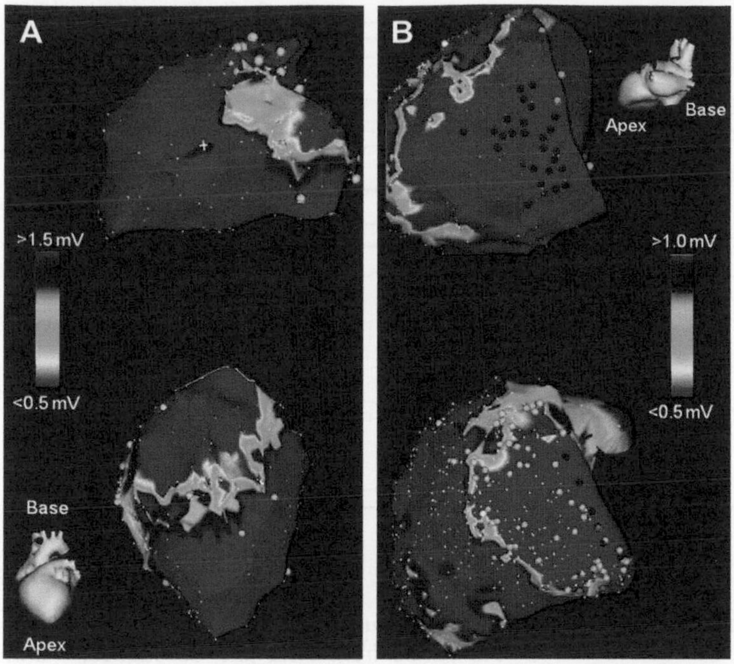

Fig. 1. (*A*) Top and bottom left of panel depicting 2 examples of the common endocardial substrate pattern in LVCM. The low-voltage region defined by the red color originates from the mitral annulus in the vast majority of cases. (*B*) Top and bottom right of panel shows the typical basal lateral epicardial substrate distribution present in 2 different patients with VT and nonischemic LV cardiomyopathy.

The authors' group recently described the epicardial EGM characteristics in 30 patients presenting with VT of suspected epicardial origin.[24] Normal epicardial bipolar voltage was described in 8 patients with structurally normal hearts and idiopathic VT; in these patients, 95% of bipolar signals were greater than 1.0 mV. The idiopathic VT patients also demonstrated a paucity of abnormal electrograms with only 2.2% of signals being wide (>80 milliseconds), 0.9% being split (EGM with 2 or more distinct components and greater than 20-millisecond isoelectric segment between individual components), and none with late potentials. Given the uniform presence of epicardial fat around the coronary vasculature, the regions within 1.5 cm of the coronary vessels (verified by angiography) were excluded from the voltage measurements. These low-voltage areas surrounding the coronary vasculature rarely demonstrated wide, split, or late potentials that are characteristic of the epicardial VT substrate in patients with LVCM.

Compared with the endocardium, the epicardial low-voltage regions in these 22 patients were significantly larger (55.3 ± 33.5 vs 22.9 ± 32.4 cm^2, $P<.01$) and more confluent (82% vs 54%). An average of 49.7% of EGMs sampled from the epicardial low-voltage regions demonstrated signals that were wide, split, or late. The most common epicardial low-voltage region was the basal lateral LV, involving 72% of patients. Patients varied in the degree of apical extension of the basal lateral low-voltage abnormality. In all 12 patients with endocardial confluent low-voltage regions from this series, the regions were located in proximity to the aortic and mitral valve annuli. (see **Fig. 1**) In patients with endocardial and epicardial low-voltage regions, the voltage abnormalities are often adjacent to one another. A minority of patients with LVCM demonstrate scar on only the endocardium or the epicardium, which has important implications when planning an ablation strategy in these patients.

ECG MORPHOLOGY AND MECHANISM OF VT

VT Morphology

The general rule when ablating LVCM-related VT is that frequently there are multiple and often unstable VTs. The typical basal, lateral LV substrate location gives rise to characteristic right bundle, right axis 12-lead ECG morphologies with an early precordial transition (**Fig. 2**). Patients with LVCM presenting with right and left bundle morphologies typically have concomitant LV septal or right ventricular (RV) involvement. Soejima and colleagues[23] found an average of 2.9 ± 17 (range 1–7) distinct VT morphologies per patient; the authors' group found similar results with 3.0 ± 1.0 (range 1–6) morphologies per patient.[22]

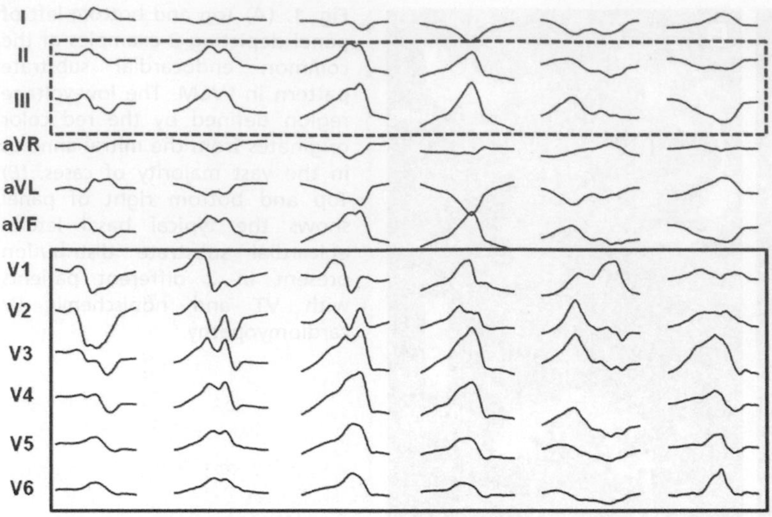

Fig. 2. Six distinct 12-lead ECG VT morphologies obtained at EP study from a 64-year-old man with LVCM. The late precordial transition for the induced VTs (solid box) reveals the typical basal LV exit site for VT in the setting of nonischemic LVCM. The variable frontal plane axis in the inferior leads (dashed box) suggests VT origin from the superior and inferior LV. This pattern of multiple induced VT morphologies with basal exit sites is pathognomonic for nonischemic LVCM.

Identifying an Epicardial VT Origin from the ECG

Several publications have assessed morphologic criteria to predict epicardial VT origin from the 12-lead ECG. Berruezo and colleagues[31] previously reported the following ECG criteria for LV epicardial sites: pseudodelta wave 34 milliseconds or greater, intrinsicoid deflection 85 milliseconds or greater, or precordial RS complex duration 121 milliseconds or greater. These criteria were derived from epicardial pacing in a cohort of patients with predominantly postinfarction VT. When Bazan and colleagues[32] prospectively applied these criteria to a cohort of patients with LVCM; only the intrinsicoid deflection greater than 85 milliseconds was consistently predictive of epicardial VT origin. Bazan and colleagues also noted that the paced QRS complexes were significantly wider from epicardial than from endocardial sites (213 ± 45 milliseconds vs 191 ± 41 milliseconds, $P<.001$). The presence of Q waves in specific leads during VT, which are not present in sinus rhythm, are also suggestive of epicardial VT origin; anterior or anterolateral epicardial LV sites of VT origin are correlated with Q waves in lead I or a QS complex in V_1 or V_2, whereas inferior LV sites are correlated with Q waves in leads II, III, and aVF.[32]

VT Mechanism

The dominant VT mechanism in LVCM is scar-based reentry. In a series of 26 patients with LVCM referred for VT ablation, Delacretaz and colleagues[33] found scar-based reentry present in 62% of patients. From the same study, 19% of patients had bundle-branch or fascicular reentry. In the series from Hsia and colleagues,[22] only 5% of patients had apical endocardial substrate, whereas 12% of induced VTs originated from apical endocardial sites.

The presence of focal VT due to abnormal automaticity or triggered activity is less commonly seen in LVCM (<20% in the series discussed earlier); however, this is probably the dominant mechanism in patients presenting with tachycardia-mediated cardiomyopathy.[34] The most common sites of origin for frequent premature ventricular contractions or VT leading to tachycardia-mediated myopathy are the RV and LV outflow tract regions. Patients presenting with this disease process are important to recognize, because they often have significant decrease in LV size and improvement in function after their arrhythmia is eliminated.[34] Patients with nonischemic cardiomyopathy presenting with an apparent focal endocardial VT mechanism may have an epicardial scar-based reentrant circuit with a focal endocardial breakthrough, giving the appearance of a focal origin (**Fig. 3**).[23]

Reentrant VT in patients with nonischemic LVCM is most commonly initiated with programmed electrical stimulation (PES).[23,33] In patients with tolerated VT, entrainment mapping is the preferred method for elucidating critical components of the arrhythmia circuit. Nonreentrant VT mechanisms are present in up to 20% of patients with LVCM.[33] Arrhythmias due to abnormal automaticity often occur spontaneously and may be incessant. Triggered rhythms may require isoproterenol infusion or burst pacing for induction and are inconsistently initiated with PES.

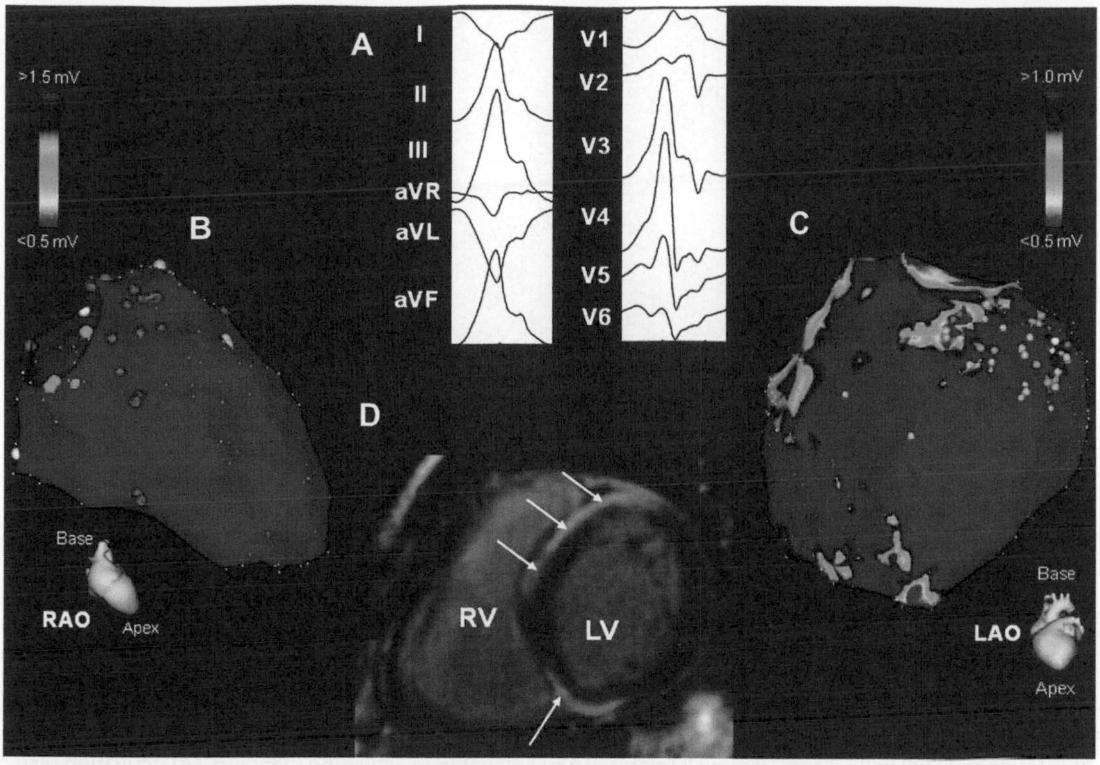

Fig. 3. (*A*) The presenting VT morphology (right bundle, right inferior axis; confidence limit 280 milliseconds) in a 35-year-old man with LVCM. He was taken to the EP laboratory where electroanatomic voltage mapping was performed, which revealed characteristics of normal endocardial (*B*) and epicardial (*C*) electrogram. (*D*) A short-axis MRI from the same patient. The MRI demonstrates a large region of midmyocardial delayed enhancement in the interventricular septum (*arrows*), which extends to the superior and inferior LV surfaces. This case illustrates the limitations of bipolar substrate mapping in patients with complex intramural substrate distributions. RAO, right anterior oblique; LAO, left anterior oblique.

GENERAL PROCEDURAL CONSIDERATIONS

The importance of preprocedural planning in nonischemic LVCM VT ablation cannot be understated. Given the heterogeneity in clinical characteristics of this population, the authors routinely obtain a detailed assessment of each of the following patient characteristics before the ablation procedure: left ventricular function, presence of obstructive coronary stenosis, clinical heart failure status, and presence of aortic or mitral valvular disease and of peripheral or aortic vascular disease. Preprocedural knowledge of potential stumbling blocks, such as impaired LV function, decompensated heart failure, obstructive valvular lesions, or significant vascular disease, may significantly alter the ablation strategy used.

The authors make a considerable effort to obtain all relevant patient imaging data including echocardiograms, computed tomography and MRIs, and coronary angiography. They often use 3-dimensional reconstructions from these datasets to facilitate their ablation procedure. Because of the complexity in substrate distribution in some patients with LVCM, the examination of preacquired tomographic images can alert the operator to the presence of epicardial or midmyocardial scar that may not be seen with endocardial electroanatomic mapping (**Fig. 4**).

The authors routinely use intracardiac echocardiography (ICE) during their LVCM ablation procedures. They have found ICE exceedingly valuable in the identification of VT substrate, the assessment/guidance of lesion creation, and the early detection of complications. They routinely assess the thickness of the basal perivalvular anatomy, the presence of ventricular noncompaction, and the presence of pericardial thickening or epicardial scar; ICE often provides valuable insight into the likelihood of epicardial VT involvement and the potential anatomic barriers to effective ablation. The authors' group has previously described acute tissue swelling and decreased fractional shortening with radial ICE during ablation.[35] They can often visualize similar acute changes during ablation using the phased array catheter. The early

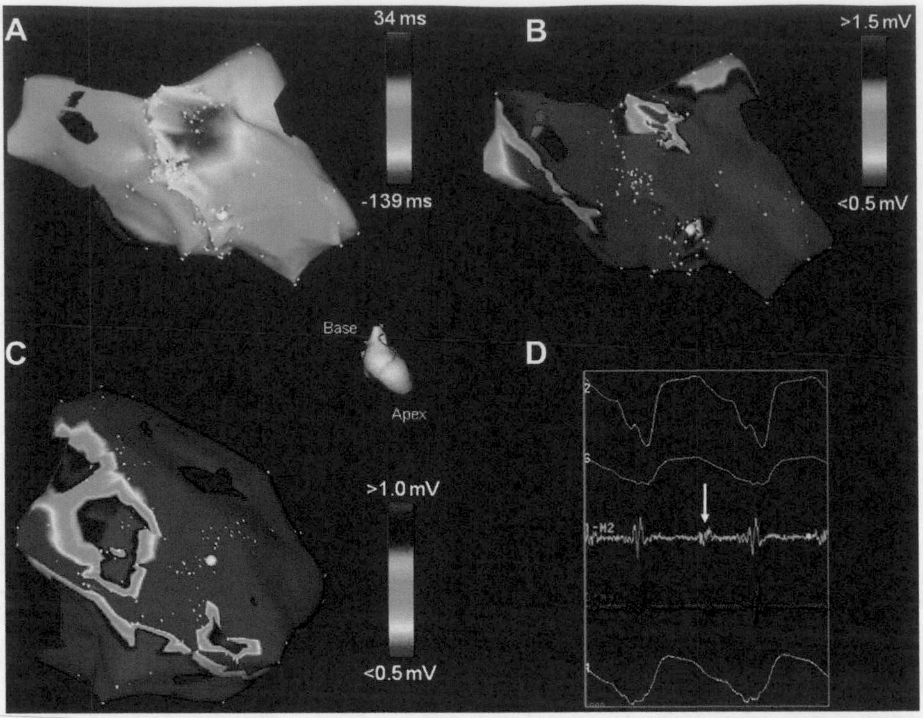

Fig. 4. A 72-year-old man with LVCM presenting with recurrent ICD shocks. The patients clinical VT (left bundle left inferior axis, 360 milliseconds) was well tolerated and amenable to activation mapping. (*A*) Activation map of the LV endocardium reveals diffusely early activation along the superior septal aspect of the LV endocardium. (*B*) A bipolar voltage map that demonstrates an area of low bipolar voltage in the region of the early endocardial activation during VT. Although at first glance, this VT may appear to originate from an area of focal reentry or automaticity from the LV endocardium, subsequent epicardial bipolar mapping (*C*) reveals a large region of low bipolar voltage involving the entire LV free wall with mid-diastolic activation during VT (*D*); location corresponds to white dot on voltage map in (*C*). This case highlights the concept that some VT with a seemingly focal mechanism may actually represent distant breakout of a scar-based, reentrant circuit from an adjacent chamber (in this case, the epicardium).

detection of intracardiac thrombus, pericardial tamponade, and worsening LV systolic function during the ablation procedure allows the operator to rapidly evaluate and treat acute hemodynamic changes and consider lytic therapy for the presence of thrombus.

Sustained VT may not be inducible in selected patients because of excessive sedation, catheter trauma, or recent antiarrhythmic drug administration. In such cases, the site of origin for focal tachycardias or the approximate exit sites for scar-based (reentrant) VTs may be approximated by comparing a paced ECG complex to the 12-lead ECG of the clinical VT. The authors have also found that correlating the stored intracardiac ICD EGMs from the patient's clinical VTs to those induced during EPS allows more efficient targeting of the relevant clinical VT morphologies when 12-lead ECG information is not available. In-hospital telemetry strips or 12-lead ECG reconstructions can also give important information about the morphologic characteristics (ie, bundle branch block pattern, frontal plane axis) and cycle lengths of the patient's arrhythmias. One may also infer the likely VT mechanism (reentrant vs focal) when repetitive VT initiation and termination is available.

PERCUTANEOUS PERICARDIAL PUNCTURE

When approaching patients with LVCM-related VT, one should always anticipate the need to use a combined endocardial and epicardial ablative approach. Specific clues to the presence of epicardial VT circuits include lack of endocardial presystolic activation during VT; late termination of VT with endocardial ablation; specific 12-lead ECG criteria (described earlier); lack of endocardial substrate on electroanatomic mapping; presence of epicardial or midmyocardial substrate on perioperative imaging studies; or failed prior endocardial procedure. Rarely, an endocardial approach may not be possible because of the presence of LV thrombus or prosthetic aortic and mitral valves; early consideration should be given to epicardial mapping and ablation in these settings.

In all VT ablation procedures on patients with nonischemic LVCM, the authors' standard patient setup includes sterile preparation of the subxiphoid region in anticipation of the need for pericardial access. Although pericardial puncture can be performed at any point during the procedure, care must be taken to ensure that previous heparin administration is reversed before access; this is easily accomplished by protamine infusion to decrease the activated clotting time to less than 150 seconds. The authors typically perform pericardial access under general endotracheal anesthesia for patient comfort; this also allows control of spontaneous tidal volumes that can significantly alter the position of the desired puncture target. Excessive respiratory motion can also be limited with transient apnea (suspending mechanical ventilation for up to 30 seconds) or by the use of high-frequency, low–tidal-volume ventilation.

The standard pericardial access technique has been previously described.[30] Potential complications of pericardial access include hemoperi cardium, inadvertent entry into the cardiac chambers, puncture of epicardial coronary vasculature, puncture of abdominal viscera/liver, or subcutaneous vascular laceration. The authors routinely place a nasogastric tube in patients after endotracheal intubation to decompress gastric air insufflation. Given the heterogeneity in the size and position of the left lobe of the liver, which can often cross the patient's midline, their puncture entry location is typically made just to the left of the midline and angled just under the rib margin. They often use biplanar fluoroscopy to guide the needle tip toward the desired puncture site; the right anterior oblique projection facilitates basal/apical orientation and the left anterior oblique projection guides appropriate needle depth. An anterior (over RV free wall) or posterior (inferior cardiac surface) access approach can be used. They commonly use a posterior approach to avoid inadvertent entry into the thin-walled RV. The needle is directed tangentially to the inferior cardiac surface, and an attempt is made to puncture the pericardium over the thicker interventricular septum or inferior LV wall. Contrast medium can also be used to delineate the tissue plane; however overuse of contrast may obscure fluoroscopic landmarks. The authors tend to probe from the needle with a floppy guidewire just after they appear to enter the pericardial space. Multiplanar fluoroscopy is recommended when entering a potential space with the guidewire, because it is often difficult to differentiate between pleural and pericardial access in a single view. Care must be taken to see the guidewire extend over the lateral border of the LV before introducing a vascular sheath. Any 8 or 9F vascular sheath can be inserted; steerable sheaths are useful in selected cases or when pericardial adhesions are present. The authors routinely aspirate from the sheath tip before removing the guidewire as an additional confirmation that the sheath is within the pericardial space. Based on the animal data from d'Avila and colleagues[36] on prevention of postablation pericarditis, they routinely instill 2 mg/kg of triamcinolone into the pericardial space after the procedure. They have noted a decrease in postoperative pericardial pain after instituting this practice.

Percutaneous pericardial access can be performed safely in selected patients with previous cardiac surgery; however, a posterior approach should be used in such patients because of the commonly present pericardial adhesions along the RV free wall.[37] Percutaneous puncture seems to be easier after valve repair or replacement surgery than prior coronary surgery. Direct surgical exposure of the pericardial space in the EP laboratory has also been described, and it may be useful in patients who fail percutaneous access or who have VT origin within an area of pericardial adhesions that are not accessible percutaneously.[38]

PITFALLS OF EPICARDIAL MAPPING AND ABLATION

Compared with LV endocardial mapping, detailed epicardial electroanatomic mapping is typically accomplished with far greater ease and with fewer requirements for fluoroscopy. The most common barriers to catheter movement in the pericardial space are pericardial reflections or adhesions. The pericardial reflections are easily navigated by redirection of the intrapericardial sheath or by deflection of the mapping catheter. It is sometimes possible to liberate chronic adhesions with blunt catheter dissection; however, care must be taken to avoid cardiac perforation with the catheter tip in these cases.

The variable thickness and distribution of epicardial LV fat has been shown to limit the efficacy of nonirrigated ablation.[39] Thus, the authors routinely use irrigated ablation in the epicardium. Fluid instilled into the pericardial space with externally irrigated catheters can rapidly accumulate and may lead to hemodynamic compromise if not periodically drained through the introducer sheath. The maintenance of small amounts of fluid within the pericardial space facilitates manipulation of the mapping catheter.

Given the commonality in substrate distribution in patients with LVCM, several important structures are frequently considered when planning an epicardial ablation strategy. First, the coronary arterial vasculature is often found adjacent to the epicardial scar. Superior LV sites may be in proximity to the left anterior descending artery and branches; lateral sites are often adjacent to branches of the circumflex artery. Ablation adjacent to the coronary vasculature has been shown in an animal model to result in intimal hyperplasia and thrombosis in only 14 days.[40] The authors' practice is to perform coronary angiography before any epicardial ablation; they also routinely obtain post ablation angiograms for comparison, whenever ablation is performed in proximity to the coronary vessels (**Fig. 5**).

The left phrenic nerve passes along the anterior LV free wall and down the midlateral LV; direct capture of the nerve is easily demonstrated with pacing. In a series of 10 consecutive patients with LVCM from the authors' institution, 8 of 10 had lateral epicardial scar; 7 of 8 patients with lateral scar also had phrenic nerve capture within the low-voltage region.[41] Various techniques have been reported to provide phrenic nerve protection by separating the visceral and parietal pericardial surfaces; these methods include air insufflation, saline infusion, or balloon inflation. A recent comparison of these methodologies found that a combination of air and saline infusion was the most reliable and tolerated method of phrenic protection.[42] When using a balloon for this purpose, the authors have found it helpful to use a deflectable pericardial sheath to more precisely position the balloon (**Fig. 6**).

Lastly, patients with nonischemic VT and LVCM often have biventricular pacing systems with coronary sinus leads; occasionally, these leads are positioned adjacent to epicardial substrate abnormalities. Little is known about the acute or chronic effect of ablation near epicardial leads; however, in the authors' experience, some patients may have an increase in pacing threshold postprocedure. The decision to proceed with ablation in this scenario must be individualized to the specific patient and clinical history.

ABLATION OUTCOMES AND COMPLICATIONS

Clinical outcomes in patients with LVCM undergoing VT ablation have greatly improved with the increased use of epicardial mapping. In the authors' recent series of 21 patients undergoing epicardial ablation, 14 of 21 patients (67%) were noninducible for any monomorphic VT after the

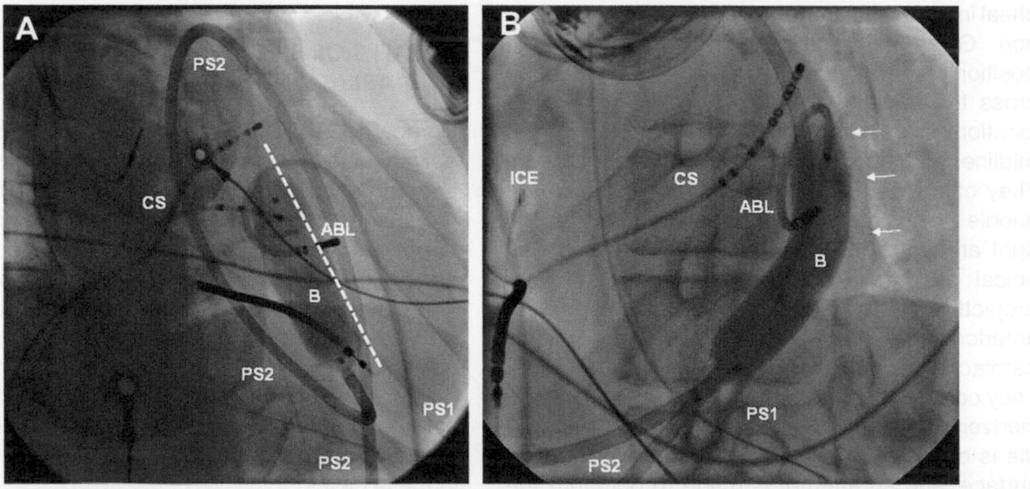

Fig. 5. A 55-year-old man with LVCM referred for epicardial VT ablation after a failed endocardial procedure. (*A*, right anterior oblique) and (*B*, left anterior oblique) demonstrate catheter positioning before epicardial ablation. The patient's VT was mapped to the mid lateral LV within an area of low bipolar voltage (not in picture). Phrenic nerve capture with high-output pacing was noted at the desired epicardial ablation site (approximate course of phrenic capture demarcated with dotted line in *A*). A second pericardial puncture was subsequently performed and a deflectable intrapericardial sheath (PS2) was inserted to facilitate placement of a 20 mm × 6 cm noncompliant balloon (*B*) along the course of the phrenic nerve. The balloon was then inflated and the ablation catheter was placed along the visceral pericardial surface. Repeat high-output stimulation was performed, which confirmed lack of phrenic nerve capture, and epicardial ablation was subsequently performed. ABL, ablation catheter; CS, coronary sinus; ICE, intracardiac echo catheter; PS, pericardial sheath.

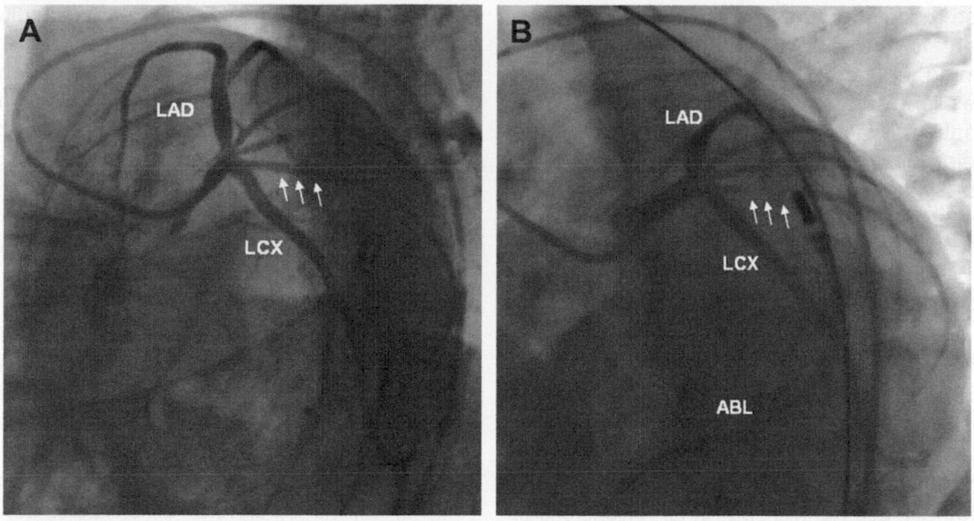

Fig. 6. Coronary artery narrowing after radiofrequency ablation lesion. These fluoroscopic images (left anterior oblique, caudal projection) were taken from a 49-year-old man with recurrent, symptomatic PVCs and LV dysfunction. (*A*) The panel was obtained during the initial ablation procedure after which, nonirrigated radiofrequency energy was delivered within the great cardiac vein. The patient had a clinical recurrence of his PVCs and was taken back to the EP laboratory 4 months later for a repeat procedure. A repeat coronary injection (*B*) before ablation revealed a long, eccentric stenosis (*arrows*) in the first marginal branch of the circumflex artery (LCX) attributable to intimal hyperplasia from the first ablation lesion. The PVC was subsequently successfully ablated from the left coronary cusp. (ABL, ablation catheter; LAD, left anterior descending artery).

procedure; in 5 of 21 patients, ablation was limited by proximity to the coronary vasculature or the phrenic nerve. At a mean follow-up of 18 ± 7 months, 15 of 21 patients remained free from recurrent VT.[24] In another series of 32 patients with a mean follow-up of 384 ± 405 days, 72% of patients undergoing epicardial ablation remained free from VT.[25]

From the Cano and colleagues[24] series, 4 of 21 patients died during follow-up; 2 deaths were due to progressive heart failure and 2 were due to noncardiac causes. Similarly, the mortality rate in the series from Grimard and colleagues[25] was 16%. These data underscore that the mortality rate remains high in this population, despite procedural success.

The complications during VT ablation depend on the approach. Major adverse events include vascular injury or spasm, cardiac perforation/tamponade, cardiac valvular injury, coronary arterial injury, phrenic nerve injury, atrioventricular block, transient ischemic attack/stroke, myocardial infarction, cardiogenic shock, and death. A multicenter study by Calkins and colleagues[43] in a predominantly ischemic population found the rate of major complications was 8%, with a periprocedural mortality rate of 2.7%. In patients undergoing epicardial procedures, the rate of pericardial tamponade has been reported to be as high as 22%.[25] Most patients from the Calkins series were older than 65 years and had significant systolic dysfunction (EF<35% in 73%). Aggressive anticoagulation monitoring, continuous ICE imaging during the procedure, and excessive catheter-tip temperature limiting during ablation may provide significant improvements in the safety of VT ablation.

SUMMARY

VT ablation in patients with nonischemic LVCM presents unique challenges. These patients are typically found to have low bipolar voltage abnormalities involving the peri-mitral valve annulus and lateral LV wall; these changes are often more striking on the LV epicardium. The low bipolar voltage areas also frequently demonstrate multicomponent, wide, and late EGMs. Adjunctive imaging modalities, such as CT, MRI, or ICE, are useful in identifying their often complex substrate distribution. At EPS, patients with nonischemic LVCM frequently have multiple inducible monomorphic VTs, and the dominant VT mechanism is scar-based reentry. Percutaneous pericardial access can be safely performed within the EP laboratory; however, special consideration should be given to patients with prior cardiac surgery. Particular attention should be given to avoiding injury to the coronary vasculature and left phrenic nerve during epicardial ablation, especially

because these structures are often found in close proximity to the bipolar substrate abnormality. Combining epicardial and endocardial ablation provides long-term success in eliminating VT in most patients with nonischemic LVCM, and the threshold for proceeding with such therapy in patients with recurrent ICD shocks should be lowered.

REFERENCES

1. de Vreede-Swagemakers JJ, Gorgels AP, Dubois-Arbouw WI, et al. Out-of-hospital cardiac arrest in the 1990's: a population-based study in the Maastricht area on incidence, characteristics and survival. J Am Coll Cardiol 1997;30(6):1500–5.
2. Bardy GH, Lee KL, Mark DB, et al. Amiodarone or an implantable cardioverter-defibrillator for congestive heart failure. N Engl J Med 2005;352(3):225–37.
3. Myerburg RJ, Kessler KM, Castellanos A. Sudden cardiac death: epidemiology, transient risk, and intervention assessment. Ann Intern Med 1993;119(12):1187–97.
4. Buxton AE, Lee KL, Hafley GE, et al. Limitations of ejection fraction for prediction of sudden death risk in patients with coronary artery disease: lessons from the MUSTT study. J Am Coll Cardiol 2007;50(12):1150–7.
5. Gehi AK, Stein RH, Metz LD, et al. Microvolt T-wave alternans for the risk stratification of ventricular tachyarrhythmic events: a meta-analysis. J Am Coll Cardiol 2005;46(1):75–82.
6. Schmidt A, Azevedo CF, Cheng A, et al. Infarct tissue heterogeneity by magnetic resonance imaging identifies enhanced cardiac arrhythmia susceptibility in patients with left ventricular dysfunction. Circulation 2007;115(15):2006–14.
7. Verberne HJ, Brewster LM, Somsen GA, et al. Prognostic value of myocardial 123I-metaiodobenzylguanidine (MIBG) parameters in patients with heart failure: a systematic review. Eur Heart J 2008;29(9):1147–59.
8. Kadish AH, Bello D, Finn JP, et al. Rationale and design for the defibrillators to reduce risk by magnetic resonance imaging evaluation (DETERMINE) trial. J Cardiovasc Electrophysiol 2009;20(9):982–7.
9. Meinertz T, Treese N, Kasper W, et al. Determinants of prognosis in idiopathic dilated cardiomyopathy as determined by programmed electrical stimulation. Am J Cardiol 1985;56(4):337–41.
10. Meinertz T, Hofmann T, Kasper W, et al. Significance of ventricular arrhythmias in idiopathic dilated cardiomyopathy. Am J Cardiol 1984;53(7):902–7.
11. Huang SK, Messer JV, Denes P. Significance of ventricular tachycardia in idiopathic dilated cardiomyopathy: observations in 35 patients. Am J Cardiol 1983;51(3):507–12.
12. Das SK, Morady F, DiCarlo L Jr, et al. Prognostic usefulness of programmed ventricular stimulation in idiopathic dilated cardiomyopathy without symptomatic ventricular arrhythmias. Am J Cardiol 1986;58(10):998–1000.
13. Poll DS, Marchlinski FE, Buxton AE, et al. Usefulness of programmed stimulation in idiopathic dilated cardiomyopathy. Am J Cardiol 1986;58(10):992–7.
14. Poole JE, Johnson GW, Hellkamp AS, et al. Prognostic importance of defibrillator shocks in patients with heart failure. N Engl J Med 2008;359(10):1009–17.
15. Pacifico A, Ferlic LL, Cedillo-Salazar FR, et al. Shocks as predictors of survival in patients with implantable cardioverter-defibrillators. J Am Coll Cardiol 1999;34(1):204–10.
16. A comparison of antiarrhythmic-drug therapy with implantable defibrillators in patients resuscitated from near-fatal ventricular arrhythmias. The Antiarrhythmics versus Implantable Defibrillators (AVID) Investigators. N Engl J Med 1997;337(22):1576–83.
17. Ellenbogen KA, Levine JH, Berger RD, et al. Are implantable cardioverter defibrillator shocks a surrogate for sudden cardiac death in patients with nonischemic cardiomyopathy? Circulation 2006;113(6):776–82.
18. Bristow MR, Saxon LA, Boehmer J, et al. Cardiac-resynchronization therapy with or without an implantable defibrillator in advanced chronic heart failure. N Engl J Med 2004;350(21):2140–50.
19. Fonarow GC, Feliciano Z, Boyle NG, et al. Improved survival in patients with nonischemic advanced heart failure and syncope treated with an implantable cardioverter-defibrillator. Am J Cardiol 2000;85(8):981–5.
20. Russo AM, Verdino R, Schorr C, et al. Occurrence of implantable defibrillator events in patients with syncope and nonischemic dilated cardiomyopathy. Am J Cardiol 2001;88(12):1444–6, A9.
21. Hohnloser SH, Dorian P, Roberts R, et al. Effect of amiodarone and sotalol on ventricular defibrillation threshold: the optimal pharmacological therapy in cardioverter defibrillator patients (OPTIC) trial. Circulation 2006;114(2):104–9.
22. Hsia HH, Callans DJ, Marchlinski FE. Characterization of endocardial electrophysiological substrate in patients with nonischemic cardiomyopathy and monomorphic ventricular tachycardia. Circulation 2003;108(6):704–10.
23. Soejima K, Stevenson WG, Sapp JL, et al. Endocardial and epicardial radiofrequency ablation of ventricular tachycardia associated with dilated cardiomyopathy: the importance of low-voltage scars. J Am Coll Cardiol 2004;43(10):1834–42.

24. Cano O, Hutchinson M, Lin D, et al. Electroanatomic substrate and ablation outcome for suspected epicardial ventricular tachycardia in left ventricular nonischemic cardiomyopathy. J Am Coll Cardiol 2009;54(9):799–808.
25. Grimard C, Lacotte J, Hidden-Lucet F, et al. Percutaneous epicardial radiofrequency ablation of ventricular arrhythmias after failure of endocardial approach: a 9-year experience. J Cardiovasc Electrophysiol 2009. [Epub ahead of print].
26. Haqqani HM, Marchlinski FE. Electrophysiologic substrate underlying postinfarction ventricular tachycardia: characterization and role in catheter ablation. Heart Rhythm 2009;6(Suppl 8):S70–6.
27. Cassidy DM, Vassallo JA, Miller JM, et al. Endocardial catheter mapping in patients in sinus rhythm: relationship to underlying heart disease and ventricular arrhythmias. Circulation 1986;73(4):645–52.
28. Hsia HH, Marchlinski FE. Characterization of the electroanatomic substrate for monomorphic ventricular tachycardia in patients with nonischemic cardiomyopathy. Pacing Clin Electrophysiol 2002;25(7):1114–27.
29. Cesario DA, Vaseghi M, Boyle NG, et al. Value of high-density endocardial and epicardial mapping for catheter ablation of hemodynamically unstable ventricular tachycardia. Heart Rhythm 2006;3(1):1–10.
30. Sosa E, Scanavacca M, d'Avila A, et al. A new technique to perform epicardial mapping in the electrophysiology laboratory. J Cardiovasc Electrophysiol 1996;7(6):531–6.
31. Berruezo A, Mont L, Nava S, et al. Electrocardiographic recognition of the epicardial origin of ventricular tachycardias. Circulation 2004;109(15):1842–7.
32. Bazan V, Gerstenfeld EP, Garcia FC, et al. Site-specific twelve-lead ECG features to identify an epicardial origin for left ventricular tachycardia in the absence of myocardial infarction. Heart Rhythm 2007;4(11):1403–10.
33. Delacretaz E, Stevenson WG, Ellison KE, et al. Mapping and radiofrequency catheter ablation of the three types of sustained monomorphic ventricular tachycardia in nonischemic heart disease. J Cardiovasc Electrophysiol 2000;11(1):11–7.
34. Bogun F, Crawford T, Reich S, et al. Radiofrequency ablation of frequent, idiopathic premature ventricular complexes: comparison with a control group without intervention. Heart Rhythm 2007;4(7):863–7.
35. Ren JF, Callans DJ, Michele JJ, et al. Intracardiac echocardiographic evaluation of ventricular mural swelling from radiofrequency ablation in chronic myocardial infarction: irrigated-tip versus standard catheter. J Interv Card Electrophysiol 2001;5(1):27–32.
36. d'Avila A, Neuzil P, Thiagalingam A, et al. Experimental efficacy of pericardial instillation of anti-inflammatory agents during percutaneous epicardial catheter ablation to prevent postprocedure pericarditis. J Cardiovasc Electrophysiol 2007;18(11): 1178–83.
37. Sosa E, Scanavacca M, D'Avila A, et al. Nonsurgical transthoracic epicardial approach in patients with ventricular tachycardia and previous cardiac surgery. J Interv Card Electrophysiol 2004;10(3): 281–8.
38. Soejima K, Couper G, Cooper JM, et al. Subxiphoid surgical approach for epicardial catheter-based mapping and ablation in patients with prior cardiac surgery or difficult pericardial access. Circulation 2004;110(10):1197–201.
39. d'Avila A, Houghtaling C, Gutierrez P, et al. Catheter ablation of ventricular epicardial tissue: a comparison of standard and cooled-tip radiofrequency energy. Circulation 2004;109(19):2363–9.
40. D'Avila A, Gutierrez P, Scanavacca M, et al. Effects of radiofrequency pulses delivered in the vicinity of the coronary arteries: implications for nonsurgical transthoracic epicardial catheter ablation to treat ventricular tachycardia. Pacing Clin Electrophysiol 2002;25(10):1488–95.
41. Fan R, Cano O, Ho SY, et al. Characterization of the phrenic nerve course within the epicardial substrate of patients with nonischemic cardiomyopathy and ventricular tachycardia. Heart Rhythm 2009;6(1): 59–64.
42. Di Biase L, Burkhardt JD, Pelargonio G, et al. Prevention of phrenic nerve injury during epicardial ablation: comparison of methods for separating the phrenic nerve from the epicardial surface. Heart Rhythm 2009;6(7):957–61.
43. Calkins H, Epstein A, Packer D, et al. Catheter ablation of ventricular tachycardia in patients with structural heart disease using cooled radiofrequency energy: results of a prospective multicenter study. Cooled RF Multi Center Investigators Group. J Am Coll Cardiol 2000;35(7):1905–14.

Epicardial Ablation of Supraventricular Tachycardia

Robert A. Schweikert, MD[a,b,*]

KEYWORDS

- Epicardial • Pericardial space • Catheter ablation
- Supraventricular tachycardia

Percutaneous pericardial instrumentation has been safely and effectively applied to a broad range of cardiac arrhythmias. Several supraventricular arrhythmia substrates have been targeted with this approach, including accessory pathways,[1–5] atrial tachycardias or flutter,[2,6,7] inappropriate sinus tachycardia,[2,8,9] and atrial fibrillation.[2,10–12] These published reports[1–12] and others documenting the experience with epicardial mapping and ablation of such arrhythmia substrates have indicated that this approach is a reasonable option, particularly for those patients in whom a standard endocardial approach has failed. The percutaneous epicardial catheter ablation option is important because it can help patients avoid a more invasive surgical approach or the prospect of suffering indefinitely with an arrhythmia or being exposed to the potential toxic side effects of antiarrhythmic drugs.

EPICARDIAL ABLATION OF VARIOUS FORMS OF SUPRAVENTRICULAR TACHYCARDIA

Accessory Pathways

Accessory pathways may have all or a portion of their course closer to the epicardial region of the myocardium. In one series examining the reasons for failure of accessory pathway catheter ablation, an epicardial location of the accessory pathway accounted for 8% of the failures.[13] Not surprisingly then, the percutaneous epicardial approach to catheter ablation of such pathways has been the most common application of this technique for supraventricular arrhythmias. This brings the interventional treatment of accessory pathways nearly full circle, as the open surgical approach for elimination of accessory pathways was the only option before the advent of catheter-based percutaneous methods. The surgical approaches to elimination of accessory pathways, which evolved from resection techniques to electrical shock ablation and then surgical ablation probes, gave way to percutaneous endocardial catheter ablation techniques. Catheter ablation of such pathways from an endocardial approach, however, may still be a difficult challenge, even with the use of the newer catheter ablation technologies, such as irrigated tip ablation systems and computerized mapping systems.

There are particular accessory pathways that are not uncommonly epicardial and may be ablated from an epicardial approach, such as certain posteroseptal and left posterior pathways[5,14–16] and right atrial appendage to right ventricular pathways.[2,4] These pathways may still be effectively ablated from an endocardial approach, but in some cases the endocardial approach may fail. In such cases an epicardial approach may be necessary. The epicardial approach to some of these pathways may include ablation from the coronary sinus or its tributaries and an approach using percutaneous instrumentation of the

Disclosures: No grants were received. Dr Schweikert receives honoraria for giving lectures for the following companies: St Jude Medical, Boston Scientific, Glaxo-Smith-Kline, and Sanofi-aventis.

[a] Department of Cardiology, Akron General Medical Center, 400 Wabash Avenue, Akron, OH 44307, USA
[b] Department of Internal Medicine, Northeast Ohio Universities College of Medicine, 4209 State Route 44, PO Box 95, Rootstown, OH 44272, USA
* Department of Cardiology, Akron General Medical Center, 400 Wabash Avenue, Akron, OH 44307.
E-mail address: rschweikert@agmc.org

Card Electrophysiol Clin 2 (2010) 105–111
doi:10.1016/j.ccep.2009.11.013

pericardial space. The epicardial approach using the coronary sinus was reported 2 decades ago, with the use of electrical shock ablation,[17] and subsequently radiofrequency (RF) catheter ablation via the coronary sinus for patients in whom endocardial approaches failed.[13,18–20]

These approaches are not always effective and some accessory pathways cannot be reached via the coronary sinus or its tributaries, so the option of a percutaneous epicardial approach via the pericardial space is important for patients. More invasive surgical operations can be avoided with these techniques. Additionally, in the past, for patients in whom an endocardial ablation technique failed and when patients were not considered candidates for a surgical approach, patients were often left with several undesirable options. These options included treatment with potentially toxic antiarrhythmic drugs, which provided mediocre efficacy and bothersome side effects; catheter ablation of the atrioventricular node with pacemaker implantation; or simply having to suffer with the arrhythmia. The percutaneous epicardial techniques for catheter ablation of these accessory pathways provide an important opportunity for such patients to avoid these suboptimal treatment options.

Published reports of experience with epicardial catheter ablation of accessory pathways have demonstrated the safety and, for some reports, efficacy of this approach.[1–5] In a series of patients undergoing percutaneous epicardial mapping and ablation for a variety of arrhythmias after failed endocardial attempts, those with accessory pathways included 10 patients.[2] There were a variety of accessory pathway locations reported in this series, including concealed left lateral (1), manifest left posterolateral (1), manifest left posteroseptal (2), concealed right midseptal (1), manifest right posterolateral (2), and right atrial appendage to right ventricular (3). Five of these pathways (the right atrial appendage to right ventricular, left posteroseptal, and right posterolateral) were found to have an epicardial earliest site. Of these five epicardial pathways, the three right atrial appendage to right ventricular accessory pathways were ablated successfully from an epicardial approach. The left posteroseptal accessory pathway, although demonstrating an earlier epicardial site, could not be ablated with epicardial lesions due to excessively high impedance, possibly due to the posterior fat pad. This pathway was associated with a large coronary sinus diverticulum and was ablated successfully from a transvenous approach at that site.[5] The right posterolateral pathway with earliest epicardial activation was only transiently affected by epicardial ablation lesions. This pathway was successfully ablated from an endocardial approach. Serious complications did not occur, and one patient had transient pericarditis that responded quickly to medical treatment. During follow-up, one patient had recurrence of tachycardia. This patient with a right atrial appendage to right ventricular accessory pathway underwent repeat percutaneous pericardial instrumentation and successful epicardial ablation a second time. The arrhythmia did not recur during the follow-up period.[2] This case illustrates the experience of the author's group and others that repeat pericardial instrumentation is feasible and generally not associated with limitations from the previous instrumentation, such as pericardial adhesions. In some patients a combined endocardial approach has been successful and avoided the need for cardiac surgery (**Fig. 1**).

There are several reasons for failure of an epicardial approach for such pathways. The epicardial fat in the posteroseptal region may prevent the application of effective ablation lesions, as illustrated in one of the failed cases (discussed previously). Another reason for failure of epicardial catheter ablation is inability to deliver lesions due to concern about damage to adjacent structures. This is particularly true for the phrenic nerve (discussed later). There may also be concern for damage to epicardial vessels, which are located nearby in the atrioventricular and interventricular grooves. Such concerns may limit the amount of power delivered to particular regions and result in failure to effectively ablate the accessory pathway.

Epicardial mapping may be beneficial even if ablation is not found necessary or feasible from that site. Epicardial mapping may be complementary to standard endocardial mapping, and this has been shown to facilitate the localization of accessory pathways.[3] The epicardial map may, therefore, provide an additional 3-D construct that facilitates localization of the accessory pathway, allowing for more effective catheter ablation even from the endocardial approach.

For some epicardial pathways, posteroseptal accessory pathways, in particular the percutaneous pericardial approach, may not be the best technique. For such pathways, an approach via the epicardial venous structures, such as the coronary sinus or its tributaries, might be a more effective technique. Some posteroseptal accessory pathways may be found to course within the middle cardiac vein[21,22] and, in some instances, be associated with a venous diverticulum.[5] Accessory pathways in other locations may also be

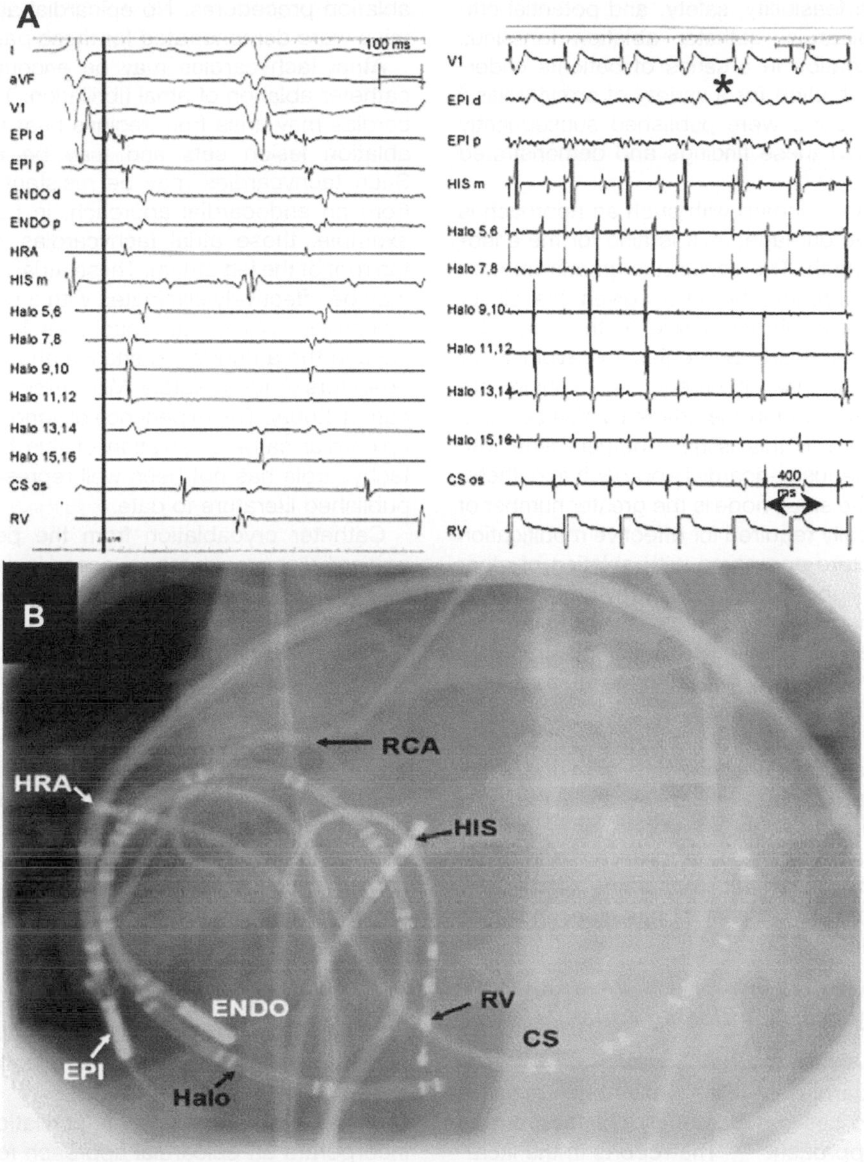

Fig. 1. Combined epicardial-endocardial accessory pathway mapping of a right-sided accessory pathway. (*A*) Electrograms made during orthodromic atrioventricular tachycardia show earliest atrial activation in the epicardial catheter (*vertical line*). RF delivery abolished retrograde accessory pathway conduction during ventricular pacing (*right panel*). (*B*) Left anterior oblique fluoroscopic view of the catheters. CS, coronary sinus catheter; ENDO, endocardial catheter; EPI, epicardial catheter through an SL1 sheath; Halo, tricuspid annulus catheter; HIS, His-bundle catheter; HRA, high right atrium; RCA, right coronary artery; RV, right ventricular catheter. (*From* Valderrábano M, Cesario DA, Ji S, et al. Percutaneous epicardial mapping during ablation of difficult accessory pathways as an alternative to cardiac surgery. Heart Rhythm 2004;1:311–6; with permission.)

ablated from an epicardial approach from within the coronary sinus.[18] Therefore, there are multiple approaches for catheter mapping and ablation of epicardial accessory pathways.

Inappropriate Sinus Tachycardia

Sinus node modification with catheter ablation for the treatment of inappropriate sinus tachycardia remains a distinct challenge. The sinus node is a relatively resilient structure compared with other cardiac ablation targets, and its subepicardial location in the atrial myocardium exacerbates the challenge from an endocardial catheter ablation approach. There are few reports of the efficacy and safety of using a percutaneous epicardial approach to catheter ablation for sinus node modification. The author and colleagues initially reported the feasibility, safety, and potential efficacy of epicardial catheter ablation for sinus node modification in a series of patients undergoing such ablation for a variety of arrhythmias,[2] and other reports were published subsequently that confirmed these findings and demonstrated better efficacy.[8,9]

The primary concern with such an approach is phrenic nerve damage, as it is also for the endocardial approach. The concern is greater from an epicardial approach, however, given the closer proximity of the phrenic nerve to the epicardial surface of the heart. Strategies for avoiding or decreasing the risk of phrenic nerve injury are discussed later and in the article by Yamada and Kay elsewhere in this issue. Another issue with the percutaneous pericardial approach to catheter ablation of the sinus node is the greater number of lesions typically required for effective modification of this structure compared with ablation of other types of supraventricular arrhythmias. This increased number of ablation lesions increases the potential for damage to adjacent structures and the creation of other undesirable issues, such as pericardial irritation.

In spite of the limitations inherent to the percutaneous epicardial catheter ablation of the sinus node for inappropriate sinus tachycardia, the technique remains an important option for patients in whom an endocardial approach fails. The technique might benefit from some of the new developments in catheter ablation technologies (discussed later).

Atrial Tachycardias, Including Atrial Fibrillation

Atrial tachycardias or flutters have been mapped and in some cases successfully ablated from an epicardial approach.[2,6,7] The reports in the literature documenting successful catheter ablation of atrial tachycardia seem to include primarily those arising from the left atrial appendage.[6,7] As with right atrial appendage to right ventricular accessory pathways, epicardial left atrial appendage tachycardias may be ablated successfully from an endocardial approach. In some cases, however, this approach is not successful and the option of a percutaneous epicardial approach is important. In the author and coworkers' published series of early experience with patients undergoing epicardial catheter ablation,[2] the three patients listed as having atrial fibrillation were mapped epicardially for the presence of an epicardial atrial tachycardia or atrial ectopic beats during a time that focal triggers of atrial fibrillation were extensively sought after and mapped for such ablation procedures. No epicardial atrial arrhythmias were demonstrated for these patients.

Atrial tachycardias may be encountered after catheter ablation of atrial fibrillation. These tachycardias may arise from regions near the previous ablation lesion sets and may be epicardial.[23] Such tachycardias may be resistant to ablation from an endocardial approach, in particular, for example, those atrial tachycardias arising from the roof of the left atrium. These atrial tachycardias may be effectively eliminated with a percutaneous epicardial ablation approach, as has been the case in the author's experience and that of other operators (Andrea Natale, MD, personal communication, 2009). The experience of various centers of epicardial catheter ablation of this type of atrial tachycardia has not been well represented in the published literature to date.

Catheter cryoablation from the percutaneous epicardial approach may succeed in cases of atrial tachycardia in which epicardial RF catheter ablation has failed.[24] This report describes for the first time the use of epicardial catheter cryoablation using percutaneous pericardial instrumentation. Also interesting is the failure of open-irrigation RF catheter ablation at this epicardial site and subsequent success of catheter cryoablation. As the investigators outline in their discussion, it is unclear whether or not this was due to "preconditioning" of the tissue by the RF energy, better positioning of the cryoablation catheter, perhaps better and more consistent contact with the ablation site by cryoadherence, or a more efficacious lesion at that site by cryothermy due to the local tissue characteristics. In any event, the feasibility and safety of epicardial catheter cryoablation in the pericardial space was demonstrated by this case.[24]

Catheter ablation for atrial fibrillation may also incorporate an epicardial approach (discussed in the article by Buch and colleagues elsewhere in this issue). Triggers for atrial fibrillation may arise from epicardial foci, such as the coronary sinus or its tributaries, including the vein of Marshall. Such epicardial triggers may be approached from the coronary sinus.[25] Pulmonary veins isolation for catheter ablation of atrial fibrillation may also be approached from a percutaneous epicardial route, primarily from the pericardial space. This is particularly appealing from the standpoint of risk, as the epicardial approach should have the advantage of a lower risk of stroke compared with that of the endocardial approach. Alternatively, the risk of injury to adjacent structures, such as the esophagus and phrenic and other nerves, might be greater from an epicardial approach. This is a concern particularly for pulmonary veins isolation, which requires the application of many ablation lesions. Additional obstacles to the use of the epicardial approach to pulmonary veins isolation include the pericardial reflections at the pulmonary veins. In spite of these limitations, there are published reports of successful catheter ablation of atrial fibrillation from a percutaneous pericardial approach, alone or as a hybrid procedure using an endocardial and epicardial approach.[10–12,26]

NEW TECHNIQUES FOR IMPROVED EFFICACY AND SAFETY

Several new techniques have been implemented to help improve the efficacy or safety of percutaneous epicardial catheter ablation of supraventricular tachycardias (SVTs). Irrigated tip RF catheter ablation systems have been increasingly used for improved efficacy of ablation lesions. This type of ablation system may provide more effective lesions in the pericardial space than standard RF catheter ablation systems.[27] The use of open-irrigation RF catheter ablation systems in the pericardial space has been shown feasible and safe.[28,29] Catheter cryoablation may be effectively applied to the epicardium.[30] As discussed previously, in some instances, the use of cryoablation lesions may be effective in cases where RF lesions, even from irrigated tip systems, have failed.[24]

Another development has been new techniques for avoidance of damage to adjacent structures. Particularly challenging has been the even greater proximity of the phrenic nerves to the ablation site on the epicardial surface of the heart. The inability to deliver ablation energy in a directional manner is a serious limitation in this regard. The use of energy sources other than RF, such as cryothermy, has not completely solved this problem. Cryothermy might not provide sufficient lesion depth to be effective, and damage to the phrenic nerve is still a potential problem.

More recently, there have been published reports of novel techniques to decrease the risk of damage to adjacent structures, such as the phrenic nerve. The general technique is to increase the distance from the ablation catheter to the adjacent structure. One approach involves inflation of a balloon within the pericardial space such that the balloon lies between the adjacent structure and the ablation catheter.[9,31] Other approaches include infusion of saline,[32] air,[32,33] or both saline and air[32] into the pericardial space to increase the distance between the epicardial ablation site and the phrenic nerve. Di Biase and colleagues[32] compared these approaches and found that a combination of saline and air was superior to the same volume of saline or air alone. For the concern of damage to the epicardial coronary arteries, a novel approach has been investigated in an animal model in which intracoronary irrigation with chilled saline was shown potentially protective from the thermal damage of epicardial RF ablation lesions.[34]

FUTURE DIRECTIONS

The catheter-based percutaneous epicardial approach to mapping and ablation of SVTs has been sufficiently efficacious and safe that it is a good option for patients, particularly for those in whom a standard endocardial approach has failed. For some patients, it might be argued that an epicardial approach might be preferred as an initial strategy, alone or as a technique complementary to an endocardial approach. For example, epicardial catheter ablation for pulmonary veins isolation in patients with atrial fibrillation might be safer from a standpoint of stroke. The anatomic obstacles of the pericardial reflections, however, may be difficult to overcome for complete isolation of the veins and the large number of ablation lesions required may limit the use of the epicardial approach with the available nonlinear ablation electrode systems.

For improved efficacy and safety of catheter ablation from the pericardial approach, better tools are required. Ablation systems capable of directional lesion delivery, such as shielded electrodes, would be important to decrease the potential for damage to adjacent structures.[27] Adherence of the ablation catheter to the myocardium would be helpful, as the pericardial space does not restrict the movement of the catheter and migration of the tip is not uncommonly encountered. Cryoablation has an advantage in this regard, and the newer cryoablation systems with larger-tip electrodes may provide the necessary increased lesion size and depth to be more effective than earlier versions of this technology.

There are RF ablation systems that are being designed for the epicardial approach, with features such as suction adherence and saline irrigation, for improved catheter stability and more effective lesions, and shielded electrodes, for directional lesion delivery.[35] Another development on the horizon is the adaptation of currently available deflectable sheaths for use in the pericardial space. Investigations and reports regarding the use of robotic tools for catheter mapping and ablation have been described and may enhance the results of this procedure.[36] In the author's experience, the use of remote magnetic navigation in the pericardial space is feasible, safe, and effective for a variety of epicardial arrhythmia substrates (discussed in the article by Burkhardt and colleagues elsewhere in this issue).

Lastly, better methods of imaging or visualization might improve the safety and efficacy of the procedure. Intrapericardial echocardiography has been demonstrated as feasible.[37,38] Direct visualization of the pericardial space and epicardial and adjacent structures has been achieved with an endoscope placed via percutaneous route in an animal model.[39] Such visualization has the potential to provide important information regarding catheter position relative to the epicardial ablation target and to adjacent structures, such as nerves and epicardial vessels.

SUMMARY

Epicardial catheter-based mapping and ablation of a variety of SVTs is feasible, safe, and effective. SVT substrates are not uncommonly epicardial, and approaches with percutaneous epicardial instrumentation or via the epicardial venous structures, such as the coronary sinus, are becoming more widely accepted. These techniques are an important treatment option as an alternative to a more invasive surgical approach or to allowing patients to suffer from an ongoing arrhythmia. New technologies and innovative techniques are being developed that hold great potential to improve the efficacy and safety of the epicardial catheter-based approach to these challenging arrhythmias.

REFERENCES

1. de Paola AA, Leite LR, Mesas CE. Nonsurgical transthoracic epicardial ablation for the treatment of a resistant posteroseptal accessory pathway. Pacing Clin Electrophysiol 2004;27:259–61.
2. Schweikert RA, Saliba WI, Tomassoni G, et al. Percutaneous pericardial instrumentation for endo-epicardial mapping of previously failed ablations. Circulation 2003;108:1329–35.
3. Valderrabano M, Cesario DA, Ji S, et al. Percutaneous epicardial mapping during ablation of difficult accessory pathways as an alternative to cardiac surgery. Heart Rhythm 2004;1:311–6.
4. Lam C, Schweikert R, Kanagaratnam L, et al. Radiofrequency ablation of a right atrial appendage-ventricular accessory pathway by transcutaneous epicardial instrumentation. J Cardiovasc Electrophysiol 2000;11:1170–3.
5. Saad EB, Marrouche NF, Cole CR, et al. Simultaneous epicardial and endocardial mapping of a left-sided posteroseptal accessory pathway associated with a large coronary sinus diverticulum: successful ablation by transection of the diverticulum's neck. Pacing Clin Electrophysiol 2002;25:1524–6.
6. Phillips KP, Natale A, Sterba R, et al. Percutaneous pericardial instrumentation for catheter ablation of focal atrial tachycardias arising from the left atrial appendage. J Cardiovasc Electrophysiol 2008;19:430–3.
7. Yamada T, McElderry HT, Allison JS, et al. Focal atrial tachycardia originating from the epicardial left atrial appendage. Heart Rhythm 2008;5:766–7.
8. Koplan BA, Parkash R, Couper G, et al. Combined epicardial-endocardial approach to ablation of inappropriate sinus tachycardia. J Cardiovasc Electrophysiol 2004;15:237–40.
9. Rubenstein JC, Kim MH, Jacobson JT. A novel method for sinus node modification and phrenic nerve protection in resistant cases. J Cardiovasc Electrophysiol 2009;20:689–91.
10. Buch E, Shivkumar K. Epicardial catheter ablation of atrial fibrillation. Minerva Med 2009;100:151–7.
11. Choi JI, Pak HN, Kim YH. Hybrid epicardial and endocardial catheter ablation in a patient with atrial fibrillation and suspicious left atrial thrombus. Circ J 2009;73:384–7.
12. Shivkumar K. Percutaneous epicardial ablation of atrial fibrillation. Heart Rhythm 2008;5:152–4.
13. Morady F, Strickberger A, Man KC, et al. Reasons for prolonged or failed attempts at radiofrequency catheter ablation of accessory pathways. J Am Coll Cardiol 1996;27:683–9.
14. Sapp J, Soejima K, Couper GS, et al. Electrophysiology and anatomic characterization of an epicardial accessory pathway. J Cardiovasc Electrophysiol 2001;12:1411–4.
15. Guiraudon GM, Klein GJ, Sharma AD, et al. "Atypical" posteroseptal accessory pathway in Wolff-Parkinson-White syndrome. J Am Coll Cardiol 1988;12:1605–8.
16. Sun Y, Arruda M, Otomo K, et al. Coronary sinus-ventricular accessory connections producing posteroseptal and left posterior accessory pathways: incidence and electrophysiological identification. Circulation 2002;106:1362–7.
17. Fisher JD, Brodman R, Kim SG, et al. Attempted nonsurgical electrical ablation of accessory pathways via the coronary sinus in the Wolff-Parkinson-White syndrome. J Am Coll Cardiol 1984;4:685–94.
18. Haissaguerre M, Gaita F, Fischer B, et al. Radiofrequency catheter ablation of left lateral accessory pathways via the coronary sinus. Circulation 1992;86:1464–8.
19. Beukema WP, Van Dessel PF, Van Hemel NM, et al. Radiofrequency catheter ablation of accessory pathways associated with a coronary sinus diverticulum. Eur Heart J 1994;15:1415–8.

20. Kleinman D, Winters SL. Successful catheter ablation of an inferoseptal accessory pathway within the coronary sinus in a patient with a previously unsuccessful attempt at surgical interruption. Coronary sinus ablation for Wolff-Parkinson-White syndrome. J Electrocardiol 1996;29:55–60.
21. Amasyali B, Kose S, Aytemir K, et al. A permanent junctional reciprocating tachycardia with an atypically located accessory pathway successfully ablated from within the middle cardiac vein. Heart Vessels 2006;21:188–91.
22. Kusano KF, Morita H, Fujimoto Y, et al. Catheter ablation of an epicardial accessory pathway via the middle cardiac vein guided by monophasic action potential recordings. Europace 2001;3:164–7.
23. Yamada T, Murakami Y, Okada T, et al. Non-pulmonary vein epicardial foci of atrial fibrillation identified in the left atrium after pulmonary vein isolation. Pacing Clin Electrophysiol 2007;30:1323–30.
24. Di Biase L, Saliba WI, Natale A. Successful ablation of epicardial arrhythmias with cryoenergy after failed attempts with radiofrequency energy. Heart Rhythm 2009;6:109–12.
25. Katritsis D, Giazitzoglou E, Korovesis S, et al. Epicardial foci of atrial arrhythmias apparently originating in the left pulmonary veins. J Cardiovasc Electrophysiol 2002;13:319–23.
26. Reddy VY, Neuzil P, D'Avila A, et al. Isolating the posterior left atrium and pulmonary veins with a "box" lesion set: use of epicardial ablation to complete electrical isolation. J Cardiovasc Electrophysiol 2008;19:326–9.
27. Fenelon G, Pereira KP, de Paola AA. Epicardial radiofrequency ablation of ventricular myocardium: factors affecting lesion formation and damage to adjacent structures. J Interv Card Electrophysiol 2006;15:57–63.
28. Pak HN, Hwang C, Lim HE, et al. Hybrid epicardial and endocardial ablation of persistent or permanent atrial fibrillation: a new approach for difficult cases. J Cardiovasc Electrophysiol 2007;18:917–23.
29. Anh DJ, Hsia HH, Reitz B, et al. Epicardial ablation of postinfarction ventricular tachycardia with an externally irrigated catheter in a patient with mechanical aortic and mitral valves. Heart Rhythm 2007;4:651–4.
30. D'Avila A, Aryana A, Thiagalingam A, et al. Focal and linear endocardial and epicardial catheter-based cryoablation of normal and infarcted ventricular tissue. Pacing Clin Electrophysiol 2008;31:1322–31.
31. Buch E, Vaseghi M, Cesario DA, et al. A novel method for preventing phrenic nerve injury during catheter ablation. Heart Rhythm 2007;4:95–8.
32. Di Biase L, Burkhardt JD, Pelargonio G, et al. Prevention of phrenic nerve injury during epicardial ablation: comparison of methods for separating the phrenic nerve from the epicardial surface. Heart Rhythm 2009;6:957–61.
33. Matsuo S, Jais P, Knecht S, et al. Images in cardiovascular medicine. Novel technique to prevent left phrenic nerve injury during epicardial catheter ablation. Circulation 2008;117:e471.
34. Thyer IA, Kovoor P, Barry MA, et al. Protection of the coronary arteries during epicardial radiofrequency ablation with intracoronary chilled saline irrigation: assessment in an in vitro model. J Cardiovasc Electrophysiol 2006;17:544–9.
35. Kiser AC, Nifong LW, Raman J, et al. Evaluation of a novel epicardial atrial fibrillation treatment system. Ann Thorac Surg 2008;85:300–3.
36. Ota T, Degani A, Zubiate B, et al. Epicardial atrial ablation using a novel articulated robotic medical probe via a percutaneous subxiphoid approach. Innovations Phila Pa 2006;1:335–40.
37. Horowitz BN, Vaseghi M, Mahajan A, et al. Percutaneous intrapericardial echocardiography during catheter ablation: a feasibility study. Heart Rhythm 2006;3:1275–82.
38. Rodrigues AC, d'Avila A, Houghtaling C, et al. Intrapericardial echocardiography: a novel catheter-based approach to cardiac imaging. J Am Soc Echocardiogr 2004;17:269–74.
39. Nazarian S, Kantsevoy SV, Zviman MM, et al. Feasibility of endoscopic guidance for nonsurgical transthoracic atrial and ventricular epicardial ablation. Heart Rhythm 2008;5:1115–9.

Epicardial Catheter Ablation of Atrial Fibrillation

Eric Buch, MD*, Shiro Nakahara, MD,
Noel G. Boyle, MD, PhD, FHRS,
Kalyanam Shivkumar, MD, PhD, FHRS

KEYWORDS

• Catheter ablation • Atrial fibrillation • Epicardial ablation

Atrial fibrillation (AF), the most common sustained arrhythmia, causes significant symptoms for many patients even when the ventricular rate is well controlled. A rhythm-control strategy to maintain sinus rhythm may be more appropriate than a rate-control strategy for such patients. However, the efficacy of antiarrhythmic drug therapy for AF is limited, and some agents cause significant side effects, including irreversible end-organ damage and life-threatening ventricular arrhythmias. Therefore nonpharmacologic therapy, including radiofrequency (RF) catheter ablation and cardiac surgical procedures, have found a growing role in the treatment of this arrhythmia.

Endocardial catheter ablation has a higher success rate than medical therapy in maintaining sinus rhythm,[1,2] and is currently recommended for treatment of patients with symptomatic drug-refractory AF.[3] This procedure carries significant risks; a wide range of serious complications have been reported, including vascular complications, perioperative stroke, pulmonary vein (PV) stenosis, phrenic nerve injury, cardiac tamponade, and atrio-esophageal fistula. The risk of periprocedural mortality from endocardial AF ablation is approximately 1 in 1000.[4]

However, the success rate of endocardial catheter ablation may be lower in real-world practice as compared with clinical trials and high-volume academic centers.[5] This may be due to differences in patient selection, follow-up, and operator experience. Concerns have been raised that the spread of AF ablation procedures to lower-volume centers might result in still lower efficacy and higher complication rates in the future.[6]

The initial epicardial procedure aimed at establishing sinus rhythm in AF patients was the surgical "maze" procedure. The original Cox maze procedure, first performed in 1987, has shown excellent results in experienced hands.[7,8] However, it requires median sternotomy and cardiopulmonary bypass, with attendant risks of stroke, cognitive impairment, renal failure, and death. Up to 20% of patients need a pacemaker following the procedure. Usually this is not performed as a standalone procedure, but rather as an adjunctive procedure at the time of another cardiac surgery, typically mitral valve surgery.

Modified, less invasive variants of the maze surgical procedure have also been developed (so-called mini-maze procedures). The approach usually involves a limited lateral thoracotomy or port access for thoracoscopic procedures. The epicardial surface of the left atrium (LA) and the PV antra are ablated using multiple energy sources including radiofrequency, laser, cryothermy, and microwave energy.[9] The goal is to mimic the traditional Cox maze procedure with transmural lesions, resulting in lines of conduction block.[10] The left atrial appendage is usually stapled and removed during these procedures. However many of the methods used may not result in transmural lesions.

Disclosure: The University of California, Los Angeles has intellectual property relating to this area of work.
Support: NIH RO1-HL084261 and HL067647 grants to Dr Shivkumar.
UCLA Cardiac Arrhythmia Center, A2-237 CHS, David Geffen School of Medicine at UCLA, 10833 Le Conte Avenue, Los Angeles, CA 90095-1679, USA
* Corresponding author.
E-mail address: ebuch@mednet.ucla.edu (E. Buch).

Card Electrophysiol Clin 2 (2010) 113–120
doi:10.1016/j.ccep.2009.11.002
1877-9182/10/$ – see front matter

Theoretical advantages include reduced operation time and lower risk of complications. Many of these newer approaches can be performed while the heart is beating, avoiding the risks of cardiopulmonary bypass. These modified versions of the maze procedure are especially attractive for stand-alone procedures.

Nonpharmacologic treatment of atrial fibrillation continues to evolve, probably favoring less invasive approaches. It is likely that a safe and effective percutaneous procedure using a subxiphoid approach will eventually be developed. Such an approach has been used successfully in the treatment of ventricular arrhythmias.[11] This will add another therapeutic option for invasive cardiac electrophysiologists experienced in the epicardial access methods.

This article discusses the background of epicardial catheter ablation, the rationale for using it to treat AF, the relevant anatomy for the approach, the challenges in performing epicardial procedures safely, and finally, the potential directions in this promising new field.

RATIONALE FOR EPICARDIAL ABLATION OF AF

Despite the superiority of endocardial catheter ablation over medical therapy, long-term clinical outcomes are still disappointing, especially for persistent AF.[12] Repeat procedures are often necessary, each subjecting the patient to the risk of complications. One reason for procedural failure is nontransmural lesions, allowing recovery of conduction across ablative lines. This occurs more often when ablating thicker parts of the left atrium, such as the tissue ridge between left superior PV and LA appendage. It is also common in areas where sufficient RF energy cannot be applied to achieve a full-thickness lesion, because of the proximity of surrounding structures, such as the esophagus or phrenic nerve. An epicardial or hybrid endocardial-epicardial ablation procedure might offer the possibility of achieving fully transmural lesions and improving procedural success with reduced risk of collateral damage to surrounding structures.

Epicardial structures themselves may be important targets for ablation of AF. Ectopic activity from the ligament (or vein) of Marshall plays a key role in AF in certain patients.[13] Other epicardial structures routinely targeted in surgical treatment of AF are ganglionated plexi,[10] discrete aggregates of cardiac neurons and neural connections[14] that may play a role in the genesis of AF.[15] These structures are currently targeted by some operators performing endocardial ablation procedures.[16,17] The ligament of Marshall and the ganglionated plexi might be ablated more safely and effectively using the percutaneous epicardial approach.

Manipulating sheaths and catheters in the LA during endocardial catheter ablation carries the risk of systemic embolism from thrombus, coagulum, or air, which can result in stroke or other end-organ damage. Energy delivery at the catheter tip combined with outwardly directed force to maintain tissue contact can cause cardiac perforation, which can result in pericardial effusion or tamponade. In theory, risks of embolism and perforation should be reduced with epicardial catheter ablation. However, thromboembolic risk might not be eliminated completely, because damage to the endothelium from a transmural epicardial lesion could still result in LA thrombus.

Some patients with drug-refractory symptomatic AF are not good candidates for endocardial ablation procedures because of increased procedural risk. For example, patients with mechanical mitral valve prosthesis, history of LA appendage thrombus, or atrial septal defect closure device have higher-than-average risk of complications with ablation by the conventional approach. Epicardial ablation that limits or eliminates endocardial LA catheter manipulation could mitigate these risks.

The proximity of other structures surrounding the LA frequently limits effective catheter ablation. The position of the esophagus may prevent creation of ablation lines in the posterior LA, because of the risk of atrio-esophageal fistula. The distance from the LA to the esophageal lumen may be only 4 mm.[18] The right phrenic nerve can lie directly adjacent to atrial tissue critical for isolating the superior right-sided PV. In these situations, key procedural endpoints may not be achievable without excessive risk of collateral damage to these surrounding structures. Another theoretical advantage of the epicardial approach is that it can allow use of protective techniques to reduce the risks of ablation. If it is possible to achieve more extensive and effective endocardial ablation, the success rate of the procedure could be higher.

Epicardial catheter ablation has the potential of combining the efficacy of surgical ablation with the less invasive approach and lower procedural risk of catheter ablation.

EPICARDIAL CATHETER ABLATION: DEVELOPMENT, CURRENT USES, AND ANATOMY

Sosa and colleagues[19] first described the technique of epicardial catheter ablation via the percutaneous subxiphoid approach in 1996. Initially, this procedure was used to treat ventricular tachycardia in patients with Chagas disease, which has a predilection for subepicardial tissue, resulting in epicardial reentrant circuits that can be difficult to treat with endocardial ablation. The technique has since been applied to the treatment of many other arrhythmias, including infarct-related ventricular tachycardia,[11] accessory pathways,[20] and other arrhythmias.[21]

The heart is invested in 2 serosal layers, the visceral and parietal pericardium. The virtual cavity between them is the pericardial space, divided into distinct pericardial sinuses through which catheters can be moved with only minimal resistance (**Fig. 1**).[22] The transverse sinus is located inferior and posterior to the aorta and main pulmonary artery (PA) and above the roof of the LA and superior PVs (**Fig. 2**).[23] The oblique sinus is a recess located behind the left ventricle and the LA and bounded by the reflection of the pericardium at the PVs. The inferoposterior left ventricle and posterior LA are accessible via the oblique sinus. The pulmonary venous pericardial recesses are particularly useful in approaching the epicardial aspect of PV ostia.[24]

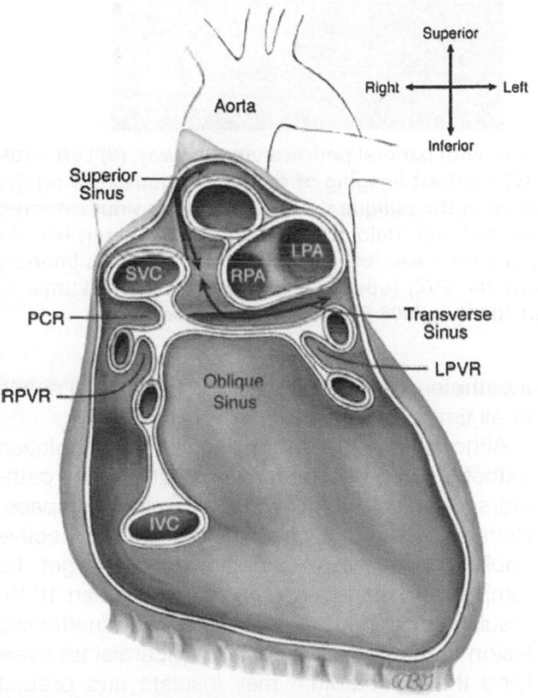

Fig. 1. Anatomy of the pericardium and its reflections. The transverse sinus is limited by pericardial reflections at the superior PVs and affords access only to the superior epicardial aspect of the PV ostia. The oblique sinus lies adjacent the posterior LA and inferoposterior left ventricle and allows access to these areas. The left PV recess (LPVR) and right PV recess (RPVR), situated just lateral to the pericardial reflection, span the upper and lower PVs. IVC, inferior vena cava; LPA, left pulmonary artery; PCR, postcaval recess; RPA, right pulmonary artery SVC, superior vena cava. (*From* D'Avila A, Scanavacca M, Sosa E, et al. Pericardial anatomy for the interventional electrophysiologist. J Cardiovasc Electrophysiol 2003;14(4):422–30; with permission.)

Catheter movement within pericardial sinuses is fairly unrestricted. However, because of pericardial reflections, complete encircling of the right-sided PVs is not possible without dissection.[23] One method of overcoming this limitation could be a hybrid endocardial-epicardial ablation procedure, in which targeted locations not reachable epicardially could be ablated from the endocardial approach. Alternatively, tools allowing dissection of these reflections from the percutaneous subxiphoid approach could be developed.

TECHNIQUE OF EPICARDIAL CATHETER ABLATION

Most equipment used for epicardial catheter ablation is also used in endocardial ablation procedures. Aside from the Tuohy needle (Smiths Medical, Norwell, MA, USA), developed to access the epidural space for anesthesia, the technology used to operate in the pericardial space is already available in most electrophysiologic laboratories.

The most common technique for subxiphoid percutaneous pericardial access has been described in detail by Sosa and colleagues.[25] Endocardial diagnostic catheters positioned in the coronary sinus and on the right ventricular (RV) septum serve as anatomic landmarks. In the authors' laboratory, epicardial access is established before systemic anticoagulation to reduce the risk of hemorrhagic complications. Before puncture, intravenous cefazolin is administered for surgical prophylaxis. After lidocaine infiltration, the skin is nicked with a #11 surgical blade 1 to 2 cm below the xiphoid process under sterile conditions. Through this opening, a Tuohy needle is inserted and directed toward the left shoulder.

The needle tip is then advanced toward the cardiac silhouette under fluoroscopic guidance in the left anterior oblique (LAO) view. When the tip of the needle reaches the pericardium, an additional resistance is usually felt, and tenting of the pericardium may be seen if a small amount of iodinated contrast is injected. If the needle tip has already punctured the pericardium, contrast will layer in the pericardial space and outline the heart. Staining of soft tissue outside the heart border generally signifies insufficient needle advancement to puncture the parietal pericardium. Rapid washout of dye or staining of muscular trabeculae usually means the needle

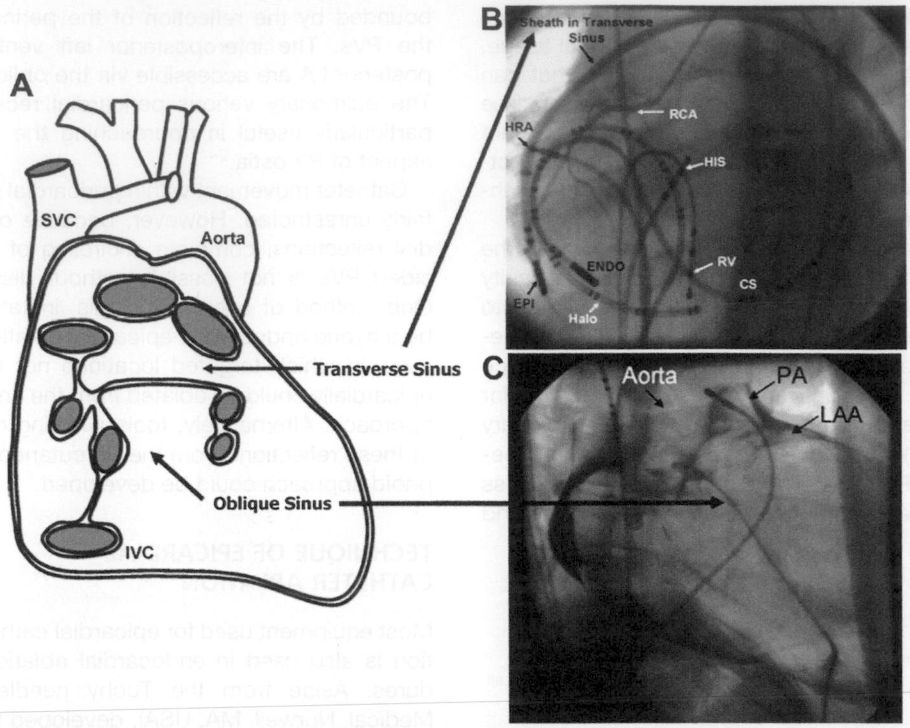

Fig. 2. Anatomy of the pericardial space. (*A*) Pericardial sinuses with parietal pericardium cut away. (*B*) Left anterior oblique view of endocardial and epicardial catheters. (*C*) Contrast imaging of the pericardium showing the oblique sinus and other structures. The pigtail catheter is deep in the oblique sinus. CS, coronary sinus catheter; ENDO, endocardial ablation catheter; EPI, epicardial ablation catheter; Halo, tricuspid annulus catheter; HIS, His bundle catheter; HRA, high right atrium; IVC, inferior vena cava; LAA, left atrial appendage; PA, pulmonary artery; RCA, right coronary artery; RV, right ventricular catheter; SVC, superior vena cava. (*From* Shivkumar K. Percutaneous epicardial ablation of atrial fibrillation. Heart Rhythm 2008;5(1):152–4; with permission.)

has passed the pericardial space and entered or penetrated the RV myocardium.

After pericardial contrast layering has been observed, a standard 0.038-in, 45-cm, J-tipped guidewire is gently advanced into the pericardial space. It should outline the left heart border in the LAO view, and wrap around the heart superiorly as it crosses into the transverse sinus. At this point, the operator must ensure fluoroscopically that the guidewire is not passing into pleural space, RV or PA with right anterior oblique (RAO) and LAO views. Next, a 5F, 20-cm dilator is used to create a passage through subcutaneous tissue. Then the 45-cm guidewire is exchanged for a long guidewire. Finally, after ensuring fluoroscopically that this guidewire is also positioned in the pericardial space, a long guiding sheath is advanced over it into the pericardial space to maintain access and facilitate catheter delivery. The authors normally use an 8F SL0 sheath (St Jude Medical, Minneapolis, MN, USA), although deflectable sheaths can also be used. Long sheaths developed specifically for epicardial ablation are currently under development. To avoid trauma from the tip of the sheath, a catheter should be kept in the pericardial space at all times.

Although virtually any diagnostic or ablation catheter can be used, conventional ablation catheters have limited utility in the pericardial space. Because of the lack of blood flow and convective cooling, noncooled catheters reach target tip temperatures at low power, often less than 10 W, resulting in limited energy delivery and ineffective lesion formation.[26] In addition, epicardial fat overlying the myocardium may insulate and protect targeted tissue. Cooled-tip catheters, whether internally or externally irrigated, allow higher power delivery (20–50 W) without temperature rise, and result in adequate lesions even when ablating through epicardial fat.[27] Irrigation flow rate is adjusted to keep catheter tip temperature at less than 42°C. Indicators of effective lesion formation include decrease in local electrogram amplitude, reduction in ablation circuit impedance, and in the case of PV isolation, dissociation or elimination of PV potentials. When using an externally irrigated ablation catheter, care must be taken to aspirate the pericardial sheath periodically to prevent fluid accumulation that could result in iatrogenic pericardial effusion or tamponade.

Electroanatomic mapping, which has proved useful in endocardial ablation procedures, can also be used in the pericardial space. In general, creating a separate map or shell prevents confusion of epicardial and endocardial points. New technologies may further improve epicardial mapping and ablation. For instance, remote navigation technology using a magnetically guided catheter has been used to create complete endocardial and epicardial substrate maps with minimal fluoroscopy exposure.[28] As manipulation of the catheter within the pericardial recesses requires precise movements, remote magnetic navigation may be especially useful in epicardial catheter ablation of AF.

SPECIAL RISKS AND CHALLENGES OF EPICARDIAL ABLATION

When planning an epicardial ablation procedure, the special risks of this technique should be considered, especially for treatment of non–life-threatening arrhythmias like AF. Although serious bleeding is rare, usually from puncture of hepatic vessels, less serious bleeding complications occurs more frequently, usually from right ventricular puncture or injury to small epicardial coronary veins. Once pericardial access is achieved, the sheath is aspirated to assess for blood in the pericardial space. If the patient has not yet been anticoagulated, bleeding is usually self-limited, and the procedure can be continued.[25] Therefore epicardial access is usually established before transseptal puncture, which requires systemic anticoagulation.

Another risk of epicardial ablation is collateral damage to structures around the heart. Although this also applies to endocardial ablation, the epicardial ablation catheter's proximity to extracardiac structures could potentially increase the risk of injury to the esophagus, phrenic nerves, or atrial branches of coronary arteries. Care should be taken to avoid ablation near these structures. This may require contrast esophagram to define esophageal location, high-output pacing to detect diaphragmatic stimulation and define the course of the phrenic nerve, and coronary angiography before epicardial energy delivery. Eventually, new technologies, such as fiberoptic pericardioscopy, might allow direct visualization of these structures to make epicardial ablation safer.[23]

Patients with a history of pericarditis, prior epicardial ablation, or previous sternotomy for cardiac surgery present special challenges. Inflammation and scarring can prevent free catheter movement within the pericardial space. Therefore, the usual percutaneous approach described earlier may not be possible. Instead,

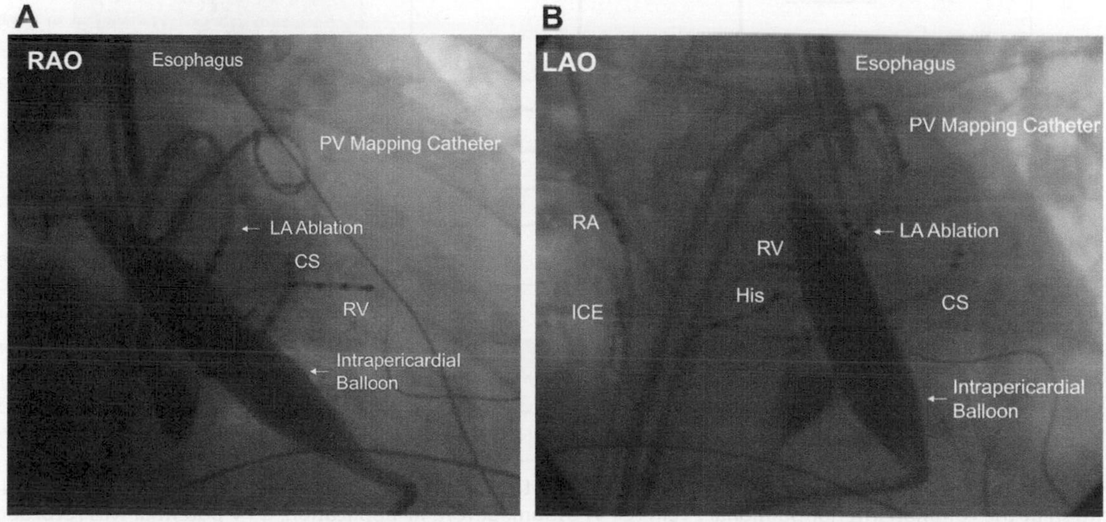

Fig. 3. Esophageal protection using intrapericardial balloon technique. (*A*) RAO and (*B*) LAO images of esophageal protection using intrapericardial balloon in the oblique sinus. The balloon was inflated to displace the esophagus and posterior LA, increasing separation between these structures, so that endocardial ablation near the antrum of the left inferior PV could be performed safely. CS, coronary sinus catheter; His, His bundle catheter; ICE, intracardiac echocardiography catheter; RA, right atrial catheter; RV, right ventricular catheter. (*From* Buch E, Nakahara S, Shivkumar K. Intra-pericardial balloon retraction of the left atrium: a novel method to prevent esophageal injury during catheter ablation. Heart Rhythm 2008;5(10):1473–5; with permission.)

some centers use a hybrid procedure with a small subxiphoid incision and pericardial dissection performed by a cardiac surgeon, to allow access to the pericardial space before epicardial mapping and ablation.[29] This technique has been described for the treatment of ventricular tachycardia, but not yet for atrial arrhythmias.

PRELIMINARY STUDIES ON EPICARDIAL AF ABLATION

Given the convincing rationale for an epicardial approach to ablation of AF and the techniques that have been developed to increase the safety and efficacy of epicardial ablation, it is not surprising that preliminary reports of such procedures have been published. In a series of 5 patients with persistent AF who had failed a conventional ablation procedure, Pak and colleagues[30] showed that adjunctive epicardial ablation was feasible. To reduce the chances of damaging surrounding structures, special precautions were taken, including filling the pericardial space with saline to separate the esophagus from the LA. In this small series of procedures, one case of hemopericardium was the only reported complication. In a case report presented by Reddy and coworkers,[31] PV isolation was not achieved despite extensive endocardial ablation. Epicardial mapping and ablation was performed at the breakthrough site, with immediate PV isolation and no apparent complications.

A case report published from the authors' center describes a hybrid epicardial-endocardial procedure, in which a balloon catheter (18 mm × 4 cm; Meditech, Boston Scientific, Natick, MA, USA) was positioned in the pericardial space between the LA and esophagus to allow safe and effective endocardial ablation.[32] This patient had a previous failed an ablation procedure in which proximity of the esophagus to PV ostia precluded adequate energy delivery. Inflation of the balloon increased separation between the esophagus and left atrium and allowed application of endocardial energy without esophageal injury (**Fig. 3**).

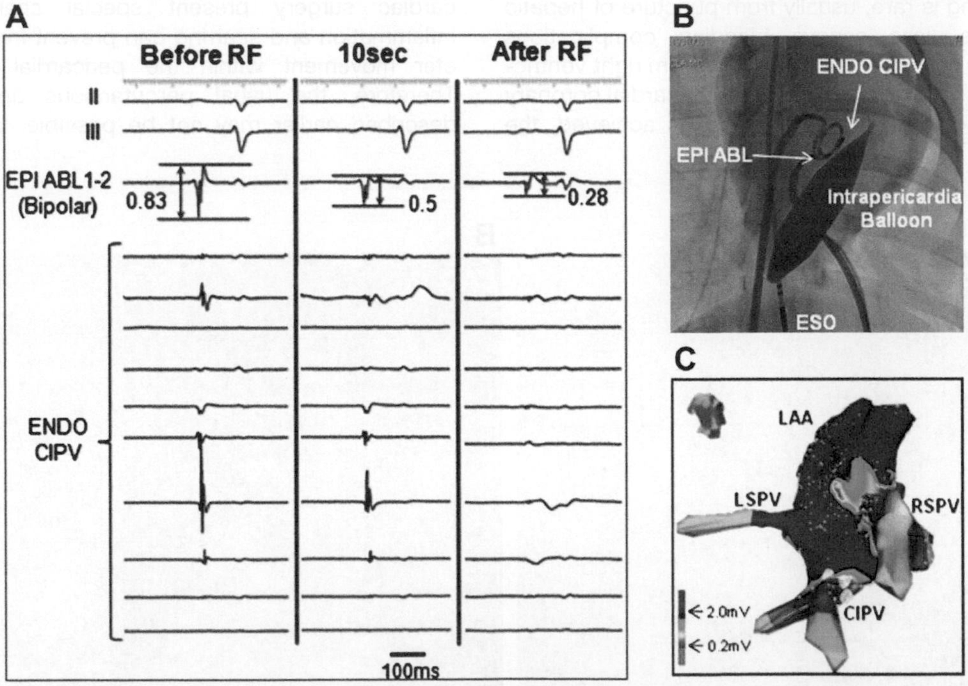

Fig. 4. Epicardial PV isolation in a porcine model. (*A*) PV potentials were eliminated by epicardial RF energy application at the common inferior pulmonary vein (CIPV) ostium. Before RF application, a PV potential was recorded from the epicardial ablation catheter (EPI ABL1-2). After RF application, endocardial PV potentials were eliminated. (*B*) RAO fluoroscopic images of the successful PV isolation sites. A 16-mm × 4-cm balloon was successfully positioned within the oblique sinus using a deflectable sheath guidance. An acute increase in temperature was observed when the same RF energy was applied without the balloon inflation. (*C*) The voltage map of the endocardial LA and PV surfaces in the same porcine heart show a low-voltage area within the CIPV after epicardial CIPV isolation. The white circles indicate the 3 ablation sites around the CIPV ostium. ENDO, endocardial ablation catheter; LAA, left atrial appendage; LSPV, left superior pulmonary vein; RSPV, right superior pulmonary vein.

The authors' group has investigated this strategy systematically in a series of animal experiments.[33] Using a porcine model, an intrapericardial balloon was inflated behind the LA during endocardial and epicardial catheter ablation. Subxiphoid epicardial access to the oblique sinus adjacent to the posterior LA wall allowed positioning of an intrapericardial balloon (12–18 mm × 4 cm; Meditech, Boston Scientific, Natick, MA, USA) over a guidewire in all 5 pigs (**Fig. 4**). Balloon inflation increased the distance between the esophagus and posterior LA by 12.8 ± 4.5 mm. Complete PV isolation was achieved in all animals with no esophageal temperature increase in the presence of the inflated balloon (+0.02 ± 0.04°C, P = not significant). In contrast, 3 control RF applications without balloon protection caused acute temperature increase (+1.2 ± 0.3°C, P<.0001). A hybrid epicardial catheter ablation procedure using intrapericardial balloon protection in conjunction with endocardial or epicardial RF application might offer improved efficacy with a lower chance of esophageal injury.

FUTURE DIRECTIONS

Despite promising preliminary communications on epicardial ablation for AF, the approach has not yet been proven safe or effective, and more studies are required to establish its role in the spectrum of procedures available for AF. New technologies under development, particularly for working within the pericardial space, should make the procedure more effective and safer in the future. Using these new tools and techniques, it may be possible to achieve the success rate of surgical treatment for AF with a catheter-based percutaneous procedure. The authors expect the role of epicardial ablation in the treatment of AF to develop at a rapid pace in the next decade.

REFERENCES

1. Oral H, Pappone C, Chugh A, et al. Circumferential pulmonary-vein ablation for chronic atrial fibrillation. N Engl J Med 2006;354(9):934–41.
2. Novak PG. Effectiveness of catheter ablation versus antiarrhythmic drug therapy for atrial fibrillation. Curr Opin Cardiol 2009;24(1):9–17.
3. Calkins H, Brugada J, Packer DL, et al. HRS/EHRA/ECAS expert Consensus Statement on catheter and surgical ablation of atrial fibrillation: recommendations for personnel, policy, procedures and follow-up. A report of the Heart Rhythm Society (HRS) Task Force on catheter and surgical ablation of atrial fibrillation. Heart Rhythm 2007;4(6):816–61.
4. Cappato R, Calkins H, Chen SA, et al. Prevalence and causes of fatal outcome in catheter ablation of atrial fibrillation. J Am Coll Cardiol 2009;53(19):1798–803.
5. Cappato R, Calkins H, Chen SA, et al. Worldwide survey on the methods, efficacy, and safety of catheter ablation for human atrial fibrillation. Circulation 2005;111(9):1100–5.
6. Quinn FR, Rankin AC. Atrial fibrillation ablation in the real world. Heart 2005;91(12):1507–8.
7. Cox JL, Schuessler RB, D'Agostino HJ Jr, et al. The surgical treatment of atrial fibrillation. III. Development of a definitive surgical procedure. J Thorac Cardiovasc Surg 1991;101(4):569–83.
8. Damiano RJ Jr, Gaynor SL, Bailey M, et al. The long-term outcome of patients with coronary disease and atrial fibrillation undergoing the Cox maze procedure. J Thorac Cardiovasc Surg 2003;126(6):2016–21.
9. Bakir I, Casselman FP, Brugada P, et al. Current strategies in the surgical treatment of atrial fibrillation: review of the literature and Onze Lieve Vrouw Clinic's strategy. Ann Thorac Surg 2007;83(1):331–40.
10. Edgerton JR, Edgerton ZJ, Weaver T, et al. Minimally invasive pulmonary vein isolation and partial autonomic denervation for surgical treatment of atrial fibrillation. Ann Thorac Surg 2008;86(1):35–8 [discussion: 39].
11. Sosa E, Scanavacca M, d'Avila A, et al. Nonsurgical transthoracic epicardial catheter ablation to treat recurrent ventricular tachycardia occurring late after myocardial infarction. J Am Coll Cardiol 2000;35(6):1442–9.
12. O'Neill MD, Wright M, Knecht S, et al. Long-term follow-up of persistent atrial fibrillation ablation using termination as a procedural endpoint. Eur Heart J 2009;30(9):1105–12.
13. Doshi RN, Wu TJ, Yashima M, et al. Relation between ligament of Marshall and adrenergic atrial tachyarrhythmia. Circulation 1999;100(8):876–83.
14. Armour JA, Murphy DA, Yuan BX, et al. Gross and microscopic anatomy of the human intrinsic cardiac nervous system. Anat Rec 1997;247(2):289–98.
15. Scherlag BJ, Po S. The intrinsic cardiac nervous system and atrial fibrillation. Curr Opin Cardiol 2006;21(1):51–4.
16. Pokushalov E, Romanov A, Shugayev P, et al. Selective ganglionated plexi ablation for paroxysmal atrial fibrillation. Heart Rhythm 2009;6(9):1257–64.
17. Lemery R. How to perform ablation of the parasympathetic ganglia of the left atrium. Heart Rhythm 2006;3(10):1237–9.
18. Lemola K, Sneider M, Desjardins B, et al. Computed tomographic analysis of the anatomy of the left atrium and the esophagus: implications for left atrial catheter ablation. Circulation 2004;110(24):3655–60.

19. Sosa E, Scanavacca M, d'Avila A, et al. A new technique to perform epicardial mapping in the electrophysiology laboratory. J Cardiovasc Electrophysiol 1996;7(6):531–6.
20. Valderrabano M, Cesario DA, Ji S, et al. Percutaneous epicardial mapping during ablation of difficult accessory pathways as an alternative to cardiac surgery. Heart Rhythm 2004;1(3):311–6.
21. Schweikert RA, Saliba WI, Tomassoni G, et al. Percutaneous pericardial instrumentation for endo-epicardial mapping of previously failed ablations. Circulation 2003;108(11):1329–35.
22. D'Avila A, Scanavacca M, Sosa E, et al. Pericardial anatomy for the interventional electrophysiologist. J Cardiovasc Electrophysiol 2003;14(4):422–30.
23. Shivkumar K. Percutaneous epicardial ablation of atrial fibrillation. Heart Rhythm 2008;5(1):152–4.
24. Truong MT, Erasmus JJ, Gladish GW, et al. Anatomy of pericardial recesses on multidetector CT: implications for oncologic imaging. AJR Am J Roentgenol 2003;181(4):1109–13.
25. Sosa E, Scanavacca M. Epicardial mapping and ablation techniques to control ventricular tachycardia. J Cardiovasc Electrophysiol 2005;16(4):449–52.
26. Aliot EM, Stevenson WG, Almendral-Garrote JM, et al. EHRA/HRS Expert Consensus on Catheter Ablation of Ventricular Arrhythmias: developed in a partnership with the European Heart Rhythm Association (EHRA), a Registered Branch of the European Society of Cardiology (ESC), and the Heart Rhythm Society (HRS); in collaboration with the American College of Cardiology (ACC) and the American Heart Association (AHA). Heart Rhythm 2009;6(6):886–933.
27. d'Avila A, Houghtaling C, Gutierrez P, et al. Catheter ablation of ventricular epicardial tissue: a comparison of standard and cooled-tip radiofrequency energy. Circulation 2004;109(19):2363–9.
28. Aryana A, d'Avila A, Heist EK, et al. Remote magnetic navigation to guide endocardial and epicardial catheter mapping of scar-related ventricular tachycardia. Circulation 2007;115(10):1191–200.
29. Soejima K, Couper G, Cooper JM, et al. Subxiphoid surgical approach for epicardial catheter-based mapping and ablation in patients with prior cardiac surgery or difficult pericardial access. Circulation 2004;110(10):1197–201.
30. Pak HN, Hwang C, Lim HE, et al. Hybrid epicardial and endocardial ablation of persistent or permanent atrial fibrillation: a new approach for difficult cases. J Cardiovasc Electrophysiol 2007;18(9):917–23.
31. Reddy VY, Neuzil P, Ruskin JN. Extra-ostial pulmonary venous isolation: use of epicardial ablation to eliminate a point of conduction breakthrough. J Cardiovasc Electrophysiol 2003;14(6):663–6.
32. Buch E, Nakahara S, Shivkumar K. Intra-pericardial balloon retraction of the left atrium: a novel method to prevent esophageal injury during catheter ablation. Heart Rhythm 2008;5(10):1473–5.
33. Nakahara S, Buch E, Ramirez J, et al. Intrapericardial balloon placement for preventing collateral injury and effective epicardial ablation of atrial fibrillation. Heart Rhythm 2009;6(Suppl I):S13.

Remote Navigation and Electroanatomic Mapping in the Pericardial Space

J. David Burkhardt, MD[a,b], Luigi Di Biase, MD[a,c,d], Rodney Horton, MD[a,c,e], Robert A. Schweikert, MD[e], Andrea Natale, MD[a,c,f,g,h,*]

KEYWORDS

- Remote magnetic navigation • Ablation • Epicardial
- Robotic • Mapping

Mapping in the pericardial space has been shown to be beneficial in a variety of arrhythmias. Atrial fibrillation, accessory pathways, ventricular tachycardia, inappropriate sinus tachycardia, and atrial tachycardias have been found to be successfully ablated from the pericardial space.[1–6] The percutaneous subxiphoid approach to the pericardial space has been developed, and interventional cardiac electrophysiologists now use this approach to map and ablate arrhythmias within this space.[7,8]

The current tool set for mapping and ablation in this space is limited. Access to this area is performed using available epidural needles and standard sheaths. Catheters that are designed for endocardial and endovascular mapping and ablation have traditionally been used for mapping and ablation in this space. Although these catheters are usable, the lack of specifically designed catheters is a limitation. The pericardial space is generally open and without obstacles. Catheters can move freely in this space, which makes movement easy; however, navigation proves difficult sometimes. Catheters designed for endovascular manipulation and endocardial mapping use vascular and cardiac structures as torque points, allowing the catheter to be directed to an area when it is not attainable by a direct approach or through manipulation of the catheter handle. For example, the tricuspid valve can be used to direct the tip of an ablation catheter to the right ventricular apex. In the pericardial space, the only available torque points are the pericardial reflections. To reach some areas, looping of the catheter around the heart is necessary to direct the tip. The curves available in deflectable catheters usually do not translate well to movement in the pericardial space. Deflectable sheaths have been used to aide navigation in the space. These sheaths allow lateral directionality, but they are less useful for anterior and posterior movements. In addition, the angle of pericardial access and the anterior or posterior entrance of the access point may limit the utility of these sheaths.

[a] Texas Cardiac Arrhythmia Institute at St David's Medical Center, 1015 East 32nd Street, #516, Austin, TX78705, USA
[b] Stereotaxis, 4320 Forest Park Avenue, Suite 100, St Louis, MO #63108, USA
[c] Department of Biomedical Engineering, University of Texas, 1 University Station CO 800, Austin, TX78712, USA
[d] Department of Cardiology, University of Foggia, viale L Pinto, 1 71100, Foggia, Italy
[e] Akron General Hospital, Department of Cardiology, 400 Wabash Avenue, Akron, OH 44307, USA
[f] Division of Cardiology, Stanford University, 300 Pasteur Drive, Stanford, CA 94305, USA
[g] Department of Cardiovascular Medicine, Case Western Reserve University, 11100 Euclid Avenue, Cleveland, OH 44106, USA
[h] EP Services, California Pacific Medical Center, 2333 Buchanan Street, San Francisco, CA 94115, USA
* Corresponding author. Texas Cardiac Arrhythmia Institute at St David's Medical Center, 1015 East 32nd Street, #516, Austin, TX 78705.
E-mail address: dr.natale@gmail.com (A. Natale).

Card Electrophysiol Clin 2 (2010) 121–125
doi:10.1016/j.ccep.2009.11.010
1877-9182/10/$ – see front matter

Remote magnetic navigation has been developed to allow the navigation of magnetically enabled devices such as ablation catheters. These catheters can be controlled remotely via a computer interface. Two large composite rare earth magnets are positioned on the lateral sides of a patient. The magnets can rotate, tilt, and move toward and away from the patient. The movement of the magnets creates a composite magnetic vector inside the chest of a patient. A magnetically enabled catheter will align with this vector. The vector can be oriented in any direction in the x, y, and z axis. When combined with a remote catheter advancing and retracting system, an ablation catheter can be remotely directed to locations within the heart. Unlike manual catheters, magnetic navigation catheters have no pull wires. This allows the catheter to have a very floppy design. Unlike conventional catheters in which the tip is controlled through pull wires and rotational manipulation of the handle that is three feet away from the tip, magnetic navigation catheters are controlled by the tip. This allows contortions and movement of catheters that are not possible with conventional catheters. In addition, various curves are not necessary to direct the tip to desired locations.[9]

Magnetically enabled ablation catheters appear to have different ablation properties than standard catheters. The contact forces of magnetic catheters tend to be in the 10 to 20 g range compared with forces that may exceed 100 g in manual catheters. Magnetic catheters appear to maintain more stable contact, unlike manual catheters that may lose contact during the cardiac cycle. With non-irrigated magnetic catheters, this may increase the risk of carbonization at the tip. It appears that the lesions made with magnetic catheters are superior at lower contact forces; however, the very deep lesions that are possible with high contact forces are not possible. Ablation with these catheters does appear to be safe. In general, the lack of high contact forces appears to reduce the risk of steam pops or perforations.[10,11]

Remote magnetic navigation has been used in the pericardial space. Navigation appears to be easier than with manual navigation. Since the catheter is controlled at the tip, it can be directed to an area of interest without the need for using the pericardial reflections as torque points. This may allow for navigation that is more direct without looping of the catheter. The catheter tip can also be directed toward the epicardial surface, which is not possible with conventional catheters. This may improve epicardial lesions and reduce the risk of collateral damage.[12]

In a case series of four patients that had arrhythmias originating from the tip of the left atrial appendage, Di Biase and colleagues[12] describe using remote magnetic navigation to perform the endocardial and epicardial mapping, although a manual irrigated tip catheter was used for ablation. An irrigated magnetic ablation catheter was not available at the time the mappings were performed. No further comments were made about the magnetic catheter in this series, but it was also used to map the appendage as reported (**Figs. 1** and **2**).

In a relatively large series of patients with ventricular arrhythmias, Aryana and colleagues[13] describe remote magnetic navigation in endocardial and epicardial mapping and ablation. In this group of 24 patients with ventricular arrhythmias associated with ischemic heart disease, non-ischemic cardiomyopathy, cardiac sarcoid,

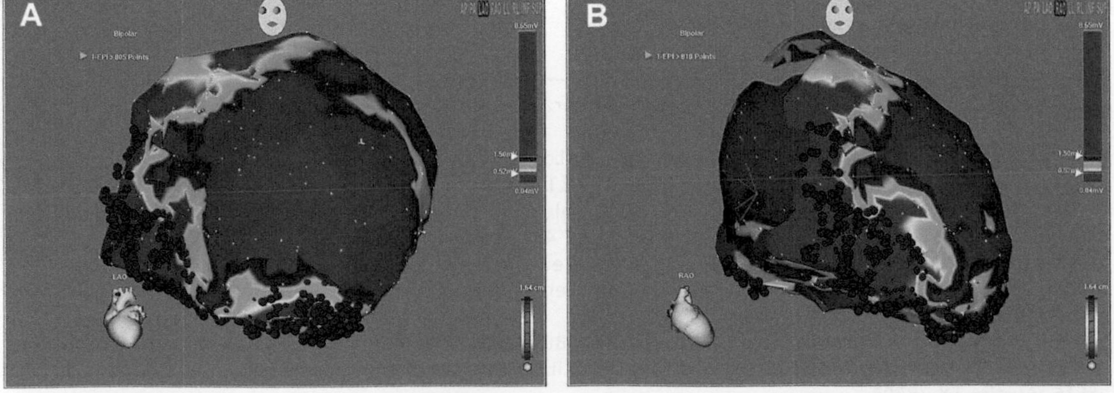

Fig. 1. Left anterior oblique (*A*) and right anterior oblique (*B*) of a 3-dimensional epicardial mapping obtained with magnetic navigation in a patient with ischemic ventricular tachycardia. Red dots indicate ablation points in the apical and anteroseptal wall of the left ventricle.

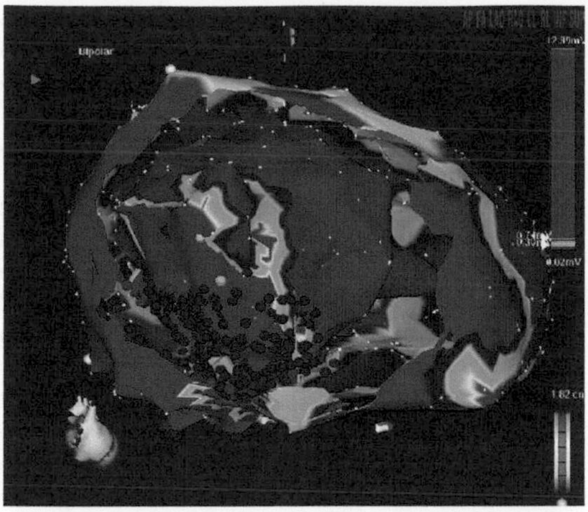

Fig. 2. Endo-epi 3-dimensional map of the left ventricle created with magnetic navigation. Red dots indicate ablation points at the level of the inferolateral epicardial wall.

arrhythmogenic right ventricular dysplasia, and hypertrophic cardiomyopathy, 12 patients underwent epicardial mapping and ablation using the magnetic navigation system. Fluoroscopy times were very short for the epicardial mapping, averaging 18 seconds plus or minus 18 seconds. In some cases, no fluoroscopy was used for the mapping. An average of 122 plus or minus 34 points was collected on the epicardial maps. Epicardial ablation was performed using the system with solid-tipped catheters in a minority of cases. In most cases, open irrigated manual catheters were also used, whether endocardial or epicardial.

According to the investigators, the main limitations of the system were the lack of irrigated ablation catheters available at the time and the limited fluoroscopic view of the entire ventricle. When the magnets were in place, table movement was limited and the small detector plate used with the system was frequently inadequate to visualize the entire ventricle in patients with enlarged chambers. The investigators felt that this limitation was minor because fluoroscopy was barely used for that portion.

The investigators report that the magnetic catheter is able to map adequately and perform all of the necessary maneuvers. They state that the catheter has enhanced maneuverability and allowed access to difficult-to-reach areas, which may obviate the need for operator skill in challenging cases.

Recently, Di Biase and colleagues[14] reported on the use of the solid-tipped magnetic catheters in the ablation of ventricular arrhythmias. The success of ablation between the 4 mm- and 8 mm-tipped catheters available at that time is described. Sixty-five patients were included in the study, and 18 patients underwent epicardial mapping and ablation. The study reported that these solid-tipped catheters were mostly ineffective in terminating ventricular tachycardia and required an open irrigated catheter to achieve the endpoint of noninducible ventricular arrhythmias. The success rates are not shown in reference to epicardial ablation; however, both catheters were very successful in patients without structural heart disease. In patients with structural heart disease, the 4 mm-tipped catheter demonstrated 22% success compared with 59% success with the 8 mm-tipped catheter. All maps were created with the 4 mm-tipped catheter owing to the ability to map the myocardial surface finely. The investigators generated very detailed 300-point maps, on average, for the patients with structural heart disease.

The investigators thought that the main limitation of the system was the lack of an irrigated ablation catheter; however, they thought that the remote navigation system enhanced the mapping of ventricular arrhythmias and the reduced fluoroscopy exposure was beneficial.

Burkhardt and colleagues[15] reported on a series of patients that underwent mapping and ablation with solid-tipped magnetic catheters in the pericardial space. This included patients with ventricular tachycardia and accessory pathways. In this series, all patients were completely mapped using the magnetic navigation system. Navigation in the pericardial space was not difficult and seemed to require less looping of the catheter. Only four of these patients underwent ablation in the pericardial space, and all of these ablations were unsuccessful. Considering the limitations of solid-tipped catheters in this space, this was not necessarily unexpected. Although the system was used to map the arrhythmia, for most cases an irrigated catheter was used for ablation. Most operators did not feel that the solid-tipped catheters were able to deliver adequate power in this space. All of the unsuccessful ablations exhibited limited power delivery due to high electrode temperatures during ablation. Once again, the open irrigated magnetic catheter was not available for use in this group. The operators felt that the benefits of mapping with the system—including precision, the ability to actively interact with the electroanatomic mapping system, and reduced radiation exposure—were worth the need to use a manual irrigated catheter for ablation.

After these articles were published, the open irrigated magnetic catheter was approved and has been available for use in the United States since

March 2009. The authors have used this catheter for mapping and ablation in the pericardial space. From a navigation perspective, the catheter performs identically to the 4 mm solid-tipped catheter. It is able to course throughout the pericardial space without limitation, and the magnetic system allows for more direct approaches to target areas. The 8 mm solid-tipped catheter is much stiffer and less pliable and rarely used for navigation. From an ablation perspective, the open irrigated magnetic catheter is a significant improvement. Power delivery in the pericardial space is usually not limited by temperature rises, and the success rates appear to be at least equal to manual open irrigated catheters in the same area. The ability to direct the tip of the catheter toward the epicardial surface appears to be a significant advantage over the manual counterpart. One limitation of the system is that the software is designed for endocardial navigation. The vectors are centered in the middle of the chamber of interest. Although this does not impair navigation, when one desires to force the catheter tip against the heart, the vector must be directed away from the surface of choice. For example, if the catheter is along the anterior surface, the vector must be directed posteriorly to cause the catheter tip to face the epicardial surface. Perhaps future software updates will address this issue and allow for navigation based on epicardial geometry.

Remote magnetic navigation and ablation in the pericardial space appears to be feasible. All of the necessary maneuvers are possible, and the system allows navigation to difficult-to-reach areas with minimal effort. Considering that navigation in the pericardial space is new to some operators, magnetic navigation may assist in making the learning curve more manageable. Considering that making large loops in a catheter is mostly foreign to operators who do not perform epicardial ablation, magnetic navigation may be of benefit. In addition, the ability to direct the catheter tip toward the epicardial surface may be beneficial. Fluoroscopy exposure to the operator is decreased and the increased interaction with the electroanatomic mapping system may reduce the radiation exposure to the patient. Most investigators report that the magnetic navigation system is particularly beneficial in mapping complex arrhythmias, including those that require mapping in the pericardial space. The main limitations appear the lack of an irrigated ablation catheter in these studies. Most investigators felt that the solid-tipped catheters were not appropriate for ablation, particularly in ventricular tachycardia in the setting of structural heart disease. Now that an irrigated magnetic catheter is available, it will be interesting to see how this catheter performs compared with the manual irrigated catheter in the pericardial space. The results of these studies are encouraging regarding the use of remote magnetic navigation in the pericardial space; however, more studies are needed with the newest generation of catheters to fully determine the usefulness of this system in these complex cases.

REFERENCES

1. Burkhardt JD, Saliba WI, Schweikert RA, et al. Remote magnetic navigation to map and ablate left coronary cusp ventricular tachycardia. J Cardiovasc Electrophysiol 2006;17:1142.
2. Chun JK, Ernst S, Matthews S, et al. Remote-controlled catheter ablation of accessory pathways: results from the magnetic laboratory. Eur Heart J 2007;28:190.
3. Di Biase L, Fahmy TS, Patel D, et al. Remote magnetic navigation: human experience in pulmonary vein ablation. J Am Coll Cardiol 2007;50:868.
4. Katsiyiannis WT, Melby DP, Matelski JL, et al. Feasibility and safety of remote-controlled magnetic navigation for ablation of atrial fibrillation. Am J Cardiol 2008;102:1674.
5. Pappone C, Vicedomini G, Manguso F, et al. Robotic magnetic navigation for atrial fibrillation ablation. J Am Coll Cardiol 2006;47:1390.
6. Schneider MA, Neuser H, Koller ML, et al. Automatic magnetic-guided electroanatomical mapping and remote-controlled ablation of atypical and typical atrial flutter. Pacing Clin Electrophysiol 2008;31:1355.
7. Schweikert RA, Saliba WI, Tomassoni G, et al. Percutaneous pericardial instrumentation for endo-epicardial mapping of previously failed ablations. Circulation 2003;108:1329.
8. Sosa E, Scanavacca M, D'Avila A, et al. Endocardial and epicardial ablation guided by nonsurgical transthoracic epicardial mapping to treat recurrent ventricular tachycardia. J Cardiovasc Electrophysiol 1998;9:229.
9. Ernst S. Magnetic and robotic navigation for catheter ablation: "joystick ablation". J Interv Card Electrophysiol 2008;23:41.
10. Di Biase L, Natale A, Barrett C, et al. Relationship between catheter forces, lesion characteristics, "popping," and char formation: experience with robotic navigation system. J Cardiovasc Electrophysiol 2009;20:436.
11. Okumura Y, Johnson SB, Bunch TJ, et al. A systematical analysis of in vivo contact forces on virtual catheter tip/tissue surface contact during cardiac mapping and intervention. J Cardiovasc Electrophysiol 2008;19:632.

12. Di Biase L, Schweikert RA, Saliba WI, et al. Left atrial appendage tip: an unusual site of successful ablation after failed endocardial and epicardial mapping and ablation. J Cardiovasc Electrophysiol 2009. [Epub ahead of print].
13. Aryana A, d'Avila A, Heist EK, et al. Remote magnetic navigation to guide endocardial and epicardial catheter mapping of scar-related ventricular tachycardia. Circulation 2007;115:1191.
14. Di Biase L, Burkhardt JD, Lakkireddy D, et al. Mapping and ablation of ventricular arrhythmias with magnetic navigation: comparison between 4- and 8-mm catheter tips. J Interv Card Electrophysiol 2009. [Epub ahead of print].
15. Burkhardt JD, Di Biase L, Lakkireddy D, et al. Remote magnetic navigation to map and ablate arrhythmias in the pericardial space. J Cardiovasc Electrophysiol. [Epub ahead of print].

Recognition and Prevention of Complications During Epicardial Ablation

Takumi Yamada, MD, PhD*, G. Neal Kay, MD

KEYWORDS

• Complication • Recognition • Prevention
• Epicardial • Catheter ablation

Transthoracic epicardial mapping and ablation has been proven to be a useful supplemental or even preferable strategy to eliminate cardiac arrhythmias in the electrophysiology laboratory.[1–4] The indication of this technique has extended to a diverse range of cardiac arrhythmias, including scar-related ventricular tachycardia (VT),[2,3,5–8] atrial fibrillation,[9,10] accessory pathways,[11–13] atrial tachycardias,[14,15] and idiopathic VTs.[16,17] Although previous studies have reported that significant complications have been infrequent with this technique,[1–17] it should be emphasized that those reports generally have come from highly experienced centers with highly skilled personnel. Electrophysiologists who attempt epicardial catheter ablation should know the potential complications associated with this technique, how to minimize their occurrence, and how to rapidly recognize and treat the complications that they encounter. As with almost all invasive procedures, complications can and do occur during epicardial ablation, during pericardial access, epicardial mapping and ablation, or after the procedure. This review describes the details of how to recognize, prevent, and manage the complications that occur during each of these 3 periods (pericardial access, mapping and ablation, and postprocedure).

COMPLICATIONS RELATED TO THE PERICARDIAL ACCESS

Transthoracic epicardial puncture is the most important step of the whole procedure. Although this process can be safely and efficiently undertaken in the electrophysiology laboratory as previously described,[18–20] inadvertent puncture of a coronary artery or vein or a cardiac chamber may sometimes occur. The subxiphoid approach involves blindly passing an 18-gauge needle from the skin, through the subcutaneous fat, rectus muscle, and usually through the diaphragm. In patients with congestive heart failure, the left lobe of the liver may also be punctured. Thus, arterial vessels in any of these structures may be punctured. Because of this, monitoring of blood pressure, heart rate, and 12-lead electrocardiogram is mandatory during the entire procedure. To minimize these complications, systemic anticoagulation with heparin should not be administered or must be reversed if already administered before the epicardial access is safely attempted. Without systemic anticoagulation, bleeding is usually self-limited and does not usually preclude mapping and catheter ablation. Patients anticoagulated with warfarin should have their oral anticoagulants discontinued or reversed before attempting elective epicardial ablation.

Inadvertent puncture of the right ventricle (RV) is relatively common. A "dry" puncture of the RV may be observed in 10% to 20% of patients. However, in a patient who is not anticoagulated, perforation of the RV is usually benign if only the needle or guidewire has entered the chamber. Therefore, it is important to recognize RV perforation before introducing the pericardial sheath. The

Division of Cardiovascular Disease, University of Alabama at Birmingham, VH B147, 1670 University Boulevard, 1530 3rd Avenue South, Birmingham, AL 35294-0019, USA
* Corresponding author.
E-mail address: takumi-y@fb4.so-net.ne.jp (T. Yamada).

Card Electrophysiol Clin 2 (2010) 127–134
doi:10.1016/j.ccep.2009.11.012
1877-9182/10/$ – see front matter

authors' practice is to routinely inject contrast through the needle before advancing a guidewire. In this way, RV perforation may be easily recognized by the ejection of contrast into the pulmonary artery. If the needle is within the RV, it should be slightly retracted and then a little more contrast can be injected until it is seen to surround the heart within the pericardial space. At this point, an attempt to feed the guidewire into the pericardial space may be made, rather than withdrawing the needle completely and starting anew. However, even with this precaution it is still possible that a soft floppy-tip guidewire may be introduced into the RV through the needle. The first sign that suggests this may be arrhythmias, usually a run of premature ventricular contractions that come from the RV outflow tract because the guidewire is likely to advance through the body of the RV to the pulmonary artery (**Fig. 1**). The second sign may be the lack of the typical appearance of the guidewire in the pericardial space on the fluoroscopic images as more guidewire is advanced.[20] It is essential to observe the guidewire in the left anterior oblique projection, observing that it hugs the cardiac silhouette, crossing more than one chamber, circumferential to both the right and left heart (**Fig. 2**). Observation in the right anterior oblique or antero-posterior projection alone can be misleading, as a guidewire that enters the RV and passes into the right atrium or pulmonary artery can be misinterpreted as being intrapericardial (see **Fig. 2**). In addition, if the guidewire is outside the cardiac silhouette, congenital absence of the pericardium may be suspected. This rare situation can be demonstrated by introducing the sheath and demonstrating that contrast fills the left pleural space. It should be noted that the fluoroscopic appearance of the cardiac silhouette is quite abnormal in the setting of congenital absence of the pericardium, and suspicion of this anomaly should result in postponing the procedure until this diagnosis can be confirmed by computed tomography or magnetic resonance imaging.

After successful cannulation of the pericardial space with a guidewire, a pericardial catheter with

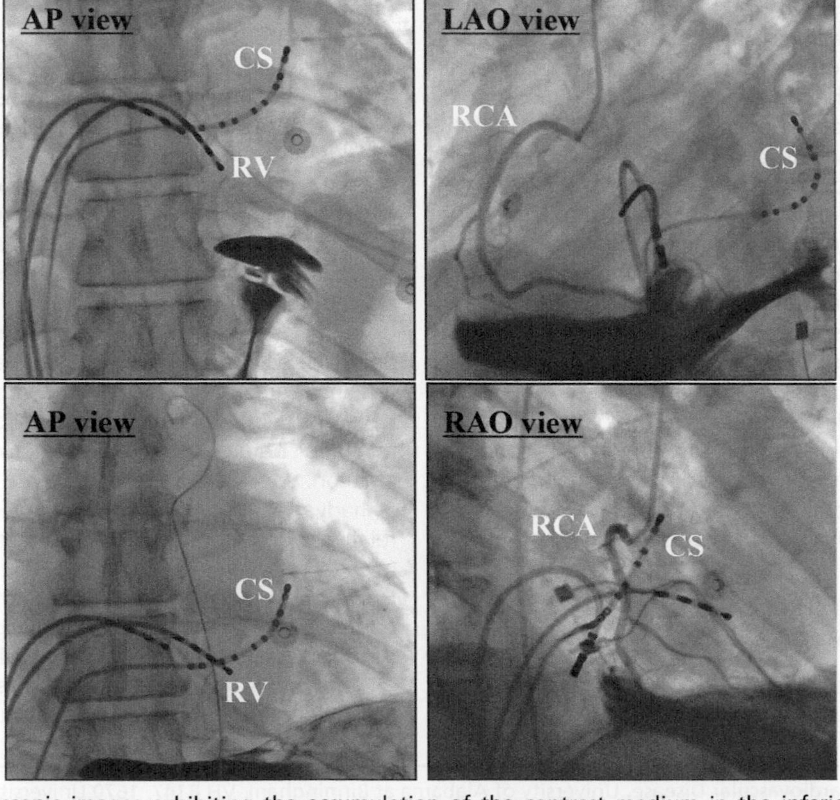

Fig. 1. Fluoroscopic images exhibiting the accumulation of the contrast medium in the inferior wall in the repeated epicardial procedure that suggested a pericardial adhesion (*left upper and right panels*) and the course of the guidewire introduced into the right ventricular outflow tract inadvertently (*left lower panel*). AP, antero-posterior; CS, coronary sinus; LAO, left anterior oblique; RAO, right anterior oblique; RCA, right coronary artery; RV, right ventricle.

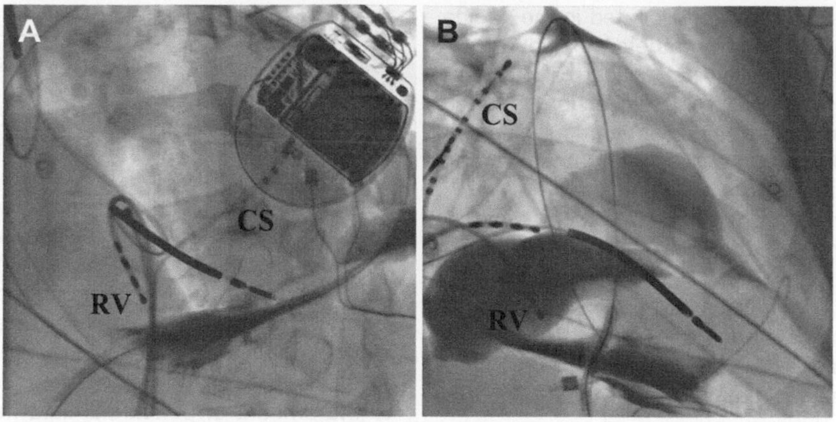

Fig. 2. Fluoroscopic images exhibiting the guidewire correctly introduced into the pericardial space. (*A*) Left anterior oblique projection. (*B*) Right anterior oblique projection. CS, coronary sinus; RV, right ventricle.

multiple side holes or a percutaneous sheath must be advanced into the pericardium. Because the pericardium can offer considerable resistance to advancing a drain or sheath, it is best to use a guidewire with a very soft tip but a relatively stiff proximal segment. To maximize the chances of recognizing bleeding within the pericardial space, it is author's practice to initially place a soft pericardial drainage catheter with multiple side holes. The pericardium is aspirated to determine the nature of the pericardial fluid. Approximately 10% to 30% of patients experience some degree of pericardial bleeding that can be managed with percutaneous drainage from the pericardial catheter. It is not uncommon to aspirate 10 to 30 mL of bloody drainage from the pericardial catheter early in the procedure; however, if a large amount of blood is present in the pericardial space, it can be autotransfused through a venous sheath until hemostasis is confirmed. Generally, bleeding ceases within 5 to 10 minutes and is self-limited. If inadvertent damage to the epicardial veins occurs, hemostasis may not be obtained. It is important to quantify the rate of bleeding by measuring the amount of blood that is removed every 60 seconds. If the rate of bleeding does not decrease by 20 minutes, surgical consultation should be requested. In this situation, surgical repair should be considered without delay. If the sheath had been introduced into the RV by mistake, a second attempt to obtain the correct pericardial access leaving the first sheath in place should be performed. The sheath may be surgically removed after the epicardial catheter ablation has been completed.

Pericardial adhesions that occur after cardiac surgery and prior transthoracic epicardial catheter ablation may significantly increase the difficulty of pericardial access, although pericardial bleeding is unlikely to be a major problem in this situation. Because pericardial adhesions are anticipated to be denser in the anterior wall, the nonsurgical transthoracic epicardial puncture may have to be directed to the inferior wall of the left ventricle. Accumulation of contrast medium in the inferior wall instead of spreading around the cardiac silhouette during the epicardial puncture procedure may suggest pericardial adhesions (see **Fig. 1**). If the epicardial puncture procedure is not successful, a direct surgical subxiphoid epicardial approach in the electrophysiology laboratory may be feasible.[21,22]

Infrequently (0.5% in one case series),[18] intra-abdominal bleeding may occur during the epicardial puncture. Hemoperitoneum can occur after injuring a diaphragmatic vessel and may require a blood transfusion and surgery to control the intra-abdominal bleeding. Bleeding within the liver may occur when the needle penetrates the liver, which is likely to be large enough to cover the course of the puncture needle in patients with heart failure. The first sign suggesting these complications may be abdominal pain, and Blumberg sign may lead to the diagnosis. Therefore, during epicardial puncture with sheath placement, conscious sedation may be preferred so that this finding may be detected early. Abdominal echocardiography may be helpful to confirm and monitor any intra-abdominal bleeding.

When positioning the pericardial sheath and introducing a mapping catheter through the pericardial sheath, air may be inadvertently aspirated into the pericardial space (**Fig. 3**).[23] Aspirated pericardial air may be easily recognized in the apex on the fluoroscopic images. Air in the pericardial space may rarely cause cardiac tamponade. However, that may elevate the defibrillation threshold by a transthoracic defibrillator especially because the air is likely to stay in the apical site, which is the most anteriorly located in the supine position (see **Fig. 3**).[23] In catheter ablation of VT, an epicardial approach via a pericardial puncture is sometimes used and cardioversion is often required for rescue from VT or ventricular fibrillation. Therefore, during epicardial catheterization via a pericardial puncture, careful attention should be paid to prevent entry of air into the pericardial space and any aspirated air should be evacuated from the pericardial space, especially before the induction of ventricular arrhythmias that may require electrical cardioversion. A pericardial sheath with side holes may be helpful for preventing entry of air into the pericardial space.

COMPLICATIONS DURING MAPPING AND ABLATION

Once the ablation catheter is introduced into the pericardial space, extensive mapping may be performed without increasing the procedure risk because there are no anatomical structures (except for the presence of pericardial reflections and sinuses) in the normal pericardial sac to restrict catheter movement.[24] However, the risk of several potential complications should still be kept in mind.

Pericardial Effusion

Epicardial radiofrequency (RF) ablation usually has to be done with an irrigated-tip catheter because there are no cooling effects by blood flow in the pericardial space and irrigated-tip RF ablation appears to be of particular benefit in ablating areas with overlying epicardial fat.[25] An internally or externally irrigated ablation catheter may be used,[26] although an externally irrigated ablation catheter may be required if an electroanatomic mapping system requires an integrated magnetic sensor. However, the use of an externally irrigated ablation catheter requires attention to the amount of pericardial fluid that is instilled within the closed pericardial space because pericardial tamponade may result with impaired hemodynamics. Thus, to safely map and deliver repeated RF applications with adequate power using an externally irrigated ablation catheter, the fluid in the pericardial space should be continuously aspirated through the sheath or a second standard pericardial sheath.[20] The pericardial space should be aspirated intermittently, for example, after every few RF applications or after every 50 mL has been instilled. Continuous low-level suction may also be used. Use of lower external irrigation flow rates, such as 1 mL/min

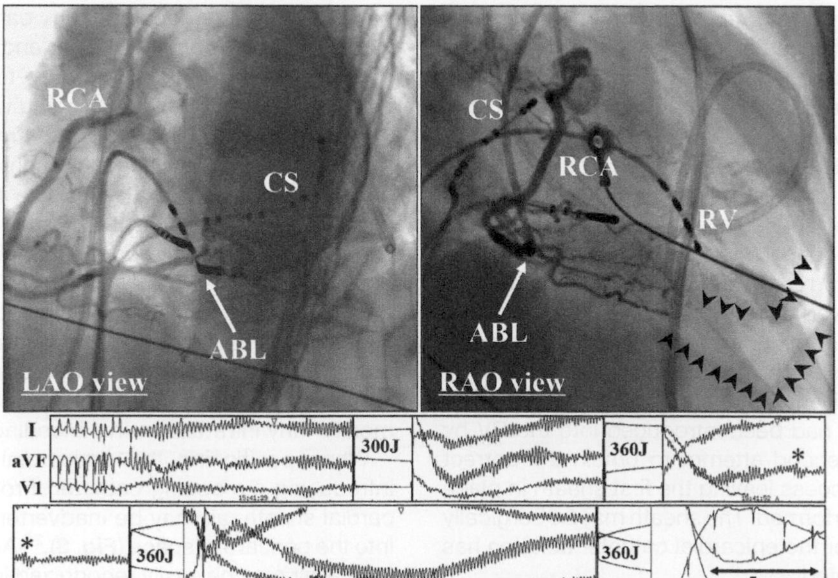

Fig. 3. Fluoroscopic images exhibiting the close relationship between the ablation catheter and right coronary artery (RCA) and demonstrating air aspirated into the pericardial space (*arrowheads*) (*upper panels*), and cardiac tracings exhibiting induction of ventricular fibrillation by programmed ventricular stimulation and multiple extrathoracic cardioversions (*lower panels*). ABL, ablation catheter; CS, coronary sinus; LAO, left anterior oblique; RAO, right anterior oblique; RV, right ventricle.

during mapping and10 to 17 mL/min during ablation, may help to control fluid accumulation in the pericardial space where thrombus formation does not pose a risk of embolization.

Damage to the Epicardial Vessels

In the percutaneous epicardial approach without the aid of visualization of all the major epicardial surfaces, there is a potential risk of damaging the epicardial vessels, coronary artery, or coronary venous system. The damage to epicardial vessels includes laceration of vessels, acute coronary artery spasms, and coronary artery occlusions.

To avoid damaging the epicardial vessels, it is important when introducing large, stiffer sheaths into the epicardial space to lead with a wire or ablation catheter before advancing or moving the curl of the sheath. It may be undesirable to leave a large sheath in the pericardial space without a catheter in place because this may cause the edges of the sheath to lacerate a pericardial structure.

According to early animal work by Sosa and colleagues,[4] when the RF energy was delivered adjacent to the coronary artery, the effects were limited to the media, but when delivered above the coronary artery, severe intimal hyperplasia and intravascular thrombus formation occurred. The susceptibility to coronary artery damage was inversely proportional to the proximity of the ablating electrode and the vessel size probably because larger vessels are protected by greater blood flow. It may be important to maintain a distance of more than 10 mm between the coronary artery and distal electrode of the ablating catheter at any point of the cardiac cycle during angiography to reduce the risk of damaging the coronary arteries during the RF energy delivery. In consideration of these rules, a prior coronary angiography evaluation must be done to determine a safer area for the RF energy delivery. Because the base and anterior and posterior septal areas are considered as the more dangerous zones, coronary angiography should be performed before and during the RF energy delivery in these areas with the ablation catheter positioned at the target site. When considering the site of the VT substrate, this step may be necessary more frequently in idiopathic VTs than VTs associated with structural heart disease. When RF energy is delivered adjacent to the coronary arteries, the ST-T segment should be monitored during the recording of the simultaneous 12-lead electrocardiogram to detect any possible lesions in the coronary arteries. Chronic damage can occur to coronary arteries even if acute effects are not observed. Therefore, in some patients, follow-up with nuclear perfusion studies may be required over a period of several months. When the target ablation site is located adjacent to the coronary arteries, cryothermal ablation may be an alternative because absence of circulating blood in the pericardial space may favor creation of cryolesions on the epicardium[27] and cryoablation may be less likely to injure the coronary arteries.[28] However, further study is warranted to assess its safety and efficacy.

Phrenic Nerve Injury

Injury to the left phrenic nerve and consequent diaphragmatic paralysis is a well-recognized complication of epicardial catheter ablation. A limitation of epicardial ablation for VT in nonischemic cardiomyopathy is the potential proximity of the left phrenic nerve to the VT substrate, which may limit the safety and efficacy of RF ablation. Anatomic and electroanatomic reconstruction studies have suggested that the course of the left phrenic nerve is in the vicinity of the left atrial appendage and the high and posterolateral left ventricular wall at the level of the mitral valve annulus and variable along the basal border of the left ventricle.[29–32] The phrenic nerve is vulnerable to heat and to cold, and cryothermal ablation seems unlikely to prevent this complication.[33,34] Strategies to identify and protect the phrenic nerve are important.

Pacing maneuvers can assist in identifying the phrenic nerve course and ensuring an apparent safe distance for ablation. Phrenic nerve points can be delineated by pacing at an output of 10 mA and a pulse width of 2 milliseconds to assess for diaphragmatic stimulation, and electroanatomic maps can incorporate tags at these sites to help the operator avoid the left phrenic nerve. Before epicardial ablation at the dangerous areas described previously, pacing is usually performed at a high output of 20 mA at a pulse width of 2 milliseconds to ensure lack of phrenic nerve capture. In fact, the pacing output that would indicate a safe distance for epicardial ablation is not known, and further investigation is needed to define the exact limits of the efficacy and safety. In addition, if patients are paralyzed under general anesthesia, diaphragmatic motion with phrenic nerve stimulation during pacing may not occur to warn of the proximity. Therefore, conscious sedation may be a better choice during epicardial ablation with an expected risk of phrenic nerve injury.

When catheter ablation has to be performed adjacent to the left phrenic nerve, left phrenic nerve injury may be avoided by interposing a sheath, balloon,[35,36] or even air[37] and saline[38] in the pericardium between the ablation site and the nerve. No matter what material is used, lack of phrenic nerve capture should be confirmed to ensure sufficient separation; monitoring of diaphragmatic movement is necessary during the ablation. Air and/or saline should be gradually injected via a hemostatic sheath into the pericardium until loss of phrenic nerve capture with careful monitoring of blood pressure to prevent any iatrogenic cardiac tamponade. Because pericardial air may elevate the defibrillation threshold by a transthoracic defibrillator, separation with air should not be performed during VT that may require electrical cardioversion and air should be evacuated from the pericardial space before the induction of ventricular arrhythmias to verify the effect of the ablation. A limitation of the technique of using a balloon catheter in the pericardial space to mechanically separate the left phrenic nerve from the ablation catheter is the inability to steer the balloon catheter. To overcome this, a steerable outer sheath may be helpful for guiding balloon placement and providing additional support and stability.

Damage to the Esophagus, Vagus Nerve, and Lungs

During epicardial ablation, there is also a potential risk of collateral damage to structures that surround the heart such as the esophagus, vagus nerve, and lungs. Ablation of the left atrial posterior wall may damage the esophagus and the left branch of the vagus nerve, which runs along the esophageal anterior wall toward the stomach, resulting in critical complications such as atrioesophageal fistula formation[38] and delayed gastric emptying.[9] Atrioesophageal fistula formation is an especially devastating complication that usually results in major morbidity or death. Real-time visualization of the esophagus with barium[39] or a radiopaque marker,[40] esophageal temperature monitoring,[41] and avoidance of ablation over the esophagus may help to eliminate inadvertent injury around the esophagus. Although small pulmonary lesions can be anticipated, no clinical significance has been reported. Care should be given to complaints of dyspnea or pleural friction rubs during the follow-up.

Development of Technologies to Prevent Collateral Damage

To prevent collateral damage, interventional electrophysiologists working in the pericardial space have relied on the fluoroscopic anatomy, electrocardiogram and pacing guidance, intracardiac echocardiography, electroanatomic mapping systems, and, in selected instances, directional ultrasound imaging from the pericardial space.[42] Technologies for visualization of the epicardial structures have been recently developed and may be helpful in preventing collateral damage. Integration of coronary artery angiograms into a 3-dimensional electroanatomic map[13,43] may facilitate safe epicardial mapping and ablation. Endoscopic guidance may allow for direct visualization of epicardial structures, catheters, and lesions and may improve the safety and efficacy of epicardial catheter ablation and reduce staff and patient radiation exposure.[44]

POSTPROCEDURAL COMPLICATIONS

Late Pericardial Effusion and Cardiac Tamponade

If bloody fluid is still aspirated through the pericardial sheath and echocardiographic examination demonstrates pericardial effusion at the end of the epicardial procedure, the pericardial sheath should be left in place and intermittent aspiration through the sheath, serial echocardiographic examinations, and continuous monitoring of blood pressure and heart rate should be performed to detect any possible late cardiac tamponade. When hemostasis is confirmed and echocardiographic examination demonstrates no pericardial effusion, the pericardial sheath may be removed, but monitoring the patient with serial transthoracic echocardiography 24 hours afterward is recommended. When a surgical pericardial window is used, the pericardial sheath is removed and the surgical incision may be closed after the insertion of an intrapericardial chest tube, which is removed the next day if there is no active drainage.

Pericarditis

Symptomatic pericarditis is a common complication of epicardial ablation. The clinical sign suggesting this complication may be precordial distress and a pericardial friction rub. This complication is usually mild, of limited duration, and often responds well to nonsteroidal anti-inflammatory medications given orally, such as ketorolac and ibuprofen; however, the intensity of the pericardial inflammatory reaction varies considerably.[45] In general, the longer the procedure and the larger the number of epicardial applications, the more severe the epicardial inflammatory reaction. However, there also appears to be considerable individual variation in the susceptibility to develop postprocedure pericarditis. To prevent pericarditis, several measures may be recommended. First, all pericardial sheaths should be removed at the end of the procedure unless there is continued bleeding. Second, 0.5 to 1.0 mg/kg of methylprednisolone or 2.0 mg/kg of intermediate-acting corticosteroid (triamcinolone) should be injected intrapericardially. This treatment may prevent postprocedural inflammatory adhesion formation especially if a repeat procedure is necessary. Third, a cephalosporin antibiotic should be administered as long as the pericardial drain is in place.

Pleuritis

Symptomatic pleuritis may occur. The clinical sign suggesting this complication may be dyspnea and a pleural friction rub. This complication may be similar in its clinical course to pericarditis and respond well to nonsteroidal anti-inflammatory medications given orally, such as ketorolac and ibuprofen.

SUMMARY

Although the transthoracic epicardial mapping and ablation technique is a relatively safe procedure, complications can and do occur. The possible complications associated with this technique should be well understood before the procedure. If these complications are recognized early and managed appropriately, the outcome is usually excellent.

REFERENCES

1. Sosa E, Scanavacca M, D'Avila A, et al. A new technique to perform epicardial mapping in the electrophysiology laboratory. J Cardiovasc Electrophysiol 1996;7:531–6.
2. Sosa E, Scanavacca M, D'Avila A, et al. Endocardial and epicardial ablation guided by nonsurgical transthoracic epicardial mapping to treat recurrent ventricular tachycardia. J Cardiovasc Electrophysiol 1998;9:229–39.
3. Sosa E, Scanavacca M, d'Avila A, et al. Nonsurgical transthoracic epicardial catheter ablation to treat recurrent ventricular tachycardia occurring late after myocardial infarction. J Am Coll Cardiol 2000;35:1442–9.
4. Sosa E, Scanavacca M, d'Avila A. Transthoracic epicardial catheter ablation to treat recurrent ventricular tachycardia. Curr Cardiol Rep 2001;3:451–8.
5. Soejima K, Stevenson WG, Sapp JL, et al. Endocardial and epicardial radiofrequency ablation of ventricular tachycardia associated with dilated cardiomyopathy: the importance of low-voltage scars. J Am Coll Cardiol 2004;43:1834–42.
6. Cesario DA, Vaseghi M, Boyle NG, et al. Value of high-density endocardial and epicardial mapping for catheter ablation of hemodynamically unstable ventricular tachycardia. Heart Rhythm 2006;3:1–10.
7. Koplan BA, Soejima K, Baughman K, et al. Refractory ventricular tachycardia secondary to cardiac sarcoid: electrophysiologic characteristics, mapping, and ablation. Heart Rhythm 2006;3:924–9.
8. Sosa E, Scanavacca M. Images in cardiovascular medicine. Percutaneous pericardial access for mapping and ablation of epicardial ventricular tachycardias. Circulation 2007;115:e542–4.
9. Scanavacca M, Pisani CF, Hachul D, et al. Selective atrial vagal denervation guided by evoked vagal reflex to treat patients with paroxysmal atrial fibrillation. Circulation 2006;114:876–85.
10. Pak HN, Hwang C, Lim HE, et al. Hybrid epicardial and endocardial ablation of persistent atrial fibrillation. A new approach for difficult cases. J Cardiovasc Electrophysiol 2007;18:917–23.
11. Schweikert RA, Saliba WI, Tomassoni G, et al. Percutaneous pericardial instrumentation for endo-epicardial mapping of previously failed ablations. Circulation 2003;108:1329–35.
12. Valderrábano M, Cesario DA, Ji S, et al. Percutaneous epicardial mapping during ablation of difficult accessory pathways as an alternative to cardiac surgery. Heart Rhythm 2004;1:311–6.
13. Ho I, d'Avila A, Ruskin J, et al. Images in cardiovascular medicine. Percutaneous epicardial mapping and ablation of a posteroseptal accessory pathway. Circulation 2007;115:e418–21.
14. Phillips KP, Natale A, Sterba R, et al. Percutaneous pericardial instrumentation for catheter ablation of focal atrial tachycardias arising from the left atrial appendage. J Cardiovasc Electrophysiol 2008;19:430–3.
15. Yamada T, McElderry HT, Allison JS, et al. Focal atrial tachycardia originating from the epicardial left atrial appendage. Heart Rhythm 2008;5:766–7.
16. Daniels DV, Lu YY, Morton JB, et al. Idiopathic epicardial left ventricular tachycardia originating remote from the sinus of Valsalva: electrophysiological characteristics, catheter ablation, and identification from the 12-lead electrocardiogram. Circulation 2006;113:1659–66.
17. Doppalapudi H, Yamada T, Ramaswamy K, et al. Idiopathic focal epicardial ventricular tachycardia originating from the crux of the heart. Heart Rhythm 2009;6:44–50.
18. Sosa E, Scanavacca M. Epicardial mapping and ablation techniques to control ventricular tachycardia. J Cardiovasc Electrophysiol 2005;16:449–52.
19. d'Avila A. Epicardial catheter ablation of ventricular tachycardia. Heart Rhythm 2008;5:S73–5.
20. Tedrow U, Stevenson WG. Strategies for epicardial mapping and ablation of ventricular tachycardia. J Cardiovasc Electrophysiol 2009;20:710–3.

21. Sosa E, Scanavacca M, D'Avila A, et al. Nonsurgical transthoracic epicardial approach in patients with ventricular tachycardia and previous cardiac surgery. J Interv Card Electrophysiol 2004;10:281–8.
22. Soejima K, Couper G, Cooper JM, et al. Subxiphoid surgical approach for epicardial catheter-based mapping and ablation in patients with prior cardiac surgery or difficult pericardial access. Circulation 2004;110:1197–201.
23. Yamada T, McElderry HT, Platonov M, et al. Aspirated air in the pericardial space during epicardial catheterization may elevate the defibrillation threshold. Int J Cardiol 2009;135:e34–5.
24. Shivkumar K. Percutaneous epicardial ablation of atrial fibrillation. Heart Rhythm 2008;5:152–4.
25. d'Avila A, Houghtaling C, Gutierrez P, et al. Catheter ablation of ventricular epicardial tissue: a comparison of standard and cooled-tip radiofrequency energy. Circulation 2004;109:2363–9.
26. Demazumder D, Mirotznik MS, Schwartzman D. Comparison of irrigated electrode designs for radiofrequency ablation of myocardium. J Interv Card Electrophysiol 2001;5:391–400.
27. D'Avila A, Aryana A, Thiagalingam A, et al. Focal and linear endocardial and epicardial catheter-based cryoablation of normal and infarcted ventricular tissue. Pacing Clin Electrophysiol 2008;31: 1322–31.
28. Skanes AC, Jones DL, Teefy P, et al. Safety and feasibility of cryothermal ablation within the mid- and distal coronary sinus. J Cardiovasc Electrophysiol 2004;15:1319–23.
29. Sánchez-Quintana D, Cabrera JA, Climent V, et al. How close are the phrenic nerves to cardiac structures? Implications for cardiac interventionalists. J Cardiovasc Electrophysiol 2005;16:309–13.
30. Sacher F, Jais P, Stephenson K, et al. Phrenic nerve injury after catheter ablation of atrial fibrillation. Indian Pacing Electrophysiol J 2007;7:1–6.
31. Sánchez-Quintana D, Ho SY, Climent V, et al. Anatomic evaluation of the left phrenic nerve relevant to epicardial and endocardial catheter ablation: implications for phrenic nerve injury. Heart Rhythm 2009;6:764–8.
32. Fan R, Cano O, Ho SY, et al. Characterization of the phrenic nerve course within the epicardial substrate of patients with nonischemic cardiomyopathy and ventricular tachycardia. Heart Rhythm 2009;6:59–64.
33. Aupperle H, Doll N, Walther T, et al. Histological findings induced by different energy sources in experimental atrial ablation in sheep. Interact Cardiovasc Thorac Surg 2005;4:450–5.
34. Tse HF, Reek S, Timmermans C, et al. Pulmonary vein isolation using transvenous catheter cryoablation for treatment of atrial fibrillation without risk of pulmonary vein stenosis. J Am Coll Cardiol 2003; 42:752–8.
35. Buch E, Nakahara S, Shivkumar K. Intra-pericardial balloon retraction of the left atrium: a novel method to prevent esophageal injury during catheter ablation. Heart Rhythm 2008;5:1473–5.
36. Matsuo S, Jaïs P, Knecht S, et al. Images in cardiovascular medicine. Novel technique to prevent left phrenic nerve injury during epicardial catheter ablation. Circulation 2008;117:e471.
37. Di Biase L, Burkhardt JD, Pelargonio G, et al. Prevention of phrenic nerve injury during epicardial ablation: comparison of methods for separating the phrenic nerve from the epicardial surface. Heart Rhythm 2009;6:957–61.
38. Pappone C, Oral H, Santinelli V, et al. Atrio-esophageal fistula as a complication of percutaneous transcatheter ablation of atrial fibrillation. Circulation 2004;109:2724–6.
39. Ruby RS, Wells D, Sankaran S, et al. Prevalence of fever in patients undergoing left atrial ablation of atrial fibrillation guided by barium esophagraphy. J Cardiovasc Electrophysiol 2009;20:883–7.
40. Yamada T, Murakami Y, Okada T, et al. Usefulness of esophageal leads for determining the strategy of pulmonary vein ablation to avoid complications associated with the esophagus. Am J Cardiol 2006;97:1494–7.
41. Kuwahara T, Takahashi A, Kobori A, et al. Safe and effective ablation of atrial fibrillation: importance of esophageal temperature monitoring to avoid periesophageal nerve injury as a complication of pulmonary vein isolation. J Cardiovasc Electrophysiol 2009;20:1–6.
42. Horowitz BN, Vaseghi M, Mahajan A, et al. Percutaneous intrapericardial echocardiography during catheter ablation: a feasibility study. Heart Rhythm 2006;3:1275–82.
43. Zeppenfeld K, Tops LF, Bax JJ, et al. Images in cardiovascular medicine. Epicardial radiofrequency catheter ablation of ventricular tachycardia in the vicinity of coronary arteries is facilitated by fusion of 3-dimensional electroanatomical mapping with multislice computed tomography. Circulation 2006; 114:e51–2.
44. Nazarian S, Kantsevoy SV, Zviman MM, et al. Feasibility of endoscopic guidance for nonsurgical transthoracic atrial and ventricular epicardial ablation. Heart Rhythm 2008;5:1115–9.
45. d'Avila A, Neuzil P, Thiagalingam A, et al. Experimental efficacy of pericardial instillation of anti-inflammatory agents during percutaneous epicardial catheter ablation to prevent postprocedure pericarditis. J Cardiovasc Electrophysiol 2007;18: 1178–83.

Future Developments in Nonsurgical Epicardial Therapies

Christopher M. Stanton, MD[a],
Samuel J. Asirvatham, MD, FHRS[b,c], Charles J. Bruce, MD[a],
Andrew Danielsen, MS[d], Paul A. Friedman, MD, FHRS, FACC[b,*]

KEYWORDS

- Pericardial space • Left atrial appendage • Ligation
- Cardiac resynchronization

The unique anatomic position of the pericardium in juxtaposition to central cardiac structures enables it to serve as the ideal vantage point for the delivery of novel cardiovascular therapies. Since it covers the entire surface of the heart and portions of the proximal great vessels, the pericardial space offers nearly unrestricted access to nearly every region of the epicardium, in the absence of prior pericardiotomy (**Fig. 1**).[1] Additionally, as the pericardial space is not in direct communication with the central circulation, left atrial and ventricular procedures may be performed without anticoagulation. This is possible because foreign materials (catheters) are not in direct contact with circulating blood, and endothelial disruption of left-sided structures (exposing tissue factor) does not occur.[2] The lack of direct contact with circulating blood also facilitates regional delivery of devices and drugs.[3–6] The mechanical constraint provided by the pericardial sac permits navigation of catheters adjacent to the heart without direct surgical visualization.[7,8]

Since its introduction into practice by Sosa and colleagues,[9] percutaneous pericardial access has become an accepted approach for the ablation of epicardial ventricular arrhythmias and accessory pathways.[7,8,10,11] The pericardial space has also been used to deploy protective tools, so that cardiac ablation does not damage extracardiac structures, and as a means of delivering stem cell and targeted gene therapy.[5] Two therapies particularly well positioned to exploit the pericardium's relationship to the heart are cardiac resynchronization and left atrial appendage (LAA) closure. Percutaneous epicardial delivery of these two therapies is the subject of this review.

PERCUTANEOUS PERICARDIAL ACCESS AND NOVEL THERAPIES

Open surgical approaches to the epicardial surface of the heart to deliver interventions for the treatment of arrhythmias have been in use for decades.[12] Advantages of open surgical approaches include direct visualization of epicardial and surrounding structures to facilitate placement of tools and delivery of therapy while avoiding collateral damage. However, the greater degree of invasiveness, the need for general anesthesia and often lung deflation, and the extensive tissue disruption required to permit access have limited broad adoption of these techniques for patients with severe congestive heart failure and

[a] Division of Cardiovascular Diseases and Internal Medicine, Mayo Clinic, 200 1st Street SW, Rochester, MN 55905, USA
[b] Division of Cardiovascular Diseases, Department of Medicine, Mayo Clinic, 200 1st Street SW, Rochester, MN 55905, USA
[c] Department of Pediatrics and Adolescent Medicine, Mayo Clinic, 200 1st Street SW, Rochester, MN 55905, USA
[d] Mayo Clinics Health Solutions, Mayo Clinic, Rochester, MN, USA
* Corresponding author.
E-mail address: pfriedman@mayo.edu (P.A. Friedman).

Card Electrophysiol Clin 2 (2010) 135–146
doi:10.1016/j.ccep.2009.11.014
1877-9182/10/$ – see front matter

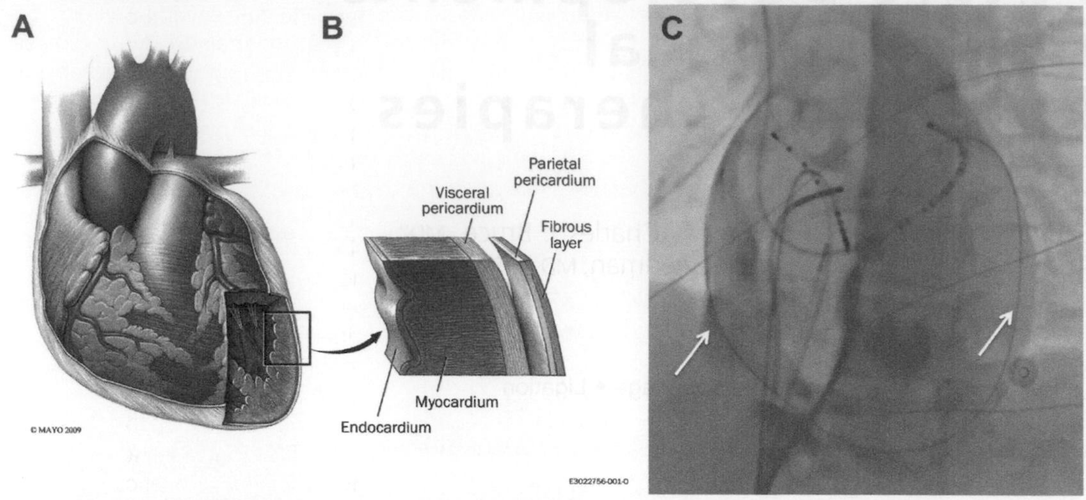

Fig. 1. Anatomic depiction of the heart and pericardium. (*A*) The pericardium extends from the apex to the great vessels, providing access to most cardiac surfaces. The pericardial space (*B*) is a "potential space" between the visceral and parietal pericardium and contains a small amount of viscous fluid. (*C*) Fluoroscopy is useful in defining this space. Contrast collects outside the heart borders and a long guide wire spans the surface of the heart from left to right in a manner incompatible with intracardiac placement. In the left anterior oblique view as shown, the wire is seen outside the right and left cardiac chambers (*arrows*). This confirms an extracardiac position. A sheath should not be advanced over the wire until an extracardiac position is confirmed. (*Courtesy of* Mayo Clinic Foundation; with permission.)

for the frail elderly, who compose the majority of the atrial fibrillation population.[13]

Percutaneous pericardial access is described in other articles in this issue. Briefly, a Tuohy needle, which is designed for entering potential spaces, is advanced toward the heart under fluoroscopy. Small puffs of contrast are used to identify the needle tip position relative to the pericardium. Tenting is seen as the needle indents the fibrous parietal pericardium, and a slight pop or relief of tension is appreciated with passage of the needle into pericardial space. Upon entry to the pericardial space, a wire is advanced, which adopts a characteristic circumcardiac conformation when within the pericardial space. This conformation confirms correct wire position when viewed from the left anterior oblique projection (see **Fig. 1**C). The right anterior oblique projection is not relied upon in isolation, as intravascular wire positions may be difficult to distinguish from pericardial space positions. Potential complications include coronary artery laceration, hemopericardium, and cardiac puncture.[7–9,14] However, with careful attention to technique, this approach has been applied to enable catheter ablation with low rates of complication.[7–9,14,15] With continued technological development of optics and surgical tools, the lines between "surgical" and percutaneous pericardial access will blur, but a common theme of small portals of entry and maintenance of an intact pericardium will differentiate these approaches from open techniques.[16–19]

Due to the limited tissue disruption associated with percutaneous access, it can be performed under conscious sedation.[20] However, by virtue of the small size of access provided, constraints are necessarily imposed on novel technologies using any percutaneous approach. First, as direct visualization is precluded, fiber-optic, radiographic, or novel forms of imaging or navigation are required to localize tools in the pericardial space.[19,21] Second, the size of tools themselves must be constrained to fit within the confines of the closed pericardial space. For many therapies, this will also require expandable tools to permit delivery through small sheaths. Third, given the limited size of the available work space, novel approaches must be applied to secure leads or to fasten sutures. Nonetheless, approaches that overcome these obstacles have the benefit of surgical access to the heart without open surgical morbidity.

CARDIAC RESYNCHRONIZATION THERAPY

In patients with depressed ventricular function and QRS prolongation greater than 120 ms, pacing the right and left ventricles simultaneously has been shown to improve quality of life, exercise tolerance, and ejection fraction, and to decrease biomarkers of heart failure, heart failure hospitalizations, and mortality.[22–24] However, at least 30% of patients in clinical trials fail to respond to cardiac resynchronization therapy, and this is likely a conservative estimate. In another 5% to 10% of patients, a left ventricular lead cannot be stably positioned.[25] The site of placement of the left ventricular lead is an important predictor of cardiac resynchronization therapy response.[25,26]

Cardiac resynchronization therapy requires that leads be placed such that the right atrium, right ventricle, and left ventricle can be paced. The left ventricle is most commonly paced by cannulation of coronary sinus branches with a pacing lead. The most frequently encountered difficulty in transvenous implantation of cardiac resynchronization therapy devices is placement of the left ventricular lead. Optimal "resynchronization" is achieved when the left ventricular pacing site corresponds to that of most delayed activation.[27] This is typically best achieved by lead placement in lateral and posterolateral positions,[28] but optimal position may also be affected by the underlying disease, and may vary over time. The preferred site is not uniformly available via the coronary sinus. The relatively distant spacing between suitable veins along the lateral left ventricle and the presence of tortuous, small-caliber veins and venous valves limits lead placement options (**Fig. 2**). In practice, ideal lateral positions are only present in 82% of patients.[29]

Epicardially placed leads—particularly if placed in a minimally invasive or percutaneous manner—have the potential to offer several benefits. Since lead position is not constrained by the course of coronary veins, any site may be accessed. Given the relatively large space within the pericardium compared with individual veins, leads could be developed that adopt a patchlike shape as opposed to a cylindrical shape. Such leads could contain multiple electrodes with a relatively broad anatomic distribution. This would permit noninvasive selection of the pacing site, long-term electronic lead "repositioning," and tailored resynchronization.[26] Moreover, multiple sites could be paced simultaneously or in sophisticated sequential patterns to optimize ventricular activation.

Epicardial patches have long been used for defibrillation, with defibrillation thresholds generally superior to that found in endovascular systems. An entirely epicardial system eliminates the need for placement of right ventricular leads. This is an advantage because right ventricular leads have been associated with symptomatic tricuspid regurgitation, and tricuspid regurgitation has been associated with increased mortality.[30,31] Conceivably, in some patients, the tricuspid regurgitation created by right ventricular leads may offset some or all of the benefits of resynchronization. Historically, unipolar nonsteroid-eluting epicardial leads and defibrillation leads have had an increased risk of threshold elevation and fracture compared with transvenous systems; small, more recent observations, suggest newer bipolar steroid-eluting designs and construction mitigate that risk.[32,33]

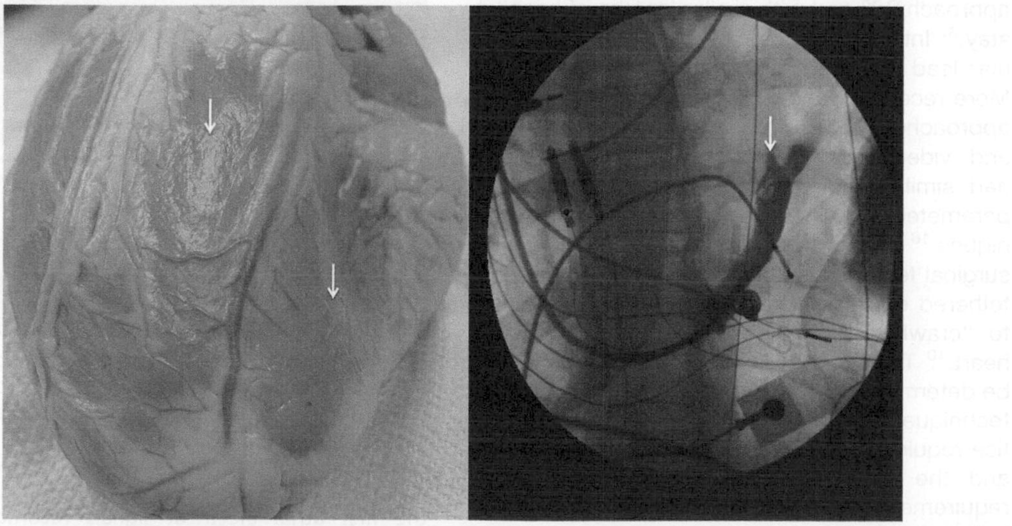

Fig. 2. Challenges in using the coronary sinus for left ventricular pacing. (*Left panel*) The wide distance between coronary veins due to their limited anatomic distribution leaves large areas of myocardium that cannot be directly accessed by a pacing lead. The arrows depict two such areas. Complex coronary venous anatomy also limits lead delivery. (*Right panel*) Arrow in venogram depicts a valve that may impede lead passage.

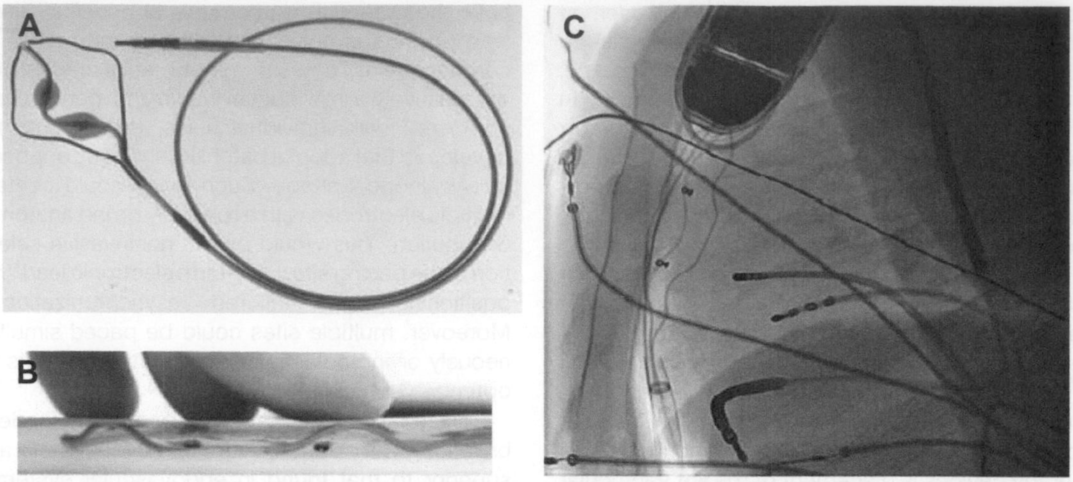

Fig. 3. Pericardial lead design for nonsurgical subxiphoid placement. (*A*) Lead depicted in expanded/deployed position. (*B*) The three-dimensional configuration of the lead applies pressure between the pericardium and epicardium to enable stable percutaneous pericardial pacing. (*C*) Radiograph showing the lead deployed in the human pericardium; lead is visible just below implantable cardioverter-defibrillator pulse generator (further details in text). (*Courtesy of* St Jude Medical, Inc, St. Paul, MN; with permission.)

Epicardial approaches for cardiac resynchronization date back to its origin, most commonly in the form of hybrid systems that joined a surgically placed left ventricular epicardial lead to an otherwise endovascular system.[34] These systems have been compared with transvenous systems in small, observational, nonrandomized studies. Surgical implantation of left ventricular leads via left thoracotomy and "minithoracotomy" in patients with advanced heart failure has similar rates of success with significantly lower procedure times than those of an endocardial coronary sinus approach[35,36] and with similar lengths of hospital stay.[37] Intermediate-term (3–6 month) left ventricular lead parameters were similar in all groups. More recent advances include minimally invasive approaches using robotics, minithoracotomy, and video-assisted thoracoscopy, which have had similar outcomes and left ventricular lead parameters to those of standard techniques.[16,17,38,39] Other novel minimally invasive surgical technologies under development include tethered epicardial crawlers that employ suction to "crawl" along the epicardial surface of the heart.[40] Their role in lead placement remains to be determined. Limitations to adoption of surgical techniques include the absence of surgical expertise required for thoracotomy in most implanters, and the greater invasiveness and anesthesia requirements of these approaches compared with those for transvenous implantation.

Recently, preliminary experience has been reported with a 6F-catheter lead deployed via a nonsurgical subxiphoid epicardial approach.[41] The lead is designed to preferentially adhere to the epicardium via passive fixation by means of a three-dimensional shape that expands in the pericardial space to maintain epicardial contact

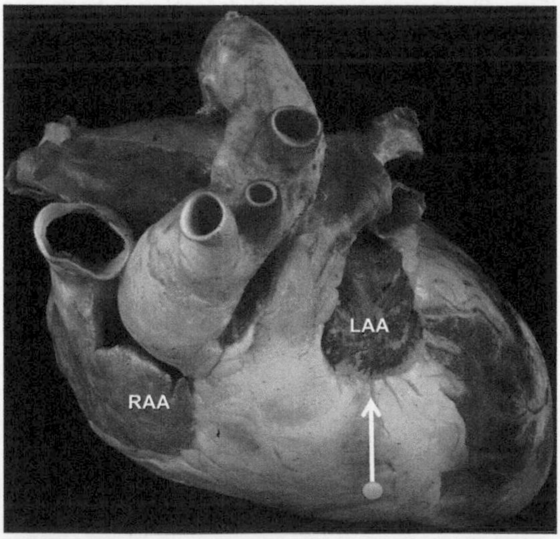

Fig. 4. Anatomic characteristics of LAA that can be exploited to permit its ligation. The circle depicts a typical point of pericardial access using an anterior subxiphoid nonsurgical approach. As the grasper is advanced superiorly from the entry site (*arrow*), the first free margin seen is that of the LAA. Similarly, the first atrial electrical signals recorded by the grasper will be those of the LAA. Further details in text. Note that both the right and left atrial appendages are largely epicardial structures. (*Courtesy of* Dr William Edwards.)

(**Fig. 3**). A stylet placed in the lead straightens it to permit passage through a 14F-catheter sheath for pericardial delivery. Within the pericardium, the hinged nature of the lead permits it to expand for stable deployment. The lead was tested in a study of nine patients undergoing epicardial ventricular tachycardia ablation. During a time period limited to 30 minutes following introducer placement, the lead was manipulated under fluoroscopic control and acute stability and pacing function was assessed. On average, 2.1 ± 0.6 locations were tested per patient, with bipolar capture thresholds of 2.0 ± 0.4 V, 2.9 ± 27 V, and 0.7 ± 0.4 V at right ventricular, left ventricular, and atrial sites, respectively. Mean ventricular R waves ranged from 11.3 to 15.0mV. To prevent air from disrupting electrode contact, suction was applied. Chronic lead function data are not currently available. In the future, this type of approach may offer the advantages of an epicardial system for pacing and defibrillation without the morbidity of traditional surgical approaches.

Percutaneous Closure of the Left Atrial Appendage

Atrial fibrillation currently affects 2.2 million Americans and this number is projected to grow to 16 million by the year 2050.[42] A clear association with thromboembolic events exists in these patients, and this risk increases with age.[43] Pharmacologic management of this risk has important limitations,[44,45] and alternative, nonpharmacologic approaches have been sought.

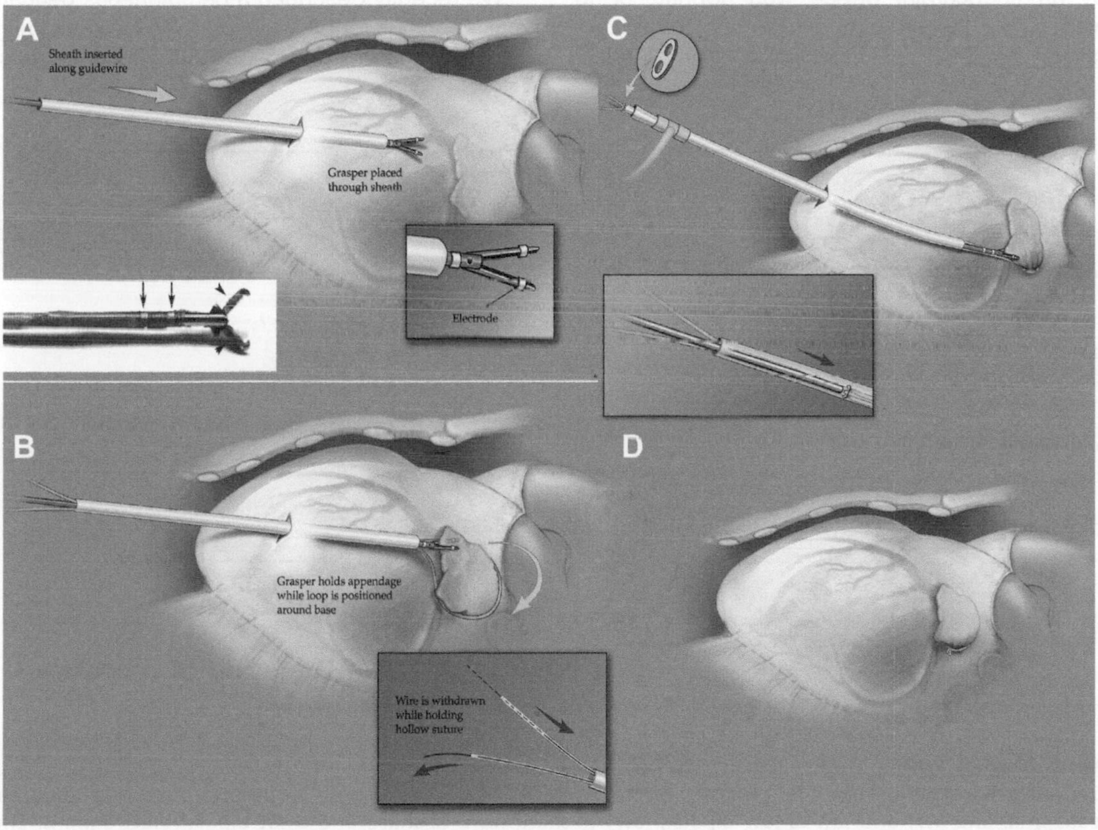

Fig. 5. LAA closure system. (*A*) The grasper has special electrodes mounted on each jaw (*arrowheads, bottom left inset photograph*) for electrical tissue characterization. This facilitates identification and control of the appendage. Inserts depict cartoon rendering (*right insert*) and actual early grasper prototype (*left insert*). (*B*) After the grasper secures the appendage, a loop of hollow suture preloaded with a radio-opaque inner support wire is advanced over the grasper to encircle the appendage. The loop can be opened, closed, and repositioned until a satisfactory position is obtained. After the loop is adequately positioned, it is tightened, and the wire is removed (*inset*). (*C*) Following removal of the wire, a suture clip is advanced over the suture to secure it. (*D*) The sutures are cut with a catheter-based tool (not shown), leaving a simple suture around the base of the appendage secured with a suture clip. (*Adapted from* Friedman PA, Asirvatham SJ, Dalegrave C, et al. Percutaneous epicardial left atrial appendage closure: preliminary results of an electrogram guided approach. J Cardiovasc Electrophysiol 2009;20:908–15; with permission.)

Due to its complex anatomy and diminished blood flow during atrial fibrillation, the LAA has been a common site of left atrial thrombi, accounting for 98% of such thrombi in transesophageal echocardiogram (TEE)–based studies comprising 1181 patients.[46,47] Consequently, strategies directed at preventing LAA thrombi from entering the circulation have been employed. While surgical exclusions of the LAA from the circulation have been performed since 1946, their role is preventing stroke is only now being investigated.[31,48,49] Many patients with atrial fibrillation have multiple potential mechanisms for thromboembolism, some of which (eg, aortic atherosclerosis) do not require LAA participation. Evidence that LAA exclusion is an effective means of stroke prevention was recently provided by the Protect AF study, which demonstrated that LAA occlusion by an endocardial device was not inferior to warfarin for the prevention of stroke, cardiovascular death, or systemic embolism.[50] Retrospective analysis of previous trials of endocardial devices further supports this observation.[48,51]

Several factors make percutaneous pericardial LAA closure attractive. The absence of sheaths in the central circulation, the lack of transseptal puncture, and absence of foreign body deposition minimize the potential for air- or thromboembolism, eliminate the need for periprocedural anticoagulation,[47] and remove the possibility of device erosion or infection.[52–54] Since effusion is the most frequently seen complication in percutaneous LAA closure, affecting 4.8% of patients, the presence of pericardial access before closure (as required for epicardial techniques) facilitates management.[50] Additionally, as shown in **Fig. 4**, the LAA is fundamentally an epicardial structure, making it amenable to epicardial approaches.

We recently described a percutaneous pericardial technique for LAA ligation.[21] To facilitate identification and closure of the LAA within the intact

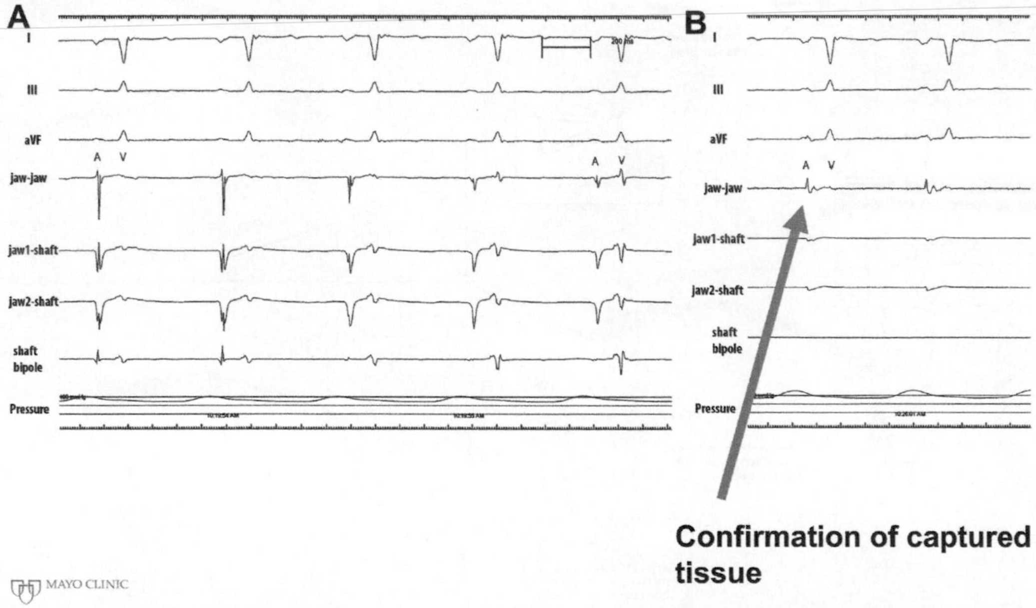

Fig. 6. Electrical navigation and confirmation of LAA capture. (*A*) Pullback of grasper from over LAA to tip just at LAA with changing electrograms. Tracings record, from top to bottom, signals from surface electrocardiogram leads I, III, and avF; and jaw-to-jaw bipolar, jaw1-to-shaft, jaw2-to-shaft, and shaft bipolar electrograms. The atrial (A) and ventricular (V) recordings of the first and last complex are labeled. The grasper is initially over the LAA so that, in the first complex, the distal recording (jaw-jaw) has a large atrial complex and a small, far-field ventricular electrogram, while the shaft bipolar electrodes are just beyond the LAA-LV junction (note "A" and "V" electrograms). As the grasper is pulled toward the left ventricle, note that the "A" electrograms progressively decline in amplitude, as the "V" electrograms increase, indicating the position of each grasper component relative to the LAA. (*B*) Confirmation of LAA capture. In this panel, recordings were obtained after LAA capture, with gentle retraction of the grasper into the sheath. Note the absence of electrogram signals on the shaft bipole recording. The jaw-jaw electrogram depicts a large "A" since viable LAA tissue is captured between the jaws. (*Adapted from* Friedman PA, Asirvatham SJ, Dalegrave C, et al. Percutaneous epicardial left atrial appendage closure: preliminary results of an electrogram guided approach. J Cardiovasc Electrophysiol 2009;20:908–15; with permission.)

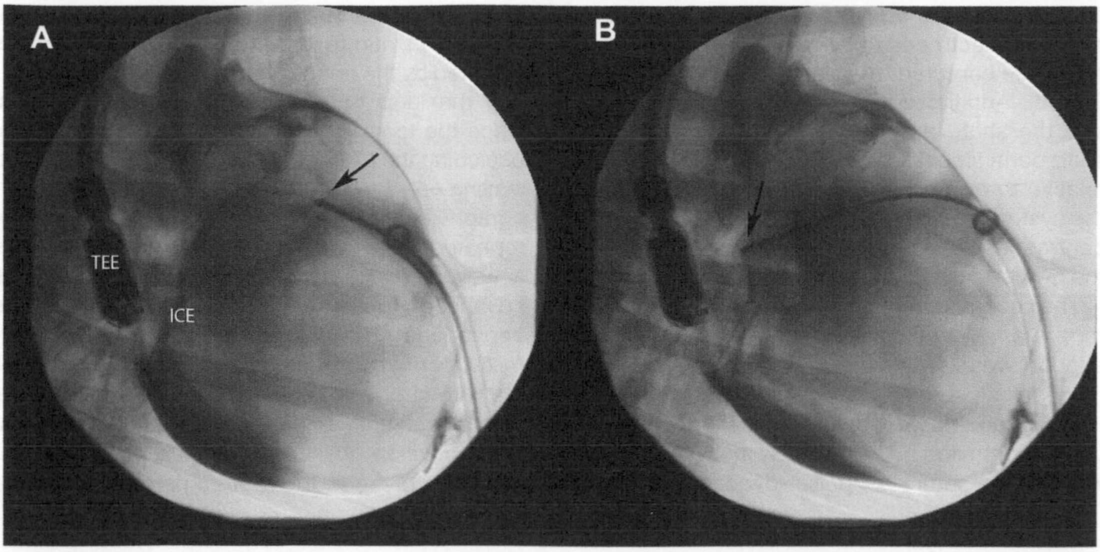

Fig. 7. Grasper controlling LAA, right anterior oblique projections during LAA ligation procedure. (*A*) The grasper's jaws (*arrow*) control the free margin of the LAA, which is outlined by contrast within the pericardium. The grasper is used to maintain and manipulate position of the LAA. ICE, intracardiac echocardiography; TEE, transesophageal echocardiography. (*B*) Grasper (*arrow*) has been advanced and corresponding movement of the LAA is seen. This type of manipulation is not needed for closure, but was performed during early experiments to confirm LAA capture. (*Adapted from* Friedman PA, Asirvatham SJ, Dalegrave C, et al. Percutaneous epicardial left atrial appendage closure: preliminary results of an electrogram guided approach. J Cardiovasc Electrophysiol 2009;20:908–15; with permission.)

pericardium, two simple anatomic characteristics of the appendage are exploited. First, as the surface of the heart is ascended following anterior pericardial access, the first free tissue margin encountered is the LAA (see **Fig. 4**). Second, the heart is electrically active, so that a device moving along its surface can use information from the underlying tissue to identify its location. The first atrial signal encountered by an ascending device along the anterior surface will be the LAA (see **Fig. 4**). This fact, combined with fluoroscopy, permits navigation without direct visualization.

The LAA closure system has two components: an appendage grasper and a ligator.[21] The grasper

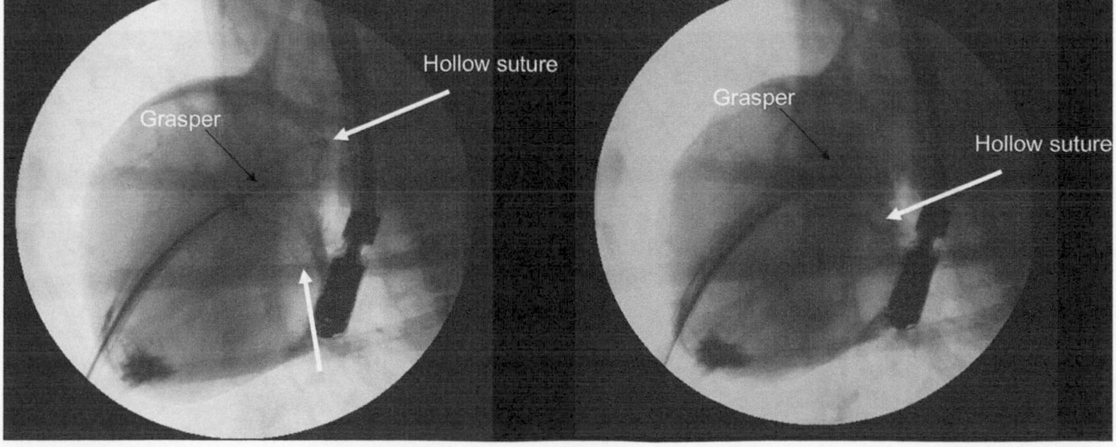

Fig. 8. Hollow suture closing around the LAA, left anterior oblique projections. The grasper position on the LAA free margin is not changed and a suture loop has been advanced to the base of the LAA and is made progressively smaller. In the left panel, the suture loop is full sized (*arrows* point to wire in loop, visible fluoroscopically) and, in the right panel, the loop is significantly smaller as closure has progressed.

(**Fig. 5**) has an articulating jaw with specially mounted electrodes to guide navigation and identify tissue captured by means of electrical signals (**Fig. 6**). Additional recordings between each jaw and the shaft, and bipolar recordings along the shaft permit identification of the grasper's position relative to electrically active cardiac tissue. Once the system is positioned near the LAA, injection of contrast at close proximity is performed to outline the LAA to facilitate and confirm its capture (**Fig. 7**).

The second component of the system—the ligator—is a hollow suture preloaded with a 0.012-in support wire. The wire in the suture provides mechanical support to permit advancement of the loop and fluoroscopic visualization. Once the LAA is controlled by the grasper, the wire-containing hollow suture loop is advanced over the grasper, around the free margin of the appendage (see **Fig. 5**), and to its base. The size of the loop is adjusted by the operator to match the LAA, permitting the loop to conform to anatomic variants. Once the loop is in position, it is cinched down, occluding the LAA, after which the wire is removed leaving only the suture behind (**Fig. 8**). Echocardiography confirms closure (**Fig. 9**). The loop can be repeatedly opened and closed until capture is achieved. Once positioned, a suture clip is advanced to secure the suture around the appendage. The sutures exit the sheath proximally, permitting operator control of the LAA until they are cut by the operator. In the event of distal loop placement (ie, the first loop is not at the most basal position possible) or if multiple appendage lobes are present, the system permits use of the

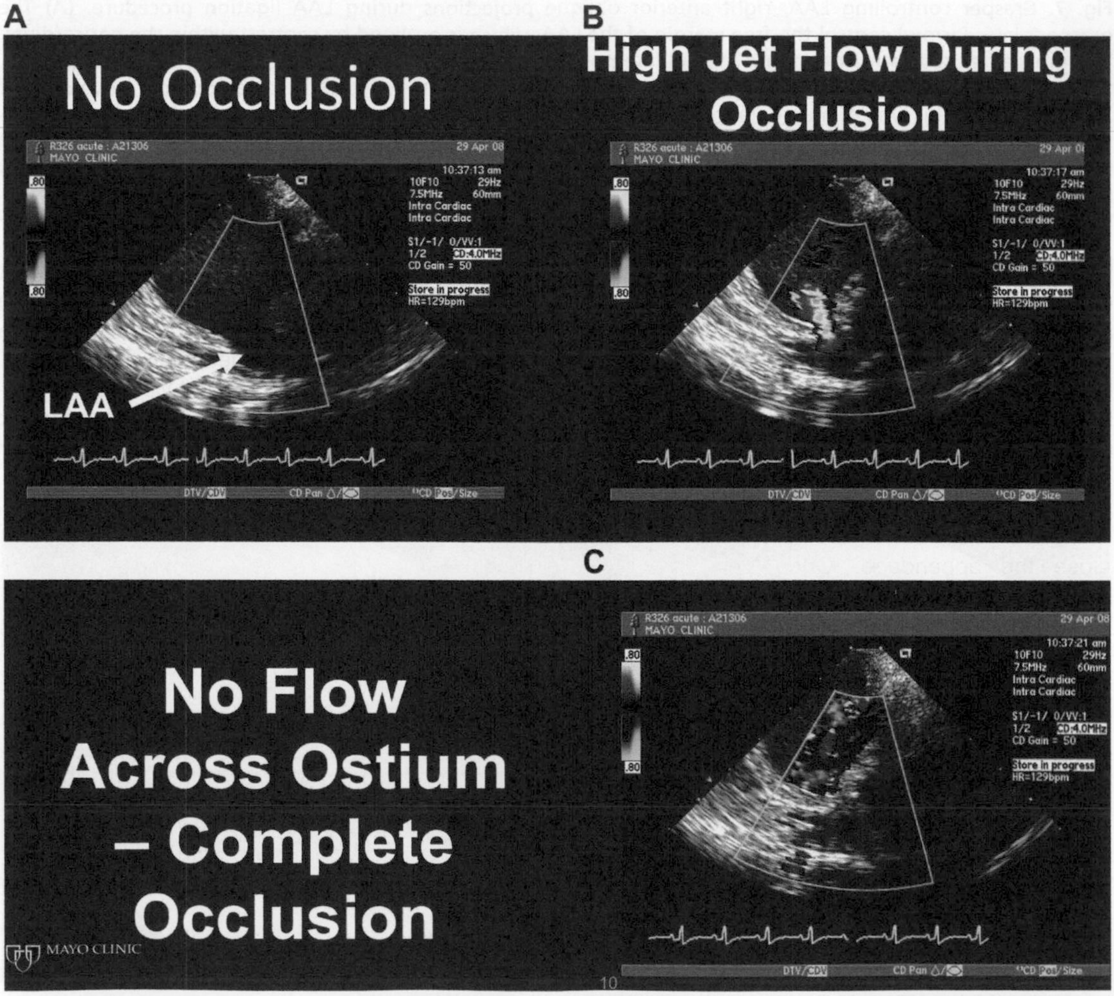

Fig. 9. Echocardiographic imaging of progressive closure. (*A*) The two-dimensional image shows a widely patent channel between the LAA and left atrium before loop deployment. As the loop is tightened around the base of the LAA, increasing emptying velocities are noted with color Doppler (*B*), until ligature is achieved and flow is no longer observed (*C*). (*Courtesy of* the Mayo Clinic Foundation; with permission.)

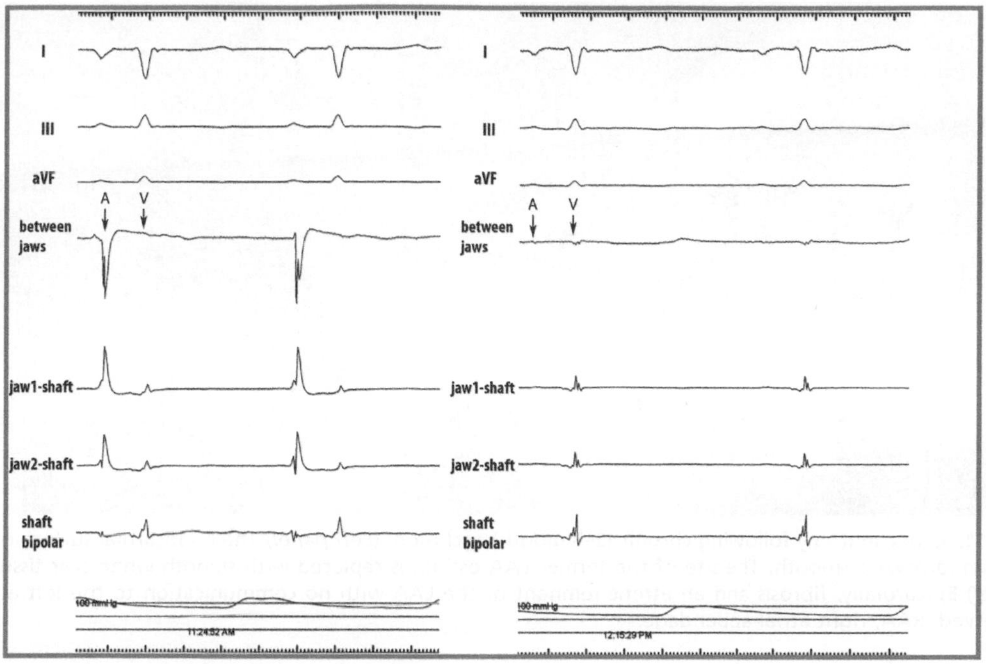

Fig. 10. Loss of electrograms following LAA occlusion. Electrograms recorded before LAA ligation (*left panel*) and after ligation (*right panel*). After ligation, the atrial electrogram is absent despite persistent capture of the LAA between the jaws of the grasper. Tracings record, from top to bottom, signals from surface electrocardiogram leads I, III, and avF; and jaw-to jaw bipolar, jaw1-to-shaft, jaw2-to-shaft, and shaft bipolar electrograms. The atrial (A) and ventricular (V) recordings of the first complex are labeled. (*Adapted from* Friedman PA, Asirvatham SJ, Dalegrave C, et al. Percutaneous epicardial left atrial appendage closure: preliminary results of an electrogram guided approach. J Cardiovasc Electrophysiol 2009;20:908–15; with permission. *Courtesy of* the Mayo Clinic Foundation; with permission.)

first suture as a guide over which subsequent, more proximal sutures can be placed to better close the appendage. Once LAA closure is completed, a catheter-based suture cutter cuts the sutures within the pericardial space.

We recently reported the results of chronic closure in six dogs. The procedure took an average of 69 minutes (range: 28–131 minutes) from the time of pericardial access to suture cutting, with last three procedures averaging 34 minutes (range 38–40 minutes).[55] The left atrial electrograms as recorded by the grasper disappeared following successful ligation in all animals (**Fig. 10**). Additionally, the surface electrocardiogram P wave acutely shortened following ligation from 70.2 $\pm$ 13.4 ms to 60.9 $\pm$ 12.9 ms ($P = .01$), presumably because of loss of LAA contribution to atrial activation. The chronic P wave duration remained shortened at 54.4 $\pm$ 0.4 ms, but did not significantly shorten beyond the acute shortening. None of the animals had pain, fever, infection, hemorrhage, or any other overt clinical sequelae either acutely or following the procedure. At autopsy, only an atretic remnant LAA with surrounding fibrosis was noted in all animals (**Fig. 11**). Paying particular attention to adjacent coronary arteries, pulmonary veins, and lung, we noted no collateral damage to adjacent structures. B-type natriuretic peptide levels and markers of inflammation (C reactive protein and sedimentation rate) were normal at baseline and at follow-up immediately presacrifice at 2 to 3 months.

The impact of closure on LAA electrical activity requires additional study, but has been consistently observed, and raises several interesting possibilities. First, the disappearance of electrograms may be a useful additional marker of successful, complete LAA closure, independent of transesophageal echocardiogram observations. This finding may minimize the risk of incomplete closure, which has been commonly observed during surgical closure in the absence of

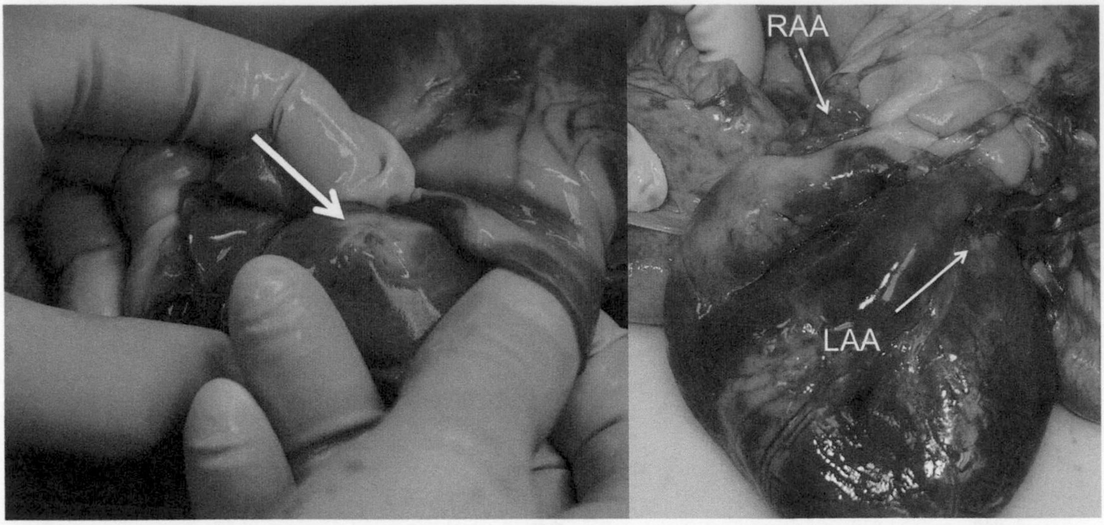

Fig. 11. Gross anatomy following chronic (2–3 month) occlusion. (*Left panel*) The endocardial surface of the left atrium (*arrow*) is smooth. The site of the former LAA ostium is replaced with smooth white scar tissue. (*Right panel*) Epicardially, fibrosis and an atretic remnant of the LAA with no communication to the left atrium are observed. RAA, right atrial appendage.

concurrent transesophageal echocardiogram closure confirmation.[56] Theoretically, electrical excision of a large mass of fibrillating atrial tissue may support efforts to restore sinus rhythm at the time of catheter ablation. Additionally, if LAA closure were combined with an atrial fibrillation ablation procedure, an epicardial approach may be advantageous, since there would be no risk of ablation catheter dislodgement of the endocardial occlusion device, of shunting current through the device, or of disruption of the endothelium adjacent to the device, inhibiting its proper endothelialization.

Other approaches have been employed to use the pericardial space, although published reports in the medical literature are currently unavailable. One system uses a hybrid approach. Following transseptal puncture, a balloon is inflated in the appendage to permit its visualization and guide placement of an epicardial loop around the LAA base. Another system uses a rigid tube scheme to control the appendage and place a suture around its base.

FUTURE DIRECTIONS

The unique anatomic position of the pericardial space clearly makes it a useful perch from which many novel therapies can be delivered. Given the rich deposition of cardiac autonomic nerves within the pericardial space, future intrapericardial therapies may modulate epicardial autonomic function to treat arrhythmias, syncope, or chest pain. The proximity to coronary arteries may enable delivery of therapy for vasospasm, and electrical stimulation of nearby phrenic nerves may prove useful for the treatment of sleep apnea, phrenic nerve injuries, or other disorders.

SUMMARY

Percutaneous pericardial access is an established technique useful for the treatment of epicardial ventricular arrhythmias and epicardial accessory. Emerging technologies may soon make it a desirable approach for cardiac resynchronization therapy and left atrial appendage closure. In the future, numerous other diagnostic and therapeutic interventions will be facilitated by this technique.

REFERENCES

1. D'Avila A, Scanavacca M, Sosa E, et al. Pericardial anatomy for the interventional electrophysiologist. J Cardiovasc Electrophysiol 2003;14:422–30.
2. Bulava A, Slavik L, Fiala M, et al. Endothelial damage and activation of the hemostatic system during radiofrequency catheter isolation of pulmonary veins. J Interv Card Electrophysiol 2004;10:271–9.
3. Waxman S, Moreno R, Rowe KA, et al. Persistent primary coronary dilation induced by transatrial delivery of nitroglycerin into the pericardial space: a novel approach for local cardiac drug delivery. J Am Coll Cardiol 1999;33:2073–7.
4. Stoll HP, Carlson K, Keefer LK, et al. Pharmacokinetics and consistency of pericardial delivery directed to coronary arteries: direct comparison with endoluminal delivery. Clin Cardiol 1999;22:I10–6.

5. Laham RJ, Simons M, Hung D. Subxyphoid access of the normal pericardium: a novel drug delivery technique. Catheter Cardiovasc Interv 1999;47:109–11.
6. Ujhelyi MR, Hadsall KZ, Euler DE, et al. Intrapericardial therapeutics: a pharmacodynamic and pharmacokinetic comparison between pericardial and intravenous procainamide delivery. J Cardiovasc Electrophysiol 2002;13:605–11.
7. Sosa E, Scanavacca M, D'Avila A, et al. Nonsurgical transthoracic epicardial approach in patients with ventricular tachycardia and previous cardiac surgery. J Interv Card Electrophysiol 2004;10:281–8.
8. Sosa E, Scanavacca M. Epicardial mapping and ablation techniques to control ventricular tachycardia. J Cardiovasc Electrophysiol 2005;16:449–52.
9. Sosa E, Scanavacca M, D'Avila A, et al. A new technique to perform epicardial mapping in the electrophysioogy laboratory. J Cardiovasc Electrophyiol 1996;7:531–6.
10. d'Avila A. Epicardial catheter ablation of ventricular tachycardia. Heart Rhythm 2008;5:S73–5.
11. Valderrabano M, Cesario DA, Ji S, et al. Percutaneous epicardial mapping during ablation of difficult accessory pathways as an alternative to cardiac surgery. Heart Rhythm 2004;1:311–6.
12. Kaltenbrunne R, Cardinal R, Dubuc M, et al. Epicardial and endocardial mapping of ventricular tachycardia in patients with myocardial infarction: Is the origin of the tachycardia always subendocardially localized? 1991;84:1058–1071. Circulation 1991;1:1058–71.
13. Miyasaka Y, Barnes M, Gersh BJ, et al. Secular trends in incidence of atrial fibrillation in Olmstod county, Minnesota, 1980 to 2000, and implications on the projections for future prevalence. Circulation 2006;114:119–25.
14. Sosa E, Scanavacca M, D'Avila A, et al. Endocardial and epicardial ablation guided by nonsurgical transthoracic epicardial mapping to treat recurrent ventricular tachycardia. J Cardiovasc Electrophysiol 1998;9:229–39.
15. Hammill SC. Epicardial ablation: reducing the risks. J Cardiovasc Electrophysiol 2006;17:550–2.
16. Mair H, Jansens JL, Lattouf OM, et al. Epicardial lead implantation techniques for biventricular pacing via left lateral mini-thoracotomy, video-assisted thoracoscopy, and robotic approach. Heart Surg Forum 2003;6:412–7.
17. Navia JL, Atik FA, Grimm RA, et al. Minimally invasive left ventricular epicardial lead placement: surgical techniques for heart failure resynchronization therapy. Ann Thorac Surg 2005;79:1536–54.
18. Shivkumar K. Percuatneous peicardial ablation of atrial fibirllation. Heart Rhythm 2008;5:152–4.
19. Nazarian S, Kantesevoy S, Zviman M, et al. Feasiblity of endoscopic guidance for nonsurgical transthoracic atrial and ventricular epicardial ablation. Heart Rhythm 2008;5:1115–9.
20. Tedrow U, Stevenson WG. Strategies for epicardial mapping and ablation of ventricular tachycardia. J Cardiovasc Electrophysiol 2009;20:710–3.
21. Friedman PA, Asirvatham SJ, Dalegrave C, et al. Percutaneous epicardial left atrial appendage closure: preliminary results of an electrogram guided approach. J Cardiovasc Electrophysiol 2009;20:908–15.
22. Bristow MR, Saxon LA, Boehmer J, et al. Comparison of Medical Therapy, Pacing, and Defibrillation in Heart Failure (COMPANION) Investigators. Cardiac-resynchronization therapy with or without an implantable defibrillator in advanced chronic heart failure. N Engl J Med 2004;350:2140–50.
23. Cleland JGDJ, Erdmann E, Freemantle N, et al. Cardiac Resynchronization–Heart Failure (CARE-HF) Study Investigators. The effect of cardiac resynchronization on morbidity and mortality in heart failure. N Engl J Med 2005;352:1539–49.
24. Rivero-Ayerza M, Theuns D, Garcia HM, et al. Effects of cardiac resynchronization therapy on overall mortality and mode of death: a meta-analysis of randomized controlled trials. Eur Heart J 2006;27:2682–8.
25. Birnie D, Tang A. The problem of non-response to cardiac resynchronization therapy. Curr Opin Cardiol 2006;21:20–6.
26. Dekker A, Phelps B, Dijkman B, et al. Epicardial left ventricular lead placement for cardiac resynchronization therapy: optimal pace site selection with pressure-volume loops. J Thorac Cardiovasc Surg 2004;127:1641–7.
27. Ansalone G, Giannantoni P, Ricci R, et al. Biventricular pacing in heart failure: back to basics in the pathophysiology of left bundle branch block to reduce the number of nonresponders. Am J Cardiol 2003;91:55f–61f.
28. Rossillo A, Verma A, Saad EB, et al. Impact of coronary sinus lead position on biventricular pacing: mortality and echocardiographic evaluation during long-term follow-up. J Cardiovasc Electrophysiol 2004;15:1120–5.
29. Meisel E, Pfeiffer D, Engelmann L, et al. Investigation of coronary venous anatomy by retrograde venography in patients with malignant ventricular tachycardia. Circulation 2001;104:442–7.
30. Nath J, Foster E, Heidenreich P. Impact of tricuspid regurgitation on long-term mortality. J Am Coll Cardiol 2004;43:405–9.
31. Healey JS, Crystal E, Lamy A, et al. Left Atrial Appendage Occlusion Study (LAAOS): results of a randomized controlled pilot study of left atrial appendage occlusion during coronary bypass surgery in patients at risk for stroke. Am Heart J 2005;150:288–93.

32. Brady P, Friedman PA, Trusty J, et al. High failure rate for an epicardial implantable cardioverter-defibrillator lead: implications for long-term follow-up of patients with an implantable cardioverter-defibrillator. J Am Coll Cardiol 1998;31:616–22.
33. Tomaske M, Gerritse B, Kretzers L, et al. A 12-year experience of bipolar steroid-eluting epicardial pacing leads in children. Ann Thorac Surg 2008; 85:1704–11.
34. Saxon LA, Kerwin WF, Cahalan MK, et al. Acute effects of intraoperative multisite ventricular pacing on left ventricular function and activation/contraction sequence in patients with depressed ventricular function. J Cardiovasc Electrophysiol 1998;9:13–21.
35. Izutani H, Quan K, Biblo LA, et al. Acute effects of intra-operative multisite ventricular pacing on left ventricular function and activation/contraction sequence in patients with depressed ventricular function versus coronary sinus lead placement. Heart Surg Forum 2002;6:E1–6.
36. Doll N, Piorkowski C, Czesla M, et al. Epicardial versus transvenous left ventricular lead placement in patients receiving cardiac resynchronization therapy: results from a randomized prospective study. Thorac Cardiovasc Surg 2008;56:256–61.
37. Mair H, Sachweh J, Meuris B, et al. Surgical epicardial left ventricular lead versus coronary sinus lead placement in biventricular pacing. Eur J Cardiothorac Surg 2005;27:235–42.
38. DeRose JJ, Ashton RC, Belsley S, et al. Robotically assisted left ventricular epicardial lead implantation for biventricular pacing. J Am Coll Cardiol 2003;41:1414–9.
39. Jutley RS, Waller DA, Loke I, et al. Video-assisted thoracoscopic implantation of the left ventricular pacing lead for cardiac resynchronization therapy. Pacing Clin Electrophysiol 2008;31:312–8.
40. Patronik N, Zenati M, Riviere C. Development of a tethered epicardial crawler for miminally invasive cardiac therapies. IEEE 2004;4:239–40.
41. Jais P, Neuzil P, D'Avila A, et al. A human acute study of a novel epicardial pacing lead for a non-surgical percutaneous subxiphoid approach. Heart Rhythm 2009;6:S417–53.
42. Chugh SS, Blackshear JL, Shen WK, et al. Epidemiology and natural history of atrial fibrillation: clinical implications. J Am Coll Cardiol 2001;37:371–8.
43. Go AS, Hylek EM, Phillips KA, et al. Prevalence of diagnosed atrial fibrillation in adults: national implications for rhythm management and stroke prevention: the AnTicoagulation and Risk Factors in Atrial Fibrillation (ATRIA) Study. JAMA 2001; 285:2370–5.
44. Preliminary report of the Stroke Prevention in Atrial Fibrillation Study. N Engl J Med 1990;322:863–8.
45. Albers GW, Diener HC, Frison L, et al. SPORTIF Executive Steering Committee for the SPORTIF V Investigators. Ximelagatran vs warfarin for stroke prevention in patients with nonvalvular atrial fibrillation: a randomized trial. JAMA 2005;293:690–8.
46. Blackshear JL, Odell JA. Appendage obliteration to reduce stroke in cardiac surgical patients with atrial fibrillation. Ann Thorac Surg 1996;61:755–9.
47. Blackshear JL, Johnson WD, Odell JA, et al. Thoracoscopic extracardiac obliteration of the left atrial appendage for stroke risk reduction in atrial fibrillation. J Am Coll Cardiol 2003;42:1249–52 [see comment].
48. Bayard YL, Ostermayer SH, Sievert H. Transcatheter occlusion of the left atrial appendage for stroke prevention. Expert Rev Cardiovasc Ther 2005;3: 1003–8.
49. Bayard YL, Ostermayer SH, Hein R, et al. Percutaneous devices for stroke prevention. Cardiovasc Revasc Med 2007;8:216–25.
50. Holmes DR, Reddy VY, Turi ZG, et al. Percutaneous closure of the left atrial appendage versus warfarin therapy for prevention of stroke in patients with atrial fibrillation: a randomised non-inferiority trial. Lancet 2009;374:534–42.
51. Ostermayer SH, Reisman M, Kramer PH, et al. Percutaneous left atrial appendage transcatheter occlusion (PLAATO system) to prevent stroke in high-risk patients with non-rheumatic atrial fibrillation: results from the international multi-center feasibility trials. J Am Coll Cardiol 2005;46:9–14 [see comment].
52. Meier B, Palacios I, Windecker S, et al. Transcatheter left atrial appendage occlusion with Amplatzer devices to obviate anticoagulation in patients with atrial fibrillation. Catheter Cardiovasc Interv 2003; 60:417–22.
53. Khumri T, Thibodeou J, Main M. Transesophageal echocardiographic diagnosis of left atrial appendage occluder device infection. Eur J Echocardiogr 2007;9:565–6.
54. Schwartzman D, Katz W, Smith A, et al. Malposition of a left atrial appendage occlusion device? A case with implications for percutaneous transcatheter left atrial appendage occlusion device therapy. Heart Rhythm 2006;4:648–50.
55. Stanton C, Friedman PA, Asirvatham SJ, et al. Percutaneous pericardial left atrial appendage ligation: intermediate-term results. Heart Rhythm 2009;6: S157–8.
56. Katz E, Tsiamtsiouris T, Applebaum R, et al. Surgical left atrial appendage ligation is frequently incomplete: a transesophageal echocardiographic study. J Am Coll Cardiol 2000;36:468–71.

Index

Note: Page numbers of article titles are in **boldface** type.

Card Electrophysiol Clin 2 (2010) 147–150
doi:10.1016/S1877-9182(09)00062-8

L

M

N

O

P

Q

R

S

Printed and bound by CPI Group (UK) Ltd, Croydon, CR0 4YY
03/10/2024
01040353-0016